Health Program Planning and Evaluation: A Practical and Systematic Approach for Community Health

Second Edition

L. Michele Issel, PhD, RN

Clinical Assistant Professor
School of Public Health
University of Illinois at Chicago

JONES AND BARTLETT PUBLISHERS

Sudbury, Massachusetts

BOSTON   TORONTO   LONDON   SINGAPORE

World Headquarters

Jones and Bartlett Publishers
40 Tall Pine Drive
Sudbury, MA 01776
978-443-5000
info@jbpub.com
www.jbpub.com

Jones and Bartlett Publishers
Canada
6339 Ormindale Way
Mississauga, Ontario L5V 1J2
Canada

Jones and Bartlett Publishers
International
Barb House, Barb Mews
London W6 7PA
United Kingdom

Jones and Bartlett's books and products are available through most bookstores and online book-sellers. To contact Jones and Bartlett Publishers directly, call 800-832-0034, fax 978-443-8000, or visit our website www.jbpub.com.

Substantial discounts on bulk quantities of Jones and Bartlett's publications are available to corporations, professional associations, and other qualified organizations. For details and specific discount information, contact the special sales department at Jones and Bartlett via the above contact information or send an email to specialsales@jbpub.com.

This publication is designed to provide accurate and authoritative information in regard to the Subject Matter covered. It is sold with the understanding that the publisher is not engaged in ren-dering legal, accounting, or other professional service. If legal advice or other expert assistance is required, the service of a competent professional person should be sought.

Production Credits
Publisher: Michael Brown
Associate Editor: Katey Birtcher
Editorial Assistant: Catie Heverling
Production Editor: Tracey Chapman
Associate Production Editor: Kate Stein
Marketing Manager: Sophie Fleck
Manufacturing and Inventory Control Supervisor: Amy Bacus
Composition: Auburn Associates, Inc.
Illustrator: Accurate Art, Inc.
Cover Design: Brian Moore
Cover Image: © Alexey Arkhipov/ShutterStock, Inc.
Printing and Binding: Malloy, Inc.
Cover Printing: Malloy, Inc.

Library of Congress Cataloging-in-Publication Data
Issel, L. Michele.
  Health program planning and evaluation : a practical and systematic approach for community health/L. Michele Issel.—2nd ed.
       p. ; cm.
  Includes bibliographical references and index.
  ISBN-13: 978-0-7637-5334-4 (pbk.)
  ISBN-10: 0-7637-5334-3 (pbk.)
  1. Health planning. 2. Community health services. I. Title.
  [DNLM: 1. Community Health Services—organization & administration—United States. 2. Health Planning—methods—United States. 3. Program Development—methods—United States. 4. Program Evaluation—methods—United States. WA 546 AA1 I86h 2009]
  RA394.9.I87 2009
  362.12—dc22
          2008028574

6048
Printed in the United States of America
13 12 11 10 09   10 9 8 7 6 5 4 3

Contributors

Arden Handler, DrPH
Professor, Community Health Sciences
School of Public Health
University of Illinois at Chicago

Deborah Rosenberg, PhD
Research Assistant Professor
Division of Epidemiology and Biostatistics
School of Public Health
University of Illinois at Chicago

Contents

LIST OF FIGURES

LIST OF TABLES

LIST OF EXHIBITS

Preface to the Second Edition

The second edition of *Health Program Planning and Evaluation* has stayed true to the purpose and intent of the first edition. This advanced-level text is written to address the needs of professionals from the variety of health disciplines who find themselves responsible for developing, implementing, or evaluating health programs. The aim of the text is to assist health professionals to become not only competent health program planners and evaluators, but also savvy consumers of evaluation reports and prudent users of evaluation consultants. To that end, the text includes a variety of practical tools and concepts necessary to develop and evaluate health programs, presenting them in language understandable to both the practicing and novice health program planner and evaluator.

Health programs are conceptualized as encompassing a broad range of programmatic interventions that can range from individual-level health education to population-level health policy programs. Examples of programs cited throughout the text are specific, yet broadly related to improving health, and reflect the breadth of public health programs. Maintaining a public health focus provides an opportunity to demonstrate how health programs can target different levels of a population, different determinants of the health problem, and different strategies and interventions to address the health problems. In addition, examples of health programs and references are selected to pique the interests of the diverse students and practicing professionals who make up multidisciplinary program teams. Thus the content and examples presented here are relevant to health administrators, medical social workers, nurses, nutritionists, pharmacists, public health professionals, physical and occupational therapists, and physicians.

The desire and idea for this textbook grew from my own teaching experiences. In teaching program planning and evaluation to both nurses and public health students, I came to appreciate the extent to which they need and want direct application of the program planning and evaluation course content to their work. In large part, the available textbooks have a social services orientation, but little direct relevance to the health programs with which nurses and public health students are more familiar. Existing texts also have very limited applicability to community-based healthcare settings, to public health issues, or to health problems at a population level. The distinction between individual patient health and behavior and population health requires special attention so that students from clinical backgrounds can learn to think and plan in terms of aggregates and populations.

In most graduate health professions programs, students are required to take a research methods course and a statistics course. Therefore, this evaluation text avoids duplicating content related to research methods and statistics, while addressing and extending that content into health program development, implementation, and evaluation. In addition, because total quality management and related methodologies are widely used in larger healthcare organizations, areas of overlap between quality improvement methodologies and traditional program evaluation approaches are discussed. This includes ways that quality improvement methodologies can complement program evaluations. Sometimes evaluations are appropriate; at other times they are not. Enthusiasm for providing health programs and doing evaluation is tempered with thoughtful notes of caution, in hopes that students will avoid potentially serious and costly program and evaluation mistakes.

UNIQUE FEATURES

Three unique features serve to distinguish this text from other program planning and evaluation textbooks: use of the public health pyramid, consistent use of a model of the program theory throughout the text, and role modeling of evidence-based practice. These features have been maintained in the second edition.

The public health pyramid explains how health programs can be developed for individuals, aggregates, populations, and service delivery systems. Use of the pyramid is also intended as a practical application of the ecological perspective that acknowledges a multilevel approach to addressing health problems. The public health pyramid contains four levels: direct services to individuals, enabling services to aggregates, services provided to entire populations, and, at the base, infrastructure. In this textbook, the pyramid is used as an organizing structure to summarize the content of each chapter in the "Across the Pyramid" sections. In that section specific attention is paid to how key concepts in the chapter might vary across the pyramid levels. This approach to summarizing the chapter content reinforces the perspective that enhancing health and well-being requires integrated efforts across the levels of the public health pyramid. That health program development and evaluation is relevant for programs targeted to individuals, aggregates, populations, and service delivery systems is a particularly germane means of tailoring program plans and evaluation designs that are congruent with the level at which the program is conceptualized. Hopefully, using the pyramid also helps health professionals begin to value their and others' contribution within and across the levels and to transcend disciplinary boundaries.

The second unique feature of this text is that one conceptual model of program planning an evaluation is used throughout the text: the program theory. The program theory is like a curricular strand, connecting content across the chapters, and activities throughout the planning and evaluation cycle. The program theory, as a conceptual model, is composed of elements. Articulating each of the component elements of the program theory sharpens the student's awareness of what must be addressed so as to create an effective health program. One element of the program theory is the effect theory, which focuses on how the intervention results in the program effects. The effect theory had its genesis in the concepts of action and intervention hypotheses described by Rossi and Freeman (1986); those concepts were dropped from later editions of their text (Rossi, Freeman, & Lipsey, 1999). I believe these authors were onto something with their effort to elucidate the various pathways leading from a problem to an effect of the program. Therefore, an adaptation, extension, and updated version of those earlier ideas is used throughout this textbook as the program theory and its elements

The pervasive use of models, program theories, and flow diagrams makes a return to Rossi and colleagues' ideas very fruitful. In this second edition, their earlier notions of hypotheses have been integrated with public health techniques and language, resulting in the effect theory portion of the program theory. The effect theory describes relationships among health antecedents, causes of health problems, program interventions, and health effects. The hypotheses that comprise the effect theory need to be understood and explicated to plan a successful health program and to evaluate the "right" elements of the program. The usefulness of the effect theory throughout the planning and evaluation cycle is highlighted throughout this text; for example, the model is used as means of linking program theory to evaluation designs and data collection. The model becomes an educational tool by serving as an example of how the program theory is manifested throughout the stages of planning and evaluation, and by reinforcing the value of carefully articulating the causes of health problems and consequences of programmatic interventions. Experience with students has shown that, while they often have an intuitive sense of the connection between their actions and outcomes, they are not skilled at articulating those connections in ways that program stakeholders can readily grasp. The effect theory and the process theory—the other main element of the program theory—provide a basis from which to identify and describe these connections.

The third unique feature of this text is the intentional role modeling of evidence-based practice. Use of published, empirical evidence as the basis for practice—whether clinical practice or program planning practice—is the professional standard. Each chapter of this book contains substantive examples drawn from the published scientific health and health-related literature. Relying on the literature for examples of programs, evaluations, and issues is consistent with the espoused preference of using scientific evidence as the basis for making programmatic decisions. Each chapter offers multiple examples from the health sciences literature that substantiate the information presented in the chapter.

ORGANIZATION OF THE BOOK

The book is organized into six sections, each covering a major phase in the planning and evaluation cycle.

Section I explores the context in which health programs and evaluations occur. Chapter 1 begins with an overview of definitions of health, followed by a historical context. The public health pyramid is introduced and presented as an ecological framework for thinking of health programs. An overview of community is provided and discussed as both the target and the context of health programs. The role of community members in health programs and evaluations is introduced, and emphasis is given to community as a context and to strategies for community participation throughout the program development and evaluation process. Chapter 2 focuses on the role of diversity in the planning and evaluation cycle and its effects on the delivery and evaluation of health programs. Although a discussion of diversity-related issues could have been added to each chapter, the sensitive nature of this topic and its importance in ensuring a successful health program warranted it being covered early in the text and as a separate chapter. Cultural competence is discussed, particularly with regard to the organization providing the health program and the program staff.

Section II contains three chapters which focus on the task of defining the health problem. Chapter 3 covers planning perspectives and the history of health program planning; it also introduces five planning systems that exist for public health, such as MAPP. Effective health program developers understand that approaches to planning are based on assumptions. These assumptions are exemplified in six perspectives that provide points of reference for understanding diverse preferences for prioritizing health needs and expenditures and, therefore, for tailoring planning actions to best fit the situation. Chapter 4 begins with a review of perspectives on conducting a community needs assessment. Building on this review, five types of assessments are discussed as foundational to decision making about the future health program. Essential steps involved in conducting a community health and needs assessment are outlined as well.

Chapter 5 expands on key elements of a community needs assessment, beginning with a review of the data collection methods appropriate for a community needs assessment. This discussion is followed by a brief overview of key epidemiological statistics. Using those statistics and the data, the reader is guided through the process of developing a causal statement of the health problem. This causal statement, which includes the notion of moderating and mediating factors in the pathway from causes to problem, serves as the basis for the effect theory of the program. Once the causal statement has been developed, prioritization of the problem is needed; four systems for prioritizing in a rational manner are reviewed in Chapter 5.

Following prioritization comes planning, beginning with the decision of how to address the health problem. In many ways, the two chapters in Section III form the heart of planning a successful health program. Unfortunately, students generally undervalue the importance of theory for selecting an effective intervention and of establishing target values for objectives. Chapter 6 explains what theory is and how it provides a cornerstone to programs and to evaluations. More importantly, the concept of intervention is discussed in detail, with attention being paid to characteristics that make an intervention ideal, including attention to intervention dosage. Program theory is introduced in Chapter 6 as the basis for organizing ideas related to the selection and delivery of the interventions in conjunction. The effect theory element of the program theory is introduced and the components of the effect theory explained. Because the effect theory is so central to having an effective program intervention and the subsequent program evaluation, it is discussed in conjunction with several examples from the Layetteville and Bowe County case. Chapter 7 goes into detail on developing goals and objectives for the program, with particular attention devoted to articulating the interventions provided by the program. A step-by-step procedure is presented for deriving numerical targets for the objectives from existing data, which makes the numerical targets more defendable and programmatically realistic.

Section IV deals with the task of implementing a health program. Chapter 8 provides an in-depth review of key elements that constitute the process theory element of the program theory—specifically, the organizational plan and services utilization plan. The distinction between inputs and outputs of the process theory is highlighted through examples and a comprehensive review of possible inputs and outputs. Budgeting for program operations is covered in this chapter as well. Chapter 9 details how to evaluate the outputs of the organizational plan and the services utilization plan. The practical application of measures of coverage is described, along with the need to connect the results of the process evaluation to programmatic changes. Program management for assuring a high-quality program that is delivering the planned intervention is the focus of Chapter 10.

Section V contains chapters that are specific to conducting the effect evaluations. These chapters present both basic and advanced research methods from the perspective of a program effect evaluation. Here, students' prior knowledge about research methods and statistics is brought together in the context of health program and services evaluation. Chapter 11 highlights the importance of refining the evaluation question and provides information on how to clarify the question with stakeholders. Earlier discussions about program theory are brought to bear on the development of the evaluation question. Key issues, such as data integrity and survey construction, are addressed with regard to the practicality of program evaluation. Chapter 12 takes a fresh approach to evaluation design by organizing the traditional experimental and quasi-experimental designs and epidemiological designs into three levels of program evaluation design based on the design complexity and purpose of the evaluation. The discussion of sampling, in Chapter 13, retains the emphasis on being practical for program evaluation, rather than taking a pure research approach. However, sample size and power are discussed, as these factors have profound relevance to program evaluation. Chapter 14 reviews statistical analysis of data, paying special attention to variables from the effect theory and their level of measurement. The data analysis is linked to interpretation, and readers are warned about potential flaws in how numbers are understood. Chapter 15 provides a review of qualitative designs and methods, especially their use in health program development and evaluation.

Chapter 16, the last chapter in Section V, addresses the topic of cost analysis. Basic comparative descriptions of cost-effectiveness, cost–benefit, cost–utility, and sensitivity analyses are given with sufficient detail so that thoughtful and realistic program and evaluation decisions can be made. There is no attempt to make the reader an expert. Rather, the goal in this chapter is to help the reader become savvy and skeptical about cost studies that might be influencing program decision making. Again, the program theory is used to organize thinking about cost evaluations.

The final section, Section VI, includes just one chapter. Chapter 17 discusses the use of evaluation results when making decisions about existing and future health programs. Practical and conceptual issues related to ethics program evaluators face are addressed. This chapter also reviews ways to assess the quality of evaluations and the professional responsibilities of evaluators.

Each chapter in the book concludes with a "Discussion Questions and Activities" section. The questions posed are intended to be provocative and to generate critical thinking. At a graduate level, students need to be encouraged to engage in independent thinking and to foster their ability to provide rationales for decisions. The discussion questions are developed from this point of view. In the new "Internet Resources" section, links are provided to websites that are related to and support the content of the chapter. These websites have been carefully chosen to be stable and reliable sources.

ADDITIONS AND REVISIONS IN THE SECOND EDITION

The second edition of *Health Program Planning and Evaluation* represents a refinement of the first edition, beginning with corrections and updated references. Classical references and references that remain state-of-the-art have been retained. In addition, there has been a surprising amount of small, but important changes in the discipline of evaluation since the publication of the first edition, requiring that references be updated. In the second edition, each chapter contains a section with at least four links to Internet resources that were chosen for their relevance to the chapter content and for their long-term accessibility.

There have also been substantive additions to the text throughout the chapters. Examples of new content include the discussions of rapid assessment, business plans, the RE-AIM model, quality improvement tools, and the Health Insurance Portability and Accountability Act of 1996 (HIPAA). Another change in the second edition is the addition of more examples using Excel to calculate basic program process evaluation statistics.

Two major additions are the use of an unfolding case study and a revision of the effect theory portion of the program theory. Chapter 1 introduces the fictitious city of Layetteville and the equally fictitious Bowe County. In subsequent chapters, chapter content is applied to the health problems of Layetteville and Bowe County so that students can learn how to use the material on an ongoing basis. In several chapters, the case study is used in the "Discussion Questions and Activities" section to further provide the student with an opportunity to practice applying the chapter content.

The revision of the effect theory stemmed directly from feedback I received about the first edition: Readers complained that the discussion of the effect theory in that edition was too complicated and difficult to understand; it was not helping students. The second edition has retained the original intent—namely, to provide students with the ability to describe a working theory of how the intervention acts upon the causes of the health problem and leads to the desired health results. In this edition, the terminology used in the effect theory has been modified to be consistent with the terms used in theory testing and statistical analyses. Specifically, the effect theory, as now presented, uses the language of moderating and mediating factors. In addition, the connection between the effect theory and process theory has been strengthened.

ACKNOWLEDGMENTS

I am indebted to the many people who supported and aided me in preparing this second edition of *Health Program Planning and Evaluation*. First and foremost, I am grateful to the numerous students over the years who asked questions that revealed the typical sticking points in their acquiring and understanding of the concepts and content, as well as where new explanations were needed. It was through their eyes that I learned there is no one way to explain a complex notion or process. Their interest and enthusiasm for planning and evaluating health programs was a great motivator for making the content of this book readily available.

I am further indebted to the colleagues with whom I have participated in program development and evaluations over the years: Shirley Fleming, Judith Levy, Agatha Lowe, Kristi Raube, Katie Merrill, Arden Handler, and Andrea McGlynn. Learning by experience and mentorship is invaluable. I am particularly grateful to former students who assisted me in preparing the first and second editions: Nicole Miller, Kusuma Madamala, Melissa Sherwin, and Sarah Forrestal. Each helped me with keeping references straight, editing, and providing insights into the understandability of the text from a student perspective.

My initial inspiration for becoming an evaluator came from Frances Marcus Lewis at the University of Washington School of Nursing. Much later, encouragement for writing this textbook came from Bernard Turnock, at the University of Illinois at Chicago School of Public Health. Several additional colleagues helped fine-tune this text. I am especially indebted to Arden Handler, at the School of Public Health, University of Illinois at Chicago, for taking time to contribute to this textbook. Her devotion to quality and clarity has added much to the richness of otherwise dry material. I am also deeply indebted to Deborah Rosenberg, also at the University of Illinois at Chicago School of Public Health, for sharing her innovative and quintessentially useful work on developing targets for program objectives. Much appreciation goes to both Arden and Deborah for being so generous with their time and contributions. Lastly, but not least, I thank Jill Hobbs and Tracey Chapman for their expert editing, and Mike Brown for his encouragement and patience.

List of Acronyms

ABCD	Asset-based community development
AEA	American Evaluation Association
AHRQ	Agency for Healthcare Research and Quality
APEX-PH	Assessment Protocol for Excellence in Public Health
APHA	American Public Health Association
BPRS	Basic Priority Rating Score
BRFSS	Behavioral Risk Factor Surveillance System
BSC	Balanced Score Card
CARF	Commission on Accreditation of Rehabilitation Facilities
CBA	Cost–benefit analysis
CBPR	Community-based participatory research
CEA	Cost-effectiveness analysis
CER	Cost-effectiveness ratio
CDC	Centers for Disease Control and Prevention
CHIP	Community Health Improvement Process
CI	Confidence interval
CQI	Continuous quality improvement
CUA	Cost–utility analysis
DALY	Disability-adjusted life-year
DHHS	U.S. Department of Health and Human Services
EBM	Evidence-based medicine
EBP	Evidence-based practice
FTE	Full-time equivalent
GAO	U.S. Government Accountability Office
GPRA	Government Performance and Results Act
HEDIS	Healthcare Effectiveness Data and Information Set
HIPAA	Health Insurance Portability and Accountability Act
HRQOL	Health-related quality of life
HRSA	Health Resources and Services Administration (part of DHHS)
IRB	Institutional review board
JCAHO	Joint Commission on the Accreditation of Healthcare Organizations
MAPP	Mobilizing for Action through Planning and Partnership
MCHB	Maternal and Child Health Bureau (part of HRSA)
NACCHO	National Association of City and County Health Officers
NAMI	National Alliance on Mental Illness
NCHS	National Center for Health Statistics
NHANES	National Health and Nutrition Examination Survey

NHIS	National Health Interview Survey
NIH	National Institutes of Health
OHRP	Office for Human Research Protections
OMB	Office of Management and Budgeting
OR	Odds ratio
PACE-EH	Protocol for Assessing Excellence in Environmental Health
PATCH	Planning Approach to Community Health
PDCA	Plan-Do-Check-Act
PEARL	Property, economic, acceptability, resource, legality system
PPIP	Putting Prevention into Prevention
PSA	Public service announcement
QALY	Quality-adjusted life-year
RAR	Rapid assessment and response
RARE	Rapid assessment and response and evaluation
RE-AIM	Reach, Effectiveness, Adoption, Implementation, and Maintenance model
RR	Relative risk
SAMHSA	Substance Abuse and Mental Health Services Adminhistration
SCHIP	State Child Health Insurance Program
SES	Socioeconomic status
TQM	Total quality management
UOS	Units of service
WHO	World Health Organization
WIC	Special Supplemental Nutrition Program for Women, Infants, and Children
YHL	Years of healthy life
YLL	Years of life lost
YPLL	Years of potential life lost

Section 1

The Context of Health Program Development and Evaluation

CHAPTER 1

Context of Health Program Development and Evaluation

Health is not a state of being that can easily be achieved through isolated, uninformed, individualistic actions. *Health* of individuals, of families, and of populations is a state in which physical, mental, and social well-being are integrated so that optimal functioning is possible. From this perspective, achieving and maintaining health across a life span is a complex, complicated, intricate affair. For some, health is present irrespective of any special efforts or intention. For most of us, health requires, at a minimum, some level of attention and specific information. It is through health programs that attention is given focus and information is provided or made available, but that does not guarantee that the attention and information are translated into actions or behaviors needed to achieve health. Thus those providing health programs, however large or small, need to understand not only the processes whereby those in need of attention and information can receive what is needed, but also the processes of learning from their experiences of providing the health program.

The processes of health program planning and evaluation are the subject of this book. The discussion begins here in Chapter 1 with a brief overview of the historical context. This background sets the stage for appreciating the growing number of publications on the topic of health program planning and evaluation that have emerged in recent years, and for acknowledging the professionalization of evaluators. The use of the term "processes" to describe the actions involved in health program planning and evaluation is intended to denote action, cycles, and open-endedness. This chapter introduces the planning and evaluation cycle, and the interactions and iterative nature of this cycle are stressed throughout the text. Because health is an individual, aggregate, and population phenomenon, health programs need to be conceptualized across those levels. The public health pyramid, introduced in this chapter, is used throughout the text as a tool for conceptualizing and actualizing health programs for individuals, aggregates, and populations.

HISTORY AND CONTEXT

An appropriate starting point for this book is reflecting on and understanding what "health" is, along with having a basic appreciation for the genesis of the fields of health program planning and evaluation. A foundation in these elements is key to becoming an evaluation professional.

Concept of Health

It is crucial to begin the health program planning and evaluation cycle by first reflecting on the meaning of health. Both explicit and implicit meanings of health can dramatically influence what is considered the health problem and the subsequent direction of a program. The most widely accepted definition of *health* is that put forth by the World Health Organization (WHO), which for the first time defined health as more than the absence of illness, but also the presence of well-being (WHO, 1947).

Since the publication of the WHO definition, health has come to be viewed across the health professions as a holistic concept that encompasses the presence of physical, mental, developmental, social, and financial capabilities, assets, and balance. This idea does not preclude each health profession from having a particular aspect of health to which it primarily contributes. For example, a dentist contributes primarily to a patient's oral health, knowing that the state of the patient's teeth and gums has a direct relationship to his or her physical and social health. Thus the dentist might say the health problem is caries. The term "health problem" is used, rather than "illness," "diagnosis," or "pathology," in keeping with the holistic view that there can be problems, deficits, and pathologies in one component of health while the other components remain "healthy." Using the term "health problem" also makes it easier to think about and plan health programs for aggregates of individuals. A community, a family, and a school can each have a health problem that is the focus of a health program intervention. The extent to which the health program planners have a shared definition of health and have defined the scope of that definition will influence the nature of the health program.

Health is a matter of concern for more than just health professionals. For many Americans, the concept of health is perceived as a right, along with civil rights and liberties. The right to health is often translated by the public and politicians into the perceived right to have or to access health care. This political aspect of health is the genesis of health policy at the local, federal, and international levels. The extent to which the political nature of health underlies the health problem of concern and is programmatically addressed will also influence the final nature of the health program.

History of Health Program Planning

The history of planning health programs has a different lineage than that of program evaluation. Only relatively recently, in historical terms, have these lineages begun to overlap, with resulting synergies. Planning for health programs has the older history, if public health is considered. Rosen (1993) argued that public health planning began approximately 4000 years ago with planned cities in the Indus Valley that had covered sewers. Particularly since the Industrial Revolution, planning for the health of populations has progressed, and it is now considered a key characteristic of the discipline of public health.

Blum (1981) related *planning* to efforts undertaken on behalf of the public well-being to achieve deliberate or intended social change, as well as providing a sense of direction and alternative modes of proceeding to influence social attitudes and actions. Others (Dever, 1980; Rohrer, 1996; Turnock, 2004) have similarly defined planning as an intentional effort to create something that has not occurred previously for the betterment of others and for the purpose of meeting desired goals. The purpose of planning is to ensure that a program has the best possible likelihood of being successful, defined in terms of being effective with the least possible resources. Planning encompasses a variety of activities undertaken to meet this purpose.

The quintessential example of planning is the development and use of the *Healthy People* goals. In 1979, *Healthy People* (U.S. Department of Health, Education, and Welfare [DHEW], 1979) was published as an outgrowth of the need to establish an illness prevention agenda for the United States. The companion publication, *Promoting Health/Preventing Disease* (U.S. Department of Health and Human Services [DHHS], 1980), marked the first time that goals and objectives regarding specific areas of the nation's health were made explicit, with the expectation that these goals would be met by the year 1990. *Healthy People* became the framework for the development of state and local health promotion and disease prevention agendas. Since its publication, the U.S. goals for national health have been revised and published as *Healthy People 2000* (DHHS, 1991), *Healthy Communities 2000* (American Public Health Association [APHA], 1991), and *Healthy People 2010* (DHHS, 2000). Efforts are currently under way to develop *Healthy People 2020*. It is worth noting that other nations also set health status goals and that international organizations, such as the World Health Organization (WHO) and Pan American Health Organization (PAHO), develop health goals applicable across nations.

The evolution of *Healthy People* goals also reflects the accelerating rate of emphasis on nationwide coordination of health promotion and disease prevention efforts and a reliance on systematic planning to achieve this coordination.

The development of the *Healthy People* publications also reflects the underlying assumption of most planners that planning is a rational activity that can lead to results. However, with regard to many health problems, the United States has not yet achieved the objectives set for 1990; this fact reflects the colossal potential for planning to fail. Given this potential, the emphasis in this book is on techniques to help future planners of health programs be more realistic in the goals set and less dependent upon a linear, rational approach to planning.

The *Healthy People 1990* objectives were developed by academics and clinician experts in illness prevention and health promotion. In contrast, the goals and health problems listed in *Healthy People 2010* were based on and incorporated ideas generated at public forums and through Internet commentary; these ideas were revised by expert panels before their final publication. The shift to a greater participation of the public in the planning stage of health programs is a major change that is now considered the norm. In keeping with the emphasis on participation, the role and involvement of stakeholders are stressed at each stage of the planning and evaluation cycle.

The history of evaluation, from which the evaluation of health programs grew, is far shorter than the history of planning, beginning roughly in the early 1900s, but it is equally rich in important lessons for future health program evaluators. The first evaluations were done in the field of education, particularly as student assessment and evaluation of teaching strategies gained interest (Patton, 1997). Assessment of student scholastic achievement is a comparatively circumscribed outcome of an educational intervention. For this reason, early program evaluators came from the disciple of education, and it was from the fields of education and educational psychology that many methodological advances were made and statistics developed.

Guba and Lincoln (1987) summarized the history of evaluations by proposing generational milestones or characteristics that typify distinct generations. Later, Swenson (1991) built on their concept of generations by acknowledging that subsequent generations will occur. Each generation incorporates the knowledge of early evaluations and extends that knowledge based on current broad cultural and political trends.

Guba and Lincoln (1987) called the first generation of evaluations in the early 1900s "the technical generation." During this time, nascent scientific management, statistics, and research methodologies were used to test interventions. Currently, evaluations continue to incorporate the rationality of this generation by using activities that are systematic, science based, logical, and sequential. Rational approaches to evaluations focus on identifying the best-known intervention or strategy given the current knowledge, measuring quantifiable outcomes experienced by program participants, and deducing the degree of effect from the program.

The second generation, which lasted until the 1960s, focused on using goals and objectives as the basis for evaluation, in keeping with the managerial trend of management by objectives. Second-generation evaluations were predominantly descriptive. With the introduction in the 1960s of broad innovation and initiation of federal social service programs, including Medicare, Medicaid, and Head Start, the focus of evaluations shifted to establishing the merit and value of the programs. Because of the political issues surrounding these and similar federal programs, there was a growing awareness of the need to determine whether the social policies were having any effect on people. Programs needed to be judged on their merits and effectiveness. The U.S. General Accounting Office (GAO) (now called the Government Accountability Office) had been established in 1921 for the purpose of studying the utilization of public finances, assisting Congress in decision making with regard to policy and funding, and evaluating government programs. The second-generation evaluation emphasis on quantifying effects was spurred, in part, by reports from the GAO that were based on the evaluations of federal programs.

Typically, the results of evaluations were not used in the "early" days of evaluating education and social programs. That is, federal health policy was not driven by whether evaluations showed the programs to be successful. Although the scientific rigor of evaluations improved, their usefulness remained minimal. Beginning in the 1980s, however, the third generation of evaluations— termed "the negotiation generation" or "the responsiveness generation" began. During this generation, evaluators began to acknowledge that they were not autonomous and that their work needed to respond to the needs of those being evaluated. As a result of this awareness, several lineages have emerged. These lineages within the responsiveness generation account for the current diversity in types, emphases, and philosophies related to program evaluation.

One lineage is utilization-focused evaluation (Patton, 1997), in which the evaluator's primary concern is with developing an evaluation that will be used by the stakeholders. Utilization-focused evaluations are built on the following premises (Patton, 1987): concern for use of the evaluation pervades the evaluation from beginning to end, evaluations are aimed at the interests and needs of the users, users of the evaluation must be invested in the decisions regarding the evaluation, and a variety of community, organizational, political, resource, and scientific factors affect the utilization of evaluations. Utilization-focused evaluation differs from evaluations that are focused on outcomes (Table 1.1).

Another lineage is participatory evaluation (Whitmore, 1998), in which the evaluation is merely guided by the expert and is actually generated by and conducted by those invested in the health problem. A participatory or empowerment approach invites a wide range of stakeholders into the activity of

Table 1.1   Comparison of Outcome-Focused and Utilization-Focused Evaluations

	Outcome-Focused Evaluations	Utilization-Focused Evaluations
Purpose	Show program effect	Get stakeholders to use evaluation findings for decisions regarding program improvements and future program development
Audience	Funders, researchers, other external audience	Program people (internal audience), funders
Method	Research methods, external evaluators (usually)	Research methods, participatory

planning and evaluation, providing those participants with the skills and knowledge to contribute substantively to the activities and fostering their sense of ownership of the product.

The fourth generation of evaluation, which emerged in the mid-1990s, seems to be meta-evaluation—that is, the evaluation of evaluations done across similar programs. This trend in program evaluation is consistent with the trend in social science toward the use of meta-analysis of existing studies to better understand theorized relationships. It is also consistent with the trend across the health professions toward the use of meta-analysis of existing research for the development of evidence-based practice.

This new generation became possible because a culture of evaluation now pervades the health services, and huge data sets are available for use in the meta-evaluations. One indicator of the evaluation culture is the mandate from United Way, a major funder of community-based health programs, for grantees to conduct outcome evaluations. To help grantees meet this mandate, United Way has published a user-friendly manual (United Way of America, 1996) that could be used by nonprofessionals in the development of basic program evaluations. The culture of evaluation is most evident in the explicit requirement of federal agencies that fund community-based health programs that such programs include evaluations conducted by local evaluators.

Despite the complexities involved in this latest stage of evaluation, most people have an intuitive sense of what evaluation is. The purpose of *evaluation* can be to measure the effects of a program against the goals set for it, in order to contribute to subsequent decision making about the program (Weiss, 1972). Alternatively, evaluation can be defined as "the use of social research methods to systematically investigate the effectiveness of social intervention programs in ways that are adapted to their political and organizational environments and are designed to inform social action to improve social conditions" (Rossi, Lipsey, & Freeman, 2004). Others (Herman, Morris, & Fitz-Gibbon, 1987) have defined evaluation as judging how well policies and procedures are working or as assessing the quality of a program. These definitions of evaluation remain relevant.

Inherent in these definitions of evaluation is an element of being judged against some criteria. This implicit understanding of evaluation leads those involved with the health program to feel as though they will be judged or found not to meet those criteria and will subsequently experience some form of repercussions. They may fear that they as individuals or as a program will be labeled a failure, unsuccessful, or inadequate. Such feelings must be acknowledged and addressed early in the planning cycle. Throughout the planning and evaluation cycle, the program planners have numerous opportunities to engage and involve program staff and stakeholders in the evaluation process. Taking advantage of these opportunities goes a long way in alleviating the concerns of program staff and stakeholders about the judgmental quality of the program evaluation.

EVALUATION AS A PROFESSION

A major development in the field of evaluation has been the professionalization of evaluators. Founded in 1986, the American Evaluation Association (AEA) serves evaluators primarily in the United States. Several counterparts to the AEA exist, such as the Society for Evaluation in the United Kingdom and the Australian Evaluation Society. The establishment of these professional organizations, whose members are evaluators, and the presence of health-related sections within these organizations demonstrate the existence of a field of expertise and of specialized knowledge regarding the evaluation of health-related programs.

As the field of evaluation has evolved, so have the number and diversity of approaches that can guide the development of evaluations. Currently, 26 different approaches to evaluation have been identified, falling into three major groups (Stufflebeam & Shinkfield, 2007). One group of evaluations is oriented toward questions and methods such as objectives-based studies and experimental evaluations. The second group of evaluations is oriented toward improvements and accountability and includes consumer-oriented and accreditation approaches. The third group of evaluations are those that have a social agenda or advocacy approach, such as responsive evaluations, democratic evaluations, and utilization-focused evaluation.

Several concepts are common across the types of evaluations—namely, pluralism of values, stakeholder constructions, fairness and equity regarding stakeholders, the merit and worth of the evaluation, a negotiated process and outcomes, and full collaboration. These concepts have been formalized into the standards for evaluations that were established by the Joint Commission on Standards for Educational Evaluation in 1975. Currently, this Joint Commission includes many organizations in its membership, such as the American Evaluation Association and the American Educational Research Association.

The four standards of evaluation established by the American Evaluation Association are utility, feasibility, propriety, and accuracy (Table 1.2; American Evaluation Association, 2002).

The utility standard specifies that an evaluation must be useful to those who requested the evaluation. An evaluation is useful when it shows ways to make improvements to the intervention, increase the efficiency of the program, or enhance the possibility of garnering financial support for the program. The feasibility standard denotes that the ideal may not be practical. Evaluations that are highly complex or costly will not be done by small

Table 1.2   Evaluation Standards Established by the Joint Commission on Standards for Educational Evaluation

Standard	Description
Utility	To ensure that the evaluation will meet the content needs of the those involved
Feasibility	To ensure that the evaluation will be realistic, prudent, diplomatic, and frugal
Propriety	To ensure that the evaluation will be conducted in a legal and unbiased way, with special attention paid to the integrity of everyone involved in the evaluation process and the implementation of its results
Accuracy	To ensure that the evaluation will communicate appropriate and accurate information concerning the standards that determine the usefulness of the program under consideration

Source: Data from American Evaluation Association (2002).

programs with limited capabilities and resources. Propriety is the ethical and politically correct component of the standards. Evaluations can invade privacy or be harmful to either program participants or program staff. The propriety standard also holds evaluators accountable for upholding all of the other standards. Accuracy is essential and is achieved through the elements that constitute scientific rigor. These established and accepted standards for evaluations reflect current norms and values held by professional evaluators and deserve attention in health program evaluations. The existence and acceptance of standards is truly an indication of the professionalism of evaluators.

Achieving these standards requires that those involved in the program planning and evaluation have experience in at least one aspect of planning or evaluation, whether that be experience with the health problem; experience with epidemiological, social, or behavioral science research methods; or skill in facilitating processes that involve diverse constituents, capabilities, and interests. Program planning and evaluation can be done in innumerable ways: there is no single "right way." This degree of freedom and flexibility can feel uncomfortable for some people. As with any skill or activity, until experience is acquired, program planners and evaluators may feel intimidated by the size of the task or by the experience of others involved. To become a professional evaluator, therefore, requires a degree of willingness to learn, to grow, and to be flexible.

Who Does Planning and Evaluations?

Many different types of health professionals and social scientists can be involved in health program planning and evaluation. At the outset of program planning and evaluation, one trepidation revolves around who ought to be the planners and evaluators. In a sense, virtually anyone with an interest and a willingness to be an active participant in the planning or evaluation process could be involved, including health professionals, businesspersons, paraprofessionals, and advocates or activists.

Planners and evaluators may be employees of the organization about to undertake the activity, or they may be external consultants hired to assist in all phases or just a specific phase of the planning and evaluation cycle. Internal and external planners and evaluators each have their advantages and disadvantages. Regardless of whether an internal or external evaluator is used, professional stakes and allegiances ought to be acknowledged and understood as factors that can affect the decision making.

Planners and evaluators from within the organization are susceptible to biases, consciously or not, in favor of the program or some aspect of the program, particularly if their involvement can positively affect their work. On the positive side, internal planners and evaluators are more likely to have insider knowledge of organizational factors that can be utilized or may have a positive effect on the delivery and success of the health program. Internal evaluators may experience divided loyalties, such as between the program and their job, between the program staff and other staff, or between the proposed program or evaluation and their view of what would be better.

A source of internal evaluators can be members of quality improvement teams, particularly if they have received any training in program development or evaluation as they relate to quality improvement. The use of total quality management (TQM), continuous quality improvement (CQI), and other quality improvement methodologies by healthcare organizations and public health agencies can be integral to achieving well-functioning programs. The quality improvement impetus of health care has been fueled by the use of standard measures of performance, such as the National Council on Quality Assurance's Healthcare Effectiveness Data and Information Set (HEDIS). The wide use of HEDIS is not only a source of data for health program planners and evaluators, but also demonstrates the social value that is currently placed on data and on the evaluation of services, albeit for competitive purposes.

External evaluators can bring a fresh perspective and a way of thinking that generates alternatives not currently in the agencies' repertoire of approaches to the health problem and program evaluation. Compared to internal evaluators, external evaluators are less likely to be biased in favor of one approach—unless, of course, they were chosen for their expertise in a particular area, which would naturally bias their perspective to some extent. External program planners and evaluators can, however, be expensive consultants. Some organizations that specialize in health program evaluations serve as one category of external evaluator. These for-profit research firms, such as Mathematica and the Alpha Center, receive contracts to evaluate health program initiatives and conduct national evaluations that require sophisticated methodology and considerable resources.

The question of who does evaluations also can be answered by looking at who funds health program evaluations. From this perspective, organizations that do evaluations as a component of their business is the answer to who does evaluations. Although most funding agencies prefer to fund health programs rather than stand-alone program evaluations, there are some exceptions. For example, the Agency for Healthcare Research and Quality (AHRQ) funds health services research about the quality of medical care, which is essentially effect evaluation research. Other federal agencies, such as the National Institutes of Health and the bureaus within the Department of Health and Human Services, fund evaluation research of pilot health programs. However, the funding priorities of these federal agencies change to be consistent with federal health policy. This is a reminder that organizations funding and conducting health program evaluations evolve over time.

Roles of Evaluators

Evaluators may be required to take on various roles, given that they are professionals involved in a process that very likely involves others. For example, as the evaluation takes on a sociopolitical process, the evaluators become mediators and change agents. If the evaluation is a learning–teaching process, evaluators become both teacher and student of the stakeholders. To the extent that the evaluation is a process that creates a new reality for stakeholders, program staff, and program participants, evaluators are reality shapers. Sometimes the evaluation may have an unpredictable outcome; at such times, evaluators are human instruments that gauge what is occurring and analyze events. Ideally, evaluations are a collaborative process, and evaluators act as collaborators with the stakeholders, program staff, and program participants. If the evaluation takes the form of a case study, the evaluators may become illustrators, historians, and storytellers.

These are but a few examples of how the roles of the professional program evaluator evolve and emerge from the situation at hand. The individual's role in the planning and evaluation activities may not be clear at the time that the project is started. Roles will develop and evolve as the planning and evaluation activities progress.

PLANNING AND EVALUATION CYCLE

Although planning and evaluation are commonly described in a linear sequential manner, they constitute a cyclical process. In this section, the cycle is described along with an emphasis on factors that enhance and detract from that process being effective.

Interdependent and Cyclic Nature of Planning and Evaluation

A major premise running through the current thinking about programs and evaluation is that the activities constituting program planning and program evaluation are cyclical and interdependent (Figure 1.1) and that the activities occur more or less in stages or sets of activities. The stages are cyclical to the extent that the end of one program or stage flows almost seamlessly into the next program or planning activity. The activities are interdependent to the extent that the learning, insights, and ideas that result at one stage are likely to influence the available information and thus the decision making and actions of another stage. Interdependence of activities and stages is ideally a result of information and data feedback loops that connect the stages.

Naturally, not all of the possible interactions among program planning, implementation, and evaluation are shown in Figure 1.1. In reality, the cyclical or interactive nature of health program planning and evaluation exists in varying degrees. In the ideal, interactions, feedback loops, and reiterations of

Figure 1.1 The Planning and Evaluation Cycle

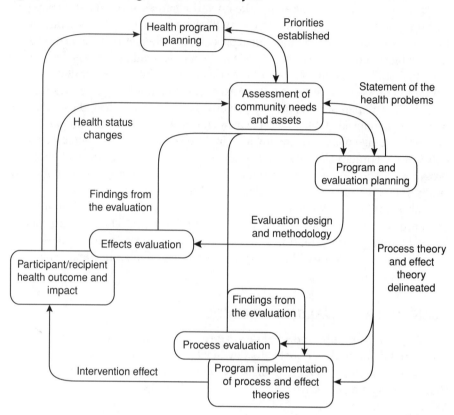

process would be reflected throughout this textbook. For the sake of clarity, however, the cycle is presented in a linear fashion in the text, with steps and sequences covered in an orderly fashion across the progression of chapters. This pedagogical approach belies the true messiness of health program planning and program evaluation. Because the planning and evaluation cycle is susceptible to and affected by external influences, to be successful as a program planner or evaluator requires a substantial degree of flexibility and creativity in recovering from these influences.

The cycle begins with a trigger event, such as awareness of a health problem, a periodic strategic planning effort, or newly available funds for a health program. This trigger event or situation leads to the collection of data about the health problem, the characteristics of the people affected, and their perceptions of the health problem. These data, along with additional data on available resources, constitute a community needs and assets assessment.

Based on the data from the needs assessment, program development begins. Problems and their solutions are prioritized. The planning phase includes developing the program theory, which explicates the connection between what is done and the intended effects of the program. Assessment of organizational and infrastructure resources for implementing the program, such as garnering resources to implement and sustain the program, is another component of the planning phase. Yet another major component of program planning is setting goals and objectives that are derived from the program theory.

After the resources necessary to implement the program have been secured and the activities that make up the program intervention have been explicated, the program can be implemented. The logistics of implementation include marketing the program to the target audience, training and managing program personnel, and delivering or providing the intervention as planned. During implementation of the program, it is critical to conduct an evaluation of the extent to which the program is provided as planned; this is the process evaluation. The data and findings from the process evaluation are key feedback items in the planning and evaluation cycle, and they can and ought to lead to revisions in the program delivery.

Ultimately, the health program ought to have an effect on the health of the individual program participants or on the recipients of the program intervention if provided to the community or a population. The evaluation can be an outcome evaluation of immediate and closely causally linked programmatic effects or an impact evaluation of more temporally and causally distal programmatic effects. Both types of evaluations provide information to the health program planners for use in subsequent program planning. The evaluation of the effect of the program provides data and information that can be used to alter the program intervention. These findings can also be used in subsequent assessments of the need for future or other health programs.

Use of Evaluation Results as the Cyclical Link

Before embarking on either a process or an effect evaluation, it is important to consider who will use the results because, in being used, evaluation results are perpetuating the program planning and evaluation cycle. The usefulness of an evaluation depends on the extent to which questions that need to be answered are, in fact, answered. Naturally, different stakeholder groups that are likely to use evaluation findings will be concerned with different questions.

One stakeholder group is the funding organizations, whether federal agencies or private foundations. Funders may use process evaluations for program accountability and effect evaluations for determining the success of broad initiatives and individual program effectiveness. Another stakeholder group is the project directors and managers, who will use both process and effect evaluation findings as a basis for seeking further funding as well as for making improvements to the health program. The program staff is another stakeholder group that is likely to use both the process and the effect evaluation as a validation of their efforts and as a justification for their feelings about their success with program participants or recipients. Scholars and health professionals constitute another stakeholder group that accesses the findings of effect evaluations through the professional literature. Members of this group are likely to use effect evaluations as the basis for generating new theories about what is effective in addressing a particular health problem, and why it is effective.

Policy makers are yet another stakeholder group that uses both published literature and final program reports regarding process and effect evaluation findings when formulating health policy and making decisions about program resource allocation. Finally, community action groups, community members, and program participants and recipients form another group of stakeholders. This stakeholder group is most likely to advocate for a community health assessment and to use process evaluation results as a basis for seeking additional resources or to hold the program accountable.

Thus far, this discussion has assumed the positive perspective that the evaluations will be used in productive ways. Of course, it is equally possible that the stakeholder groups may suppress, ignore, or discredit evaluations that are not favorable. This reality gains the most visibility in the health policy arena. An example will illustrate this point.

Mathematica, a private research firm, was hired by the Federal Maternal and Child Health Bureau (MCHB) of the Health Resources Services Administration to evaluate the effect of the Healthy Start Initiative programs funded by the MCHB (Howell et al., 1997). The Healthy Start Initiative funded local programs designed to reduce infant mortality and the rate of low birthweight births; each local Healthy Start program had a local evaluation. Mathematica evaluated a range of programmatic interventions in more than 20 locations, using much of the data from the local evaluations in addition to other data sources. The Mathematica meta-evaluation revealed a lack of evidence that the Healthy Start programs had an effect on the rates of infant mortality or low birth weight. These findings, however, were not used by the MCHB in subsequent requests to Congress for funds for the Healthy Start Initiative.

This story illustrates the tension that exists between health policy, which may be driven by contradictions between beliefs about what will work, and the "cold, hard facts" of both poorly and well done evaluations. The political considerations involved in situations like these can be problematic. Regardless of the source of the political issues, planners and evaluators will encounter the occasional unexpected "landmine."

Program Life Cycle

Feedback loops contribute to the overall development and evolution of a health program, giving it a life cycle from pilot to institutionalized. In the early stages of an idea for a health program, the program may begin as a pilot. That is, the program does not rely on any existing format or theory, so simple trial and error is used to determine whether it is feasible and might produce an effect. This is a *pilot program*. It is likely to be small and somewhat experimental because a similar type of program has not been developed or previously attempted.

If the pilot program appears to be successful and doable, as documented by both the process and effect evaluations, it may evolve into a model program. A *model program* has interventions that are formalized, or explicit, with protocols that standardize the intervention, and the program is delivered under conditions that are controlled by the program staff and developers. The model program, because it is provided under ideal rather than realistic conditions, is difficult to sustain over time. Evaluating the effects of this type of program is easier than in a pilot program, however, because more stringent procedures have been developed for enrollment and follow-up of program participants.

If the model program shows promise for addressing the health problem, it can be copied and implemented as a prototype program. A *prototype program* is implemented under realistic conditions and, therefore, is easily replicated and tailored to the organization and the specifics of the local target audience. Finally, if the prototype health program is successful and stable, it may become *institutionalized* within the organization as an ongoing part of the services provided. It is possible for successful programs that are institutionalized across a number of organizations in a community to gain wide acceptance as standard practice, with the establishment of an expectation that a "good" agency will provide the program. At this last stage, the health program has become institutionalized within health services.

Regardless of the stage in a program's life cycle, the major planning and evaluation stages of community assessment and evaluation are carried out. The precise nature and purpose of each activity vary slightly as the program matures (Table 1.3). Being aware of the stage of the program being implemented can help tailor the community assessment and evaluation.

This life cycle of a health program is reflected in the evolution of hospice care. Hospice—care for the dying in a home and family setting—began in London in 1967 as a grassroots service that entailed trial and error (pilot) about

Table 1.3   Assessment, Implementation, and Evaluation Across the Program Life Cycle

Stage of Program	Community Assessment	Program Implementation	Program Evaluation
Pilot	Generic, global information about the health problem and the target audience	Small number of participants; strict guidelines and protocols for intervention	Rigorous impact evaluation; rigorous process monitoring
Model	Greater information about the target audience	Realistic number of participants; use of previously set procedures	Outcome and impact assessment; rigorous process monitoring
Prototype	Very specific information about the local target audience and local variations on the health problem	Some flexibility and adaptation to local needs; realistic enrollment	Outcome and impact assessment; routine process monitoring
Organizationally institutionalized	More attention on assessment of organizational resources for program sustainability	Use standard operating procedures, organization specific	Outcome and impact assessment based on objectives; routine process monitoring
Professionally institutionalized	Rarely any detailed community assessment; more assessment of competitors and professional norms	Standard for professional practice, certification may be involved	Use professionally set standards as benchmarks of outcome and impact assessment

how to manage dying patients (Kaur, 2000). As its advocates saw the need for reimbursement for the service, they began to systematically control what was done and who was "admitted" to hospice. Once evaluations of these hospice programs began to yield findings that demonstrated their positive benefits, they become the model for more widespread programs that were implemented in local agencies or by new hospice organizations (prototypes). As the proto-type hospice programs became accepted as a standard of care for the dying, the hospice programs became standard, institutionalized services for the organization. Today the availability and use of hospice services for terminally ill patients are accepted as standard practice, and most larger healthcare organizations or systems have established a hospice program. The evolution of hospice is but one example of how an idea for a "better" or "needed" program can gradually become widely available as routine care.

TYPES OF EVALUATION

Several major types of activities are classified as evaluations. Each type of activity requires a specific focus, purpose, and set of skills. The types of evaluations are introduced here as an overview of the field of planning and evaluation, although each receives far greater discussion in subsequent chapters.

Community needs assessment (also known as community health assessment) is a type of evaluation that is performed to collect data about the health problems of a particular group. The data collected for this purpose are then used to tailor the health program to the needs and distinctive characteristics of that group. A community needs assessment is a major component of program planning, being done at an early stage in the program planning and evaluation cycle. In addition, community assessments may be required to be completed on a regular basis. For example, many states do five-year planning of programs based on state needs assessments.

Another type of evaluation begins at the same time that the program starts. *Process evaluations* focus on the degree to which the program has been implemented as planned and on the quality of the program implementation. Process evaluations are known by a variety of terms, such as monitoring evaluations, depending on their focus and characteristics. The underlying framework for designing a process evaluation comes from the process theory component of the overall program theory developed during the planning stage. The *process theory* delineates the logistical activities, resources, and interventions needed to achieve the health change in program participants or recipients. Information from the process evaluation is used to plan, revise, or improve the program.

The third type of evaluation seeks to determine the effect of the program—in other words, to demonstrate or identify the program's effect on those who participated in the program. *Effect evaluations* answer a key question: Did the program make a difference? The effect theory component of the program theory is used as the basis for designing this evaluation. For the most part, evaluators seek to use the most rigorous and robust designs, methods, and statistics possible and feasible when conducting an effect evaluation. Thus chapters of this text are devoted to various aspects of conducting effect evaluations with particular attention to the methods, designs, and samples needed to achieve scientific rigor, giving practical suggestions for maximizing rigor. Findings from effect evaluations are used to revise the program and may be used in subsequent initial program planning activities.

Effect evaluations are more commonly known as outcome or impact evaluations. *Outcome evaluations* focus on the more immediate effects of the program, whereas *impact evaluations* may have a more long-term focus. This language is not used consistently in the evaluation literature; indeed, the terms "impact evaluation" and "outcome evaluation" seem to be used interchangeably. Program planners and evaluators must be vigilant with regard to how they and others are using terms and should not hesitate to clarify meanings and address any underlying misconceptions or misunderstandings.

A fourth type of evaluation focuses on efficiency and the costs associated with the program. *Cost evaluations* encompass a variety of more specific cost-related evaluations—namely, cost-effectiveness evaluations, cost–benefit evaluations, and cost–utility evaluations. For the most part, cost evaluations are done by researchers because cost–benefit and cost–utility evaluations, in particular, require expertise in economics. Nonetheless, small-scale and simplified cost-effectiveness evaluations can be done if good cost accounting has been maintained by the program and a more sophisticated outcome or impact evaluation has been conducted. The similarities and differences among these three types of cost studies are reviewed in greater detail in the text so that program planners can be, at minimum, savvy consumers of published reports of cost evaluations. Because cost evaluations are performed late in the planning and evaluation cycle, their results are not likely to be available in time to make program improvements or revisions. Instead, such evaluations are generally used during subsequent planning stages to gather information for prioritizing program options.

Comprehensive evaluations, the fifth type of evaluation, involve analyzing needs assessment data, process evaluation data, effect evaluation data, and cost evaluation data as a set of data. It is not uncommon for program staff to have each of these types of data available for further analyses; it is relatively uncommon, however, for the program to use all of these data to draw more sweeping conclusions about the effectiveness and efficiency of the program. In addition, for larger, more complex health programs, a comprehensive evaluation can be quite costly and challenging and, therefore, is less likely to be planned as an evaluation activity. It is possible to create a comprehensive evaluation from existing process and effect evaluations done over time, if the data can be collated and interpreted as a complete set of information. Comprehensive evaluations are more likely to be done for model or prototype programs, as a point of reference and to document the value of the program.

A sixth type of evaluation is a *meta-evaluation*. A meta-evaluation is done by combining the findings from previous outcome evaluations of various programs for the same health problem. The purpose of a meta-evaluation is to gain insights into which of the various programmatic approaches has had the most effect and to determine the maximum effect that a particular programmatic approach has had on the health problem. This type of evaluation relies on the availability of existing information about evaluations and on the use of a specific set of methodological and statistical procedures. For these reasons, meta-evaluations are less likely to be done by program personnel; instead, they are generally carried out by evaluation researchers. Meta-evaluations that are published are extremely useful in program planning because they indicate which programmatic interventions are more likely to succeed in having an effect on the participants. Published meta-evaluations can also be valuable in influencing health policy and health funding decisions.

Summative evaluations, in the strictest sense, are done at the conclusion of a program to provide a conclusive statement regarding program effects. Unfortunately, the term "summative evaluation" is sometimes used to refer to either an outcome or impact evaluation, adding even more confusion to the evaluation terminology and vernacular language. Summative evaluations are usually contrasted with formative evaluations. The term *formative evaluation* is used to refer to program assessments that are performed early in the implementation of the program and used to make changes to the program. Formative evaluations might include elements of process evaluation and preliminary effect evaluations.

Mandated and Voluntary Evaluations

Evaluations are not spontaneous events. Rather, they are either mandated or voluntary.

A mandate to evaluate a program is always linked in some way to the funding agencies, whether a governmental body or a foundation. If an evaluation is mandated, then the contract for receiving the program funding will include language specifying the parameters and timeline for the mandated evaluation. The mandate for an evaluation may specify whether the evaluation will be done by project staff or external evaluators or both. For example, the State Child Health Insurance Program (SCHIP) was created in 1998 as a federally funded and mandated program to expand insurance coverage to children just above the federal poverty level. Congress has the authority to mandate evaluations of federal programs and did just that with the SCHIP. In 2003,

Wooldridge and associates from the Urban Institute published an interim report on the implementation of SCHIP. This is just one example of a federal program having a mandated evaluation.

Other evaluations may be linked to accreditation that is required for reimbursement of services provided, making them de facto mandated evaluations. For example, to receive accreditation from the Joint Commission on Accreditation of Healthcare Organizations (JCAHO), a health services organization must collect data over time on patient outcomes. These data are then used to develop ongoing quality improvement efforts. A similar process exists for mental health agencies. The Commission on Accreditation of Rehabilitation Facilities (CARF) requires that provider organizations conduct a self-evaluation as an early step in the accreditation process. These accreditation-related evaluations apply predominantly to direct care providers, rather than to specific programs.

Completely voluntary evaluations are initiated, planned, and completed by the project staff in an effort to make improvements. However, given the relatively low reward from, and cost associated with, doing an evaluation when it is not required, these evaluations are likely to be small with low scientific rigor. Programs that engage voluntarily in evaluations may have good intentions, but they often lack the skills and knowledge required to conduct an appropriate evaluation.

When Not to Evaluate

Situations and circumstances do exist that are not amenable to conducting an evaluation, despite a request or the requirement for having an evaluation. Specifically, it is not advisable to attempt an evaluation under the following four circumstances: when there are no questions about the program, when the program has no clear direction, when stakeholders cannot agree on the program objectives, and when there is not enough money to conduct a sound evaluation (Patton, 1997). In addition to these situations, Weiss (1972) recognized that sometimes evaluations are requested and conducted for less than legitimate purposes—namely, to postpone program or policy decisions, thereby avoiding the responsibility of making the program or policy decision; to make a program look good as a public relations effort; or to fulfill program grant requirements. As these lists suggest, those engaged in program planning and evaluation need to be purposeful in what is done and should be aware that external forces can influence the planning and evaluation processes.

Since Weiss made her observation in 1972, funders have begun to require program process and effect evaluations, and conducting these evaluations to meet that requirement is considered quite legitimate. This change has occurred as techniques for designing and conducting both program process and effect evaluations have improved, and the expectation is that even mandated evaluations will be useful in some way. Nonetheless, it remains critical to consider how to conduct evaluations legitimately, rigorously, inexpensively, and fairly. In addition, if the AEA standards of utility, feasibility, propriety, and accuracy cannot be met, it is not wise to conduct an evaluation (Patton, 1997).

Interests and the degree of influence held by stakeholders can change. Such changes affect not only how the evaluation is conceptualized, but also whether evaluation findings are used. In addition, the priorities and responsibilities of the organizations and agencies providing the program can change during the course of delivering the program, which can then lead to changes in the program implementation that have not been taken into account by the evaluation. For example, if withdrawal of resources leads to a shortened or streamlined evaluation, subsequent findings may indicate a failure of the program intervention. However, it will remain unclear whether the apparently ineffective intervention was due to the design of the program or the design of the evaluation. In addition, unanticipated problems in delivering the program interventions and the evaluation will always exist. Even rigorously designed evaluations face challenges in the real world stemming from staff turnover, potential participants' non-involvement in the program, bad weather, or any of a host of other factors that might hamper achieving the original evaluation design. Stakeholders will need to understand that the evaluator attempted to address challenges as they arose, if they are to have confidence in the evaluation findings.

THE PUBLIC HEALTH PYRAMID

As part of the Government Performance and Results Act (GPRA) of 1993, U.S. federal agencies were directed to evaluate their services and effectiveness. One agency, the Maternal and Child Health Bureau of the Health Resources Services Administration, administers several entitlement programs, including Title V, which provides funds to states for maternal and child health improvement programs. One step toward complying with the GPRA was the development of standard performance measures for the Title V programs. To address the range of health issues covered under Title V, a model was developed under the leadership of the director, Pete Van Dyke, in which the range of services could be categorized. The model became known as "the pyramid" among the state and local maternal and child health programs that received Title V funds. Although the pyramid was developed for use with state maternal and child health programs, it has applicability and usefulness as an overarching framework for public health program planning and evaluation.

Pyramids tend to be easy to understand and work well to capture tiered concepts. For these reasons, other agencies in the federal government have also relied on pyramids to depict tiered services. For example, the U.S. Public Health Service used the Health Care Pyramid (Public Health Service, 1994) to show the tiered nature of primary health care, secondary health care, and tertiary health care. At the base of that pyramid was population services, which has a corresponding level in the public health pyramid.

The public health pyramid is divided into four sections (Figure 1.2). The top section of the pyramid contains direct healthcare services, such as medical care, psychological counseling, hospital care, and pharmacy services. At this level of the pyramid, programs are delivered to individuals, whether patients, clients, or even students. Generally, programs at the direct services level have a direct, and often relatively immediate, effect on individual participants in the health program. Direct services of these types appear at the tip of the pyramid to reflect that, overall, the smallest proportion of a population receives them.

At the second level of the pyramid are enabling services, which are those health and social services that support or supplement the health of

Figure 1.2 The Public Health Pyramid

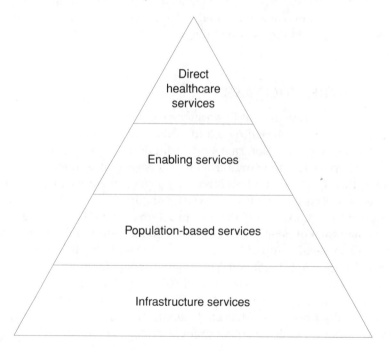

aggregates. *Aggregates* are used to distinguish between individuals and populations; they are groups of individuals who share a defining characteristic, such as mental illness or a terminal disease. Examples of enabling services include mental health drop-in centers, hospice programs, financial assistance programs that provide transportation to medical care, community-based case management for AIDS patients, nutrition education programs provided by schools, and workplace child care centers. As this list of programs demonstrates, the services at this level may directly or indirectly contribute to the health of individuals, families, and communities and are provided to aggregates.

The next, more encompassing level of the public health pyramid is population-based services. At the population level of the pyramid, services are delivered to an entire population, such as all persons residing in a city, state, or country. Examples of population services include immunization programs for all children in a county, newborn screening for all infants born in a state, food safety inspections carried out under the auspices of federal regulations, workplace safety programs, nutrition labeling on food, and the Medicaid program for pregnant women whose incomes fall below the federal poverty guidelines. As this list reflects, the distinction between an aggregate and a population can be blurry. Programs at this level typically are intended to reach an entire population, sometimes without the conscious involvement of individuals. In this sense, individuals receive a population-based health program, such as water fluoridation, rather than participating in the program, as they would in a smoking-cessation class. The terms "participant" and "recipient" are used throughout this text to denote the level of the public health pyramid at which the program was designed and delivered. Population-level programs contribute to the health of individuals and, cumulatively, to the health status of the population.

Supporting the pyramid at its base is the infrastructure of the health-care system and the public health system. The health services at the other pyramid levels would not be possible unless there were skilled, knowledgeable health professionals; laws and regulations pertinent to the health of the people; quality assurance and improvement programs; leadership and managerial oversight; health planning and program evaluation; information systems; and technological resources. The planning and evaluation of health programs at the direct, enabling, and population services levels is itself a component of the infrastructure; these are infrastructure activities. In addition, planning programs to address problems of the infrastructure, as well as to evaluate the infrastructure itself, are needed to keep the health and public health system infrastructure strong, stable, and supportive of the myriad of health programs.

Use of the Public Health Pyramid in Program Planning and Evaluation

Health programs exist across the pyramid levels, and evaluations of these programs are needed. However, at each level of the pyramid, certain issues unique to that level must be addressed in developing health programs. Accordingly, the types of health professionals and the types of expertise needed vary by pyramid level, reinforcing the need to match program, participants, and providers appropriately. Similarly, each level of the pyramid is characterized by unique challenges for evaluating programs. For this reason, the public health pyramid is an extremely useful framework to help illuminate those differences, issues, and challenges, as well as to reinforce that health programs are needed across the pyramid levels if the *Healthy People 2010* goals and objectives are to be achieved.

In a more general sense, the public health pyramid provides reminders that various aggregates of potential audiences exist for any health problem and program and that health programs are needed across the pyramid. Depending on the health discipline and the environment in which the planning is being done, direct service programs may be the natural or only inclination. The pyramid provides a rationale for thinking about only those programs needed to improve the health of the people that are appropriately at the direct services level. It is both difficult and expensive to reach the same number of persons with a direct services program as with a population services program.

The pyramid also serves as a reminder that stakeholder alignments and allegiances may be specific to a level of the pyramid. For example, a school health program (an enabling-level program) will have a different set of constituents and concerned stakeholders than a highway safety program (a population-level program). The savvy program planner considers not only the potential program participants at each level of the pyramid, but also the stakeholders who are likely to make themselves known during the planning process.

The public health pyramid has particular relevance for public health agencies concerned with addressing the three core functions of public health (Institute of Medicine, 1988): assessment, assurance, and policy. These core functions are evident, in varying forms, at each level of the pyramid. Similarly, the pyramid can be applied to the strategic plans of organizations in the private healthcare sector. For optimal health program planning, each health program being developed or implemented ought to be considered in terms of its relationship to services, programs, and health needs at other levels of the pyramid. For all of these reasons, the public health pyramid is used throughout this textbook as a framework for summarizing specific issues and applications of chapter content to each level of the pyramid. At the end of each chapter in this text, the pyramid is used as a framework to identify and discuss potential or real issues related to the topic of the chapter.

The public health pyramid has been used in the education and training of public health nutritional personnel (Mixon, 2002), for explaining services provided to children with special healthcare needs (Colorado Department of Public Health and Environment, n.d.), and for education of general health professionals (Rocky Mountain Public Health Education Consortium, 2004). Other health and human service agencies have used pyramids to help explain the organization of services. For example, the Substance Abuse and Mental Health Services Administration (SAMHSA) used a pyramid to explain expenditures for mental health services. Its Mental Health Services Pyramid was included in the agency's annual report to Congress (Center for Mental Health Services, 2000).

The Public Health Pyramid as an Ecological Model

Individual behavior and health are now understood to be influenced by the social and physical environment of individuals. This recognition is reflected in the growing use of the ecological approach to health services and public health programs. The ecological approach, which stemmed from systems theory applied to individuals and families (Bronfenbrenner, 1970, 1989), postulates that individuals can be influenced by factors in their immediate social and physical environment. The individual is viewed as a member of an intimate social network, usually a family, which is a member of a larger social network, such as a neighborhood or community. The way in which individuals are nested within these social networks has consequences for the health of the individual.

The public health pyramid, by distinguishing and recognizing the importance of enabling and population services, can be integrated with an ecological view of health and health problems. If one were to look down on the pyramid from above, the levels would appear as concentric squares (Figure 1.3)—direct services for individuals nested within enabling services for families, aggregates, and neighborhoods, which are in turn nested within population services for all residents of cities, states, or countries. This is similar to individuals being nested within the enabling environment of their family, workplace setting, or neighborhood, all of which are nested within the population environment of factors such as social norms and economic and political environments. The infrastructure of the healthcare system and public health system is the foundation and supporting environment for promoting health and preventing illnesses and diseases.

At the end of each chapter in this book, a summary of the chapter contents is presented in the form of challenges or issues related to applying the chapter content to each level of the pyramid. This feature is intended to reinforce the message that each level of the pyramid has value and importance to health program planning and evaluation. In addition, certain unique challenges are

Figure 1.3 The Pyramid as an Ecological Model

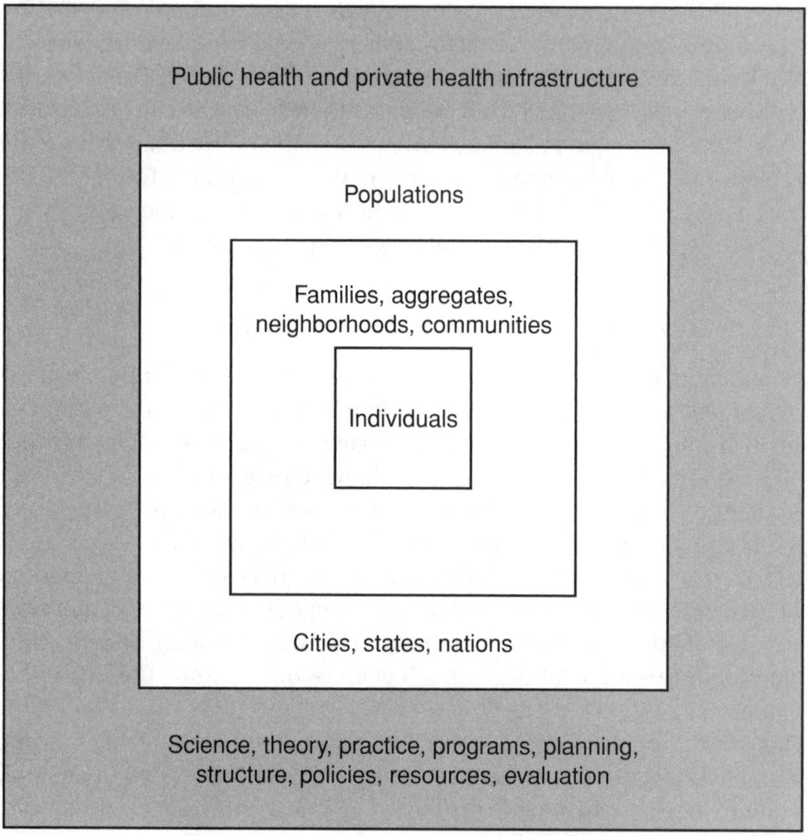

Public health and private health infrastructure

Populations

Families, aggregates, neighborhoods, communities

Individuals

Cities, states, nations

Science, theory, practice, programs, planning, structure, policies, resources, evaluation

specific to each level of the pyramid. The chapter summary by levels offers an opportunity to acknowledge and address the issues related to the levels.

Health Programs, Projects, and Services

What distinguishes a program from a project or from a service can be difficult to explain, given the fluidity of language and terms. The term *program* is fairly generic, but generally connotes a structured effort to provide a specific set of services or interventions. In contrast, a *project* often refers to a time-limited or experimental effort to provide a specific set of services or interventions through an organizational structure. In the abstract, a *service* can be difficult to define, but generally includes interaction between provider and client, an intangibility aspect to what is provided, and a non-permanence or transitory nature to what is provided. Using this definition of service, it is easy to see that what is provided in a health program qualifies as a service, although it may not be a health service.

A *health program* is a totality of an organized structure designed for the provision of fairly discrete health-focused intervention, where that intervention is designed for a specific target audience. By comparison, *health services* are the organizational structures through which providers interact with clients or patients so as to meet the needs or address the health problems of the clients or patients. Health programs, particularly in public health, tend to provide educational services, have a prevention focus, and deliver services that are not at the direct services level of the pyramid. In contrast, health services exist exclusively at the direct services level of the public health pyramid. Recognizing the distinction between health programs and health services is important for understanding the corresponding unique planning and evaluation needs of each. The approach used in this textbook considers those unique differences through the lens of the public health pyramid.

LAYETTEVILLE AND BOWE COUNTY

As an aid to understanding and assimilating the content covered in each chapter, examples are given from the literature. In addition, each chapter includes some application of content to a hypothetical town (Layetteville) in an imaginary county (Bowe County). Based on a fictional community needs assessment, subsequent prioritization leads to the identification of five health problems as foci for health program planning. These health problems are used throughout the text as opportunities to demonstrate application of the chapter content. Also, some discussion questions and activities use Layetteville and Bowe County as opportunities for the reader to practice applying the chapter content. While the town and county are fictitious, the health problems around which the program planning and evaluation occur are very real and relevant.

ACROSS THE PYRAMID

At the direct services level, health program planning and evaluation focus on individual clients or patients—that is, on developing programs that are provided to those individuals and on assessing the extent to which those programs make a difference in the health of the individuals who receive the health program. Health is defined in individual terms, and program effects are measured as individual changes. From this level of the public health pyramid, community is most likely viewed as the context affecting individual health.

At the enabling services level, health program planning and evaluation focus on the needs of aggregates of individuals and on the services that the aggregate needs to maintain health or make health improvements. Enabling services are often social, educational, or human services that have an indirect effect on health, thus warranting their inclusion in planning health programs. Health continues to be defined and measured as an individual characteristic to the extent that enabling services are provided to individual members of the aggregate. However, program planning and evaluation focus not on individuals, but rather on the aggregate as a unit. At this level of the pyramid, community can be either the aggregate that is targeted for a health program or the context in which the aggregate functions and lives. How community is viewed will depend on the health problem being addressed.

At the population-based services level, health program planning and evaluation focus on the needs of all members of a population. At this level of the pyramid, health programs are at a minimum population driven, meaning that data collected in regard to the health of the population drive the decisions about the health program. This approach results in programs that are population focused and, ideally (but not necessarily), population based. It is worth noting that population-focused programs tend to have a health promotion or health maintenance focus, rather than a focus on treatment of illnesses. At a population level, health is defined in terms of population statistics, such as mortality and morbidity rates. In this regard, the *Healthy People 2010* objectives (Table 1.4) are predominantly at the population level of the public health pyramid. Community is more likely to be the population targeted by the health program.

At the infrastructure level, health program planning and evaluation are infrastructure activities of both the public health system and the healthcare system. Infrastructure includes organizational management, acquisition of resources, and development of health policy. A significant document reflecting health policy is *Healthy People 2010*, which outlines the goals and objectives for the health of the people of the United States. These national objectives are considered when setting priorities and are used by many federal and nongovernmental funding agencies, which often require that a health program identify which *Healthy People 2010* objectives are being addressed. To the extent that health planners and evaluators are familiar with these objectives, they will be better able to design appropriate programs and then to argue in favor of the relevance of that program. At the infrastructure level, health can be defined in terms of the individual workers in the healthcare sector (an aggregate). More to the point, because program planning and evaluation are infrastructure activities, it is actually at the infrastructure level that the decisions are made on the definition of health to be used in the program. Similarly, the way that community is viewed is determined at the infrastructure level.

Table 1.4   A Summary of the *Healthy People 2010* Priority Areas

1. Access to quality health services	15. Injury and violence prevention
2. Arthritis, osteoporosis, and chronic back conditions	16. Maternal, infant, and child health
3. Cancer	17. Medical product safety
4. Chronic kidney disease	18. Mental health and mental disorders
5. Diabetes	19. Nutrition and overweight
6. Disability and secondary conditions	20. Occupational safety and health
7. Educational and community-based programs	21. Oral health
8. Environmental health	22. Physical activity and fitness
9. Family planning	23. Public health infrastructure
10. Food safety	24. Respiratory diseases
11. Health communication	25. Sexually transmitted diseases
12. Heart disease and stroke	26. Substance abuse
13. HIV	27. Tobacco use
14. Immunization and infectious diseases	28. Vision and hearing

Source: Department of Health and Human Services website, www.healthypeople.gov/about/hpfact.htm (accessed January 11, 2008)

INTERNET RESOURCES

American Evaluation Association

This international, professional organization of evaluators is devoted to the application and exploration of program evaluation, personnel evaluation, technology, and many other forms of evaluation. The AEA website (http://www.eval.org/resources.asp) includes links to professional groups, foundations, online publications, and other resources related to evaluation.

DISCUSSION QUESTIONS

1. When and under what conditions might it be advisable not to conduct an evaluation?

2. Oral health is a major health problem, especially for children living in poverty. Describe how an oral health program developed at each level of the public health pyramid would differ and how the considerations would differ.

3. Conduct a literature search using words such as "planning," "evaluation," "program," and a health condition of interest to you. Which journals publish articles about health program planning and health program evaluations? What are the current trends in the field as reflected in the published literature that you reviewed?

4. Access and review the material in the following document and compare it with the perspective given in this chapter: Centers for Disease Control and Prevention. (1999). Framework for program evaluation in public health. *Morbidity and Mortality Weekly Report*, *48*(RR-11): i–41. Retrieved January 11, 2008, from http://www.cdc.gov/mmwr/preview/mmwrhtml/rr4811a1.htm

Centers for Disease Control and Prevention

Centers for Disease Control and Prevention. (1999). Framework for program evaluation in public health. *Morbidity and Mortality Weekly Report*, *48*(RR-11): i–41. Retrieved January 11, 2008, from http://www.cdc.gov/mmwr/preview/mmwrhtml/rr4811a1.htm

This online textbook describes the steps involved in conducting an evaluation.

Evaluation Center of Western Michigan University

This organization focuses on advancing the theory and practice of program, personnel, and student/constituent evaluation, as applied primarily to education and human services. Its website (http://ec.wmich.edu/resources/) has links, which are arranged by topic, to a variety of evaluation-related resources. The glossary is a nice feature at this website.

The Evaluation Exchange

Harvard Family Research Project's evaluation periodical, *The Evaluation Exchange*, addresses current issues facing program evaluators of all levels, with articles written by the most prominent evaluators in the field. Designed as an ongoing discussion among evaluators, program practitioners, funders, and policy makers, *The Evaluation Exchange* highlights innovative methods and approaches to evaluation, emerging trends in evaluation practice, and practical applications of evaluation theory. It goes out to its subscribers free of charge four times per year. It can be accessed via the Internet at http://www.gse.harvard.edu/hfrp/eval.html.

REFERENCES

American Evaluation Association. (2002). *The program evaluation standards: Summary of the standards.* Retrieved April 28, 2008, from www.eval.org/EvaluationDocuments/progeval.html

American Public Health Association (APHA). (1991). *Healthy communities 2000: Model standards.* Washington, DC: Author.

Blum, H. L. (1981). *Planning for health: Generics for the eighties* (2nd ed.). New York: Human Sciences Press.

Bronfenbrenner, U. (1970). *Two worlds of childhood.* New York: Russell Sage Foundation.

Bronfenbrenner, U. (1989). Ecological systems theory. *Annals of Child Development, 16,* 187–249.

Center for Mental Health Services. (2000). *Annual report to Congress on the evaluation of the Comprehensive Community Mental Health Services for Children and Their Families Program, 2000.* Atlanta, GA: ORC Macro. Retrieved January 11, 2008, from http://mentalhealth.samhsa.gov/publications/allpubs/CB%2DE200/figure72.asp

Colorado Department of Public Health and Environment. (n.d.). *Core public health services delivered by the Children and Youth with Special Health Care Needs Section.* Denver, CO: Author. Retrieved November 9, 2007, from http://www.cdphe.state.co.us/ps/hcp/home/pyramid.html

Dever, G. E. (1980). *Community health analysis: A holistic approach.* Germantown, MD: Aspen.

Guba, E. G., & Lincoln, Y. S. (1987). Fourth generation evaluation. In D. J. Palumbo (Ed.), *The politics of program evaluation* (pp. 202–204). Newbury Park, CA: Sage.

Herman, J. L., Morris, L. L., & Fitz-Gibbon, C. T. (1987). *Evaluators' handbook.* Newbury Park, CA: Sage Publications.

Howell, E. M., Devaney, B., Foot, B., Harrington, M., Schettini, M., McCormick, M., et al. (1997). *The implementation of Healthy Start: Lessons for the future.* Washington, DC: Mathematica Policy Research.

Institute of Medicine, National Academy of Sciences. (1988). *The future of public health.* Washington, DC: National Academy Press.

Kaur, J. (2000). Palliative care and hospice programs. *Mayo Clinic Proceedings, 75,* 181–184.

Mixon, H. M. (2002). *Applying Bright Futures in practice: Physical activity. The 2002 continuing education program training manual for public health nutrition personnel in Region IV.* Washington, DC: U.S. Department of Health and Human Services, Maternal and Child Health Bureau.

Patton, M. Q. (1987). *How to use qualitative methods in evaluation.* Newbury Park, CA: Sage Publications.

Patton, M. Q. (1997). *Utilization-focused evaluation: The new century text* (3rd ed.). Thousand Oaks, CA: Sage Publications.

Rocky Mountain Public Health Education Consortium, Summer Institute. (2004). Salt Lake City, UT. Retrieved November 9, 2006, from http://servicdes.tacc.utah.edu/rmphec/summerinstitute2005/events.html

Rohrer, J. (1996). *Planning for community-oriented health systems.* Washington, DC: American Public Health Association.

Rosen, G. (1993). *A history of public health* (expanded ed.). Baltimore: Johns Hopkins University Press.

Rossi, P. H., Lipsey, M. W., & Freeman, H. E. (2004). *Evaluation: A systematic approach* (7th ed.). Newbury Park, CA: Sage.

Stufflebeam, D. L., & Shinkfield, A. J. (2007). *Evaluation theory, models and applications.* San Francisco: Jossey-Bass.

Swenson, M. M. (1991). Using fourth generation evaluation. *Evaluation and Health Professions, 14*(1), 79–87.

Turnock, B. (2004). *Public health: What it is and how it works* (3rd ed.). Sudbury, MA: Jones and Bartlett.

United Way of America. (1996). *Measuring program outcomes: A practical approach.* Alexandria, VA: Author.

U.S. Department of Health, Education, and Welfare (DHEW). (1979). *Healthy people: The Surgeon General's report on health promotion and disease prevention* (DHEW, PHS Publication No. 79-55071). Washington, DC: Author.

U.S. Department of Health and Human Services (DHHS). (1980). *Promoting health/preventing disease: Objectives for the nation.* Washington, DC: Author.

U.S. Department of Health and Human Services (DHHS). (1991). *Healthy people 2000: National health promotion and disease prevention objectives.* Publication No. (PHS) 91-50212. Washington, DC: Author. Retrieved August 12, 2003, from www.healthypeople.gov/publications

U.S. Department of Health and Human Services (DHHS). (2000). *Healthy people 2010: Understanding and improving health* (2nd ed.). Washington, DC: U.S. Government Printing Office.

U.S. Public Health Service. (1994). *For a healthy nation: Return on investment in public health.* Washington, DC: Author.

Weiss, C. (1972). *Evaluation.* Englewood Cliffs, NJ: Prentice Hall.

Whitmore, E. (Ed.). (1998). *Understanding and practicing participatory evaluation: New directions for evaluation.* San Francisco: Jossey-Bass.

Wooldridge, J., Hill, I., Harrington, M., Kenney, G. M., Hawkes, C., & Haley, J. M. (2003). Interim evaluation report: Congressionally mandated evaluation of the state children's health insurance program. Washington, DC: Urban Institute. Retrieved March 18, 2008, from http://www.urban.org/expert.cfm?ID=JudithWooldridge

World Health Organization. (1947). Constitution of the World Health Organization. *Chronicle of World Health Organization, 1,* 29–43.

CHAPTER 2

Relevance of Diversity and Disparities to Health Programs

The health status of individuals and populations is influenced by biological processes and by lifestyle behaviors and circumstances. The intersection of biology, lifestyle, and environmental circumstances leads to disparities in health status, with some groups having lower morbidity and mortality rates than other groups. At the root of health disparities is diversity in biological characteristics, as well as in social, cultural, ethnic, linguistic, and economic characteristics of individuals and populations.

In the late 1990s, President Bill Clinton put race, racism, and ethnic diversity on the public agenda. As a consequence, federal agencies, including the National Institutes of Health (NIH) and the Department of Health and Human Services (DHHS), began to explicitly fund research into understanding and eliminating racial and ethnic disparities in health status. Private foundations and other agencies funding health programs followed suit by requiring grantees to state explicitly how each program contributes to reducing racial and ethnic health disparities. The high level of attention given to health disparities means that program planners and evaluators must appreciate the sources of disparity—notably diversity; understand what the key aspects of diversity are and how those aspects are relevant to health programs; and know which strategies can be used to address diversity so that the health program will be successful. This chapter begins to address these issues.

A current urban legend exemplifies the influence of culture on healthcare decisions and the importance of having culturally competent staff. A woman from Africa was in labor with her first child in a U.S. hospital. Her labor was not progressing, and the physician wanted to deliver the baby by cesarean section in an effort to minimize the potential brain damage that was likely to result from a vaginal delivery. The woman and her husband refused the surgery, opting for a difficult vaginal delivery. The couple explained that they needed to make their decision based on what their life would be like when

35

they returned to Africa. In their home village, a woman with a history of a cesarean section would be in grave danger if she were to have another baby because of the lack of surgical services for delivery in her home village. The life and health of the woman were paramount. The child would be loved and cared for by the entire village, even if it were mentally retarded from the difficult delivery. Whether the story is true has been lost in the telling. Regardless of its veracity, it highlights the influence of cultural values and norms on behavior and demonstrates how critical culture, diversity, and life circumstances are to health discussions.

The topic of diversity is addressed early in this textbook because of its relevance throughout the planning and evaluation cycle (Figure 2.1) and because it has such pervasive effects on programs (Lientz & Rea, 2002). Diversity is relevant with regard to assessment of the health disparities to be addressed. It also affects the intervention choice and delivery, a component of which is the

Figure 2.1   Effects of Diversity Throughout the Planning and Evaluation Cycle

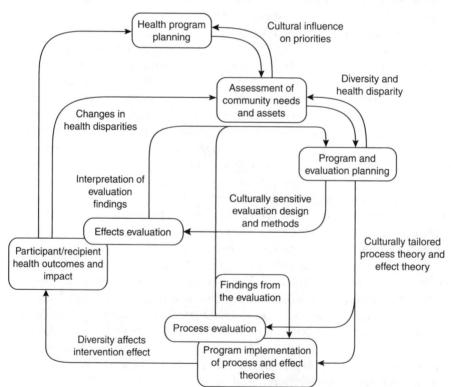

Table 2.1   Examples of Cultural Tailoring Throughout the Program Planning and Evaluation Cycle

Stage in the Planning and Evaluation Cycle	Examples of Tailoring for Cultural and Ethnic Diversity
Community needs assessment	Definitions of health and illness; willingness to reveal needs or wants; self-definition in terms of culture, race, or ethnicity; health disparities; experience of disparities in access to or quality of health care
Program theory and development	Identification of contributing and determinant factors of the health disparities; role of discrimination and culturally bound health behaviors in the disparities; culturally acceptable and appropriate interventions
Process or program implementation	Culturally and ethnically adjusted program objective targets; cultural, racial, and ethnic representations and appropriateness of materials developed or chosen, such as visual representations, colors used, language or languages, location, media used, modality of distribution, and enticement used
Program intervention delivery	Type of intervention; length of time participants receive intervention (i.e., session length); amount of intervention (i.e., number of sessions)
Program effect evaluation	Language or languages of survey questionnaires; culturally appropriate enticements to participate; access to culturally and ethnically equivalent "control" groups

issue of diversity of health providers. Table 2.1 provides examples of considerations that need to be weighed throughout the health program planning and evaluation cycle. The culture of the healthcare organization and the cultural competency of the program staff are directly related to the ability to culturally tailor programs, as is the formation of coalitions.

HEALTH DISPARITIES

Health disparities is a term denoting the important differences in health status among socioeconomic, racial, and ethnic groups. The commonly cited

definition of disparities is found in the Institute of Medicine's report on disparities in health care (Smedley, Stith, & Nelson, 2002): *Disparities* in health care
are defined as differences by race or ethnicity in the quality of health care that
are not due to the health or clinical needs or preferences of the person.

Well-documented health disparities exist. For example, blacks have higher
rates of low birthweight infants (Hamilton, Martin, & Ventura, 2007) and twice
the infant mortality as whites (Hamilton, Minino, et al., 2007). Black children
have a higher prevalence of asthma as well as a greater chance of having gone
to the emergency department as a result of their asthma (McDaniel, Paxson, &
Waldfogel, 2006). Unintentional injury mortalities are higher for non-Hispanic
whites and American Indians or Alaska Natives than for blacks (Minino,
Anderson, Fingerhut, Boudreault, & Warner, 2005). Disparities also exist for
chronic illnesses: American Indians and Alaska Natives are 2.2 times more
likely to have diabetes than non-Hispanic whites of a similar age (National Diabetes Statistics, 2005). Black women have higher mortality rates from breast
cancer than any other racial or ethnic group in the United States (National
Cancer Institute, 2007). These are a few examples of health disparities that
could be addressed by individual practitioners, but are perhaps more appropriately targeted by health programs across the public health pyramid.

The causes of health disparities remain the subject of research, but current
theories regarding health disparities posit that they have multiple, interactive
(i.e., not mutually exclusive) causes that are biological, socioeconomic, and
cultural in nature. The interactive causes of health disparities either can be primary targets for health programs or can constitute a contextual environment
for the health program. In either case, at the heart of addressing health disparities in a practical manner and developing successful health programs lies the
need to understand the relationship of diversity to health disparities.

Diversity and Health Disparities

Diversity, in the context of health, refers to the numerous ways in which
individuals and groups differ in their beliefs, behaviors, values, backgrounds,
preferences, and biology. Diversity is most often described in terms of language, culture, ethnicity, and race. Each of these aspects, along with biological
diversity within the human population, has health implications.

Culture is a learned set of beliefs, values, and norms that are shared by a
group of people; it is a design for how to live (Spector, 1991). As a set of behavioral norms or expectations, cultural beliefs influence a wide range of
behaviors, including dietary choices, hygiene practices, sexual practices, and
illness behaviors. Through such behaviors, culture has an effect on health and,
therefore, is relevant to health programs. Cultures can be difficult to define

and distinguish, particularly when subcultures rather than the dominant culture are the target of a program.

Assigning a label to a culture is less important than seeking information about unique or distinct culturally bound patterns of behavior that have health implications. For example, it is not as important to be able to identify a person as being from Hopi culture versus Navajo culture as it is to ask about daily consumption of meats and fresh vegetables and the ways in which those foods are prepared. Culture, as the sharing of similar beliefs, values, and norms, contributes to a sense of unity among the members of the culture. The cultural cohesion and sense of belonging to a cultural group is a powerful force in creating conflicts as well as in creating opportunities. Both the Hopi and the Navajo have strong cultural identities that present an opportunity for health program planners to build that cultural identity into the program. The strong cultural identity, however, also can create conflicts between program planners and the Hopi or Navajo if the program is perceived as threatening their culture or being inconsistent with their cultural beliefs.

The relationship between culture and illness is recognized as having distinct manifestations, especially in mental health. The American Psychiatric Association's *Diagnostic and Statistical Manual of Mental Disorders*, fourth edition (*DSM-IV*) includes a category for psychiatric conditions that are "culture-bound syndromes" (Tseng, 2006). *Culture-bound syndromes* are mental conditions or psychiatric conditions that are closely related to cultural factors. These syndromes or conditions are specific to specific cultures, generally indigenous peoples. The existence of culture-bound syndromes lends credence to the theory that illness is, at least in part, socially and culturally constructed. The interaction of culture and illness extends into physical illnesses: It is generally accepted that pain tolerance or intolerance is also influenced by cultural norms (cf. Vlaar et al., 2007). The message is that diversity in culture is related to diversity in illness manifestations and responses to illnesses (Edwards, Moric, Husfeldt, Buvanendran, & Ivankovich, 2005; Hastie, Riley, & Fillingim, 2005), but these differences are likely to be identified only through cross-cultural comparisons and astute observations. If program planners lack direct personal knowledge of the culture, they will need to rely on key informants and published reports of cultural influences on illness manifestations that are specific to the target audience.

Diversity also exists with regard to the economic well-being of individuals, as measured through socioeconomic status (SES). The relationship between SES and a wide variety of health status indicators has a long, well-documented history (Kosa & Zola, 1975; Polednak, 1997). More recent research is beginning to unravel the relationships among education, income, and health. For example, Herd, Goesling, and House (2007) found that education was more predictive of health than income. The correlation between SES and health status applies both across racial groups and within racial groups. For example, Shakoor-Abdullah, Kotchen, Walker, Chelius, and Hoffman (1997) compared moderate- and low-income African American communities. Compared to the moderate-SES African American community, significantly more obesity was found in the very low SES African American community and significantly more women had high blood pressure. The fact that individuals in lower-SES groups, regardless of other characteristics, have poorer health suggests that health programs may need to target specific SES groups, not just specific cultural, racial, or ethnic groups.

The attention given to cultural and ethnic diversity is driven, in part, by the numbers. In 2006, 447,016 individuals newly immigrated to the United States. Of the 1,266,264 total number of immigrants, 14% were from Mexico, 6.9% from China, 5.9% from the Philippines, and 4.8% from India (Jefferys, 2007). Of the total immigrants, 17.1% (216,454) were refugees. By 2050, the population of the United States will be 50% non-Hispanic white, 24% Hispanic, 15% African American, and 8% Asian (U.S. Census Bureau, 2004). Although these numbers reflect the continually evolving racial composition of the U.S. population, they do not reflect possible changes in the distribution of cultures or ethnicities. Changes in the cultural and ethnic composition of the United States cannot be as easily predicted, given that cultures evolve over time and ethnicity can be subsumed into the dominant culture.

Diversity and Health Programs

As this very brief introduction to health disparities suggests, the extent of diversity within a target population can have various effects on how health programs are developed and provided. The three main areas affected by diversity are measurement done during planning and evaluating the health program, design and implementation of the health program intervention, and the healthcare organization and program itself, including cultural competency and coalition formation. Each of these is addressed in some detail, in the sections that follow.

MEASUREMENT

Measurement occurs throughout the planning and evaluation cycle. Measurement of health status and of factors contributing to the health problem occurs during the community needs assessment phase. Program delivery and participation measurement occurs during the process evaluation phase. Measurement of program effects occurs during program evaluation. At each of these points in the planning and evaluation cycle, diversity in the target audience and in program participants or recipients has ramifications regarding what is measured, which data are collected, and how data are collected.

The first consideration is always the purpose of measuring an aspect of diversity. This purpose is paramount in deciding how diversity will be measured. Imagine that in a Bowe Country community assessment, an atheist born in Layetteville and a Muslim born in a neighboring town were grouped into the same ethnic category. Stated in this way, it seems strange to assign these two individuals the same ethnicity. But grouping these individuals together makes sense if the purpose of the assessment is to have data on Mexican immigrant culture. Given that *ethnicity* denotes a set of religious, racial, national, linguistic, or cultural characteristics that define a group, the ethnicity measure in this community needs assessment was based on religion as Catholic or not and on birthplace as Bowe County or not. Thus non-Bowe County born Catholics were assigned a Mexican ethnicity. This example was intentionally contrived to demonstrate the importance of purpose in developing indicators of diversity and the profound effect the variables used have on the indicator and findings.

Culture is often implicit, tacit, and not expressed as a distinct factor, making it difficult to measure. In addition, because a dominant culture exists at a societal level, measures of culture are less useful in health programs than indicators of more discrete, smaller subpopulations, such as those that might be defined by ethnicity or nationality. For these reasons, ethnicity is used as a proxy for cultural identity. The extent of language diversity and religious diversity makes constructing a comprehensive measure of ethnicity very difficult. For example, today's vast religious diversity is reflected in the large number of religions, religious sects, and churches listed in the U.S. military's *Ministry Team Handbook*, each of which has specific dietary practices, clothing, health practices, religious practices, and birth, marriage, and death rituals. Health researchers are attempting to understand the relationship between health status and mainstream religious beliefs and practices (Cotton, Zebracki, Rosenthal, Tsevat, & Drotar, 2006; Masters & Spielmans, 2007; Park, 2007). Typically, ethnicity is measured with a single item; however, using a valid and reliable measure of ethnicity is key to having good data for planning and evaluating health programs.

Nationality, which identifies the place of birth of the individual or the parents, is a more straightforward measure. Because cultural identity and ethnicity can be difficult to measure, nationality by birth or birthplace of the parents is sometimes used as an indicator of culture and ethnicity. Many countries, however, have multiple ethnic groups, making it problematic to equate nationality with ethnicity or culture. Thus, if nationality is measured, another measure, such as primary language, may be needed to have a more accurate measure of ethnicity and culture.

The following example demonstrates the importance of carefully choosing indicators of diversity, such as measures of ethnicity or culture, for planning health programs. In one neighborhood of Chicago, a large percentage of the residents belong to a specific sect of Judaism. In this neighborhood, the food stores are kosher, the women's clothing is consistent with their religion, and friendships are built around synagogue membership. Less than half a mile away is another neighborhood with a large percentage of residents with ties to the Indian subcontinent. In this neighborhood, the food stores stock food for their cuisine, the women wear the traditional sari, and the social structure is built around the dominance of the male head of the household. The health statistics for the Jewish neighborhood are relatively good, but the health statistics for the East Indian neighborhood reveal women's health problems due to high rates of domestic violence and chronic illness related to alcoholism. Unless the data from the two neighborhoods are separated, the health statistics for the area as a whole will mask some of the women's health problems and understate the males' health problems related to alcoholism.

This description of two actual neighboring ethnic groups shows the extent to which program planners need to be familiar not only with the data but, more importantly, with the community characteristics. These characteristics include the cultural beliefs of the residents and the degree to which ethnic and religious diversity coexist, rather than overlap. Having this level of understanding about the cultural and ethnic diversity of a community facilitates appropriate interpretation of community health status data.

Race has long been considered a physical characteristic. From a biological perspective, race has historically been associated with specific genetic diseases, including sickle cell anemia, thalassemia, and some forms of lactose intolerance. Race has also been used as a proxy measure of culture, ethnicity, and SES. To the extent that race can be used as a risk factor for specific genetically transmitted health conditions, it has some medical value. However, little agreement exists regarding which categories ought to be used to measure race (Table 2.2). Some (Bhopal, 2006; Lin & Kelsey, 2000; Williams, 1996) argue that the ways in which race data are collected have limited value from the perspective of health, particularly given that many indicators used to identify race are also indicators of culture or ethnicity.

As progress on the Human Genome Project continues and the field of genomics matures (Hunter, Khoury, & Drazen, 2008), researchers may identify genetic markers for diseases that are more specific than race. As tests for these more specific markers become available and affordable, race, as currently measured, may have less medical value. It is easy to imagine a future

Table 2.2 Indicators Used to Measure Race in Different Surveys

Category Used Question(s) are phrased to ask about:	2000 U.S. Census[1] Race	2001 National Birth Certificate[2] Hispanic origin; race	2003–2004 NHANES[3] Race	2004 National Hospital Discharge Survey[4] Race; ethnicity
White	✓	✓	✓	✓
Non-Hispanic white			✓	
Non-Hispanic black			✓	
Black		✓		✓
Black, African American	✓			
Hispanic or Latino			✓	✓
Mexican, Mexican American, Chicano	✓			
Mexican American			✓	
Puerto Rican	✓	✓	✓	
Cuban	✓		✓	
Other Spanish, Hispanic, Latino	✓			
Other Spanish or Hispanic		✓	✓	
American Indian or Alaska Native	✓			
Asian Indian	✓		✓	
Asian or Pacific Islander (API)		✓	✓	✓
Chinese	✓	✓	✓	
Filipino	✓	✓	✓	
Japanese	✓	✓	✓	
Korean	✓		✓	
Vietnamese	✓		✓	
Cambodian	✓		✓	
Thai	✓			
Laotian	✓			
Hmong	✓			
Native Hawaiian	✓			
Guamanian or Chamorro	✓		✓	

Table 2.2   Indicators Used to Measure Race in Different Surveys *(continued)*

Category Used	2000 U.S. Census[1]	2001 National Birth Certificate[2]	2003–2004 NHANES[3]	2004 National Hospital Discharge Survey[4]
Question(s) are phrased to ask about:	Race	Hispanic origin; race	Race	Race; ethnicity
Samoan	✓			
Other Pacific Islander	✓		✓	
Other race			✓	✓

Sources: [1]U.S. Census. Retrieved February 7, 2008, from http://www.census.gov/prod/cen2000/dp1/2kh00.pdf. [2]U.S. Standard Certificate of Live Birth. Retrieved February 7, 2008, from http://www.cdc.gov/nchs/data/dvs/birth1-acc.pdf. [3]National Health and Nutrition Examination Survey (NHANES). Retrieved February 7, 2008, from http://www.cdc.gov/nchs/data/nhanes/nhanes_05_06/demo_d.pdf. [4]Medical Abstract—National Hospital Discharge Survey. (2004). Retrieved February 7, 2008, from http://www.cdc.gov/nchs/data/series/sr_13/sr13_162.pdf#table2.

when the current self-report measures of race will no longer be medically relevant. Until the future arrives, however, race will continue to be used as a measure in planning health promotion and disease prevention programs.

The cultural and ethnic background of program participants affects the development or choice of questionnaires, as well as the interpretation of results. In the development of scientifically sound and rigorous data collection tools, the language and culture of the intended respondents must be considered. To ensure that a questionnaire is culturally and linguistically appropriate and understood requires that the questionnaire be translated from the primary language into the second language and then translated back into the primary language. The back-translated version is then compared with the original version of the questionnaire to determine the accuracy of the translation. In addition, the translation in each direction ought to be done with input from several fully bilingual experts in the content of the questionnaire. Translation of the words is not sufficient; both the ideas embodied in the questionnaire and the wording of each item need to be translated (Su & Parham, 2002; Willis & Zahnd, 2007). The questionnaire needs to be culturally equivalent, so that the ideas and the expressions are the same, not just the words.

The following is an example of the measurement challenges that program planners and evaluators could face. A questionnaire developed in the United

States for the mainstream culture regarding group functioning in a work unit was chosen for use with Taiwanese employees. The questionnaire was translated into Chinese by three Taiwanese researchers and then translated back into English by three other Taiwanese researchers. The back-translated version was considerably different from the original English version.

In trying to understand what had happened, the researchers found that two factors had come into play. First, the lack of a future tense in some Chinese languages made it impossible to directly translate the English items that asked about the future actions of the respondent. Second, the questionnaire had been designed to measure the degree of individual and group functioning, based on the American value of individualism. Thus the questionnaire was difficult to translate both linguistically because of the future tenses and conceptually because of the individualist versus collectivist values of the two cultures.

This example hints at the potential complexity of using a survey questionnaire designed for one culture with a second culture. It also highlights the potential ethnocentrism involved in thinking that what is valued in the American culture—in this example, individualism—would be relevant in other cultures. This translation story helps explain why such extensive publications exist for the SF-12, a 12-item measure of overall health that is one of the most widely translated health questionnaires. The various publications document the SF-12's psychometric properties when translated and used in different countries, demonstrating that even a widely used and thoroughly researched questionnaire requires a considerable amount of work to ensure that it is culturally and linguistically appropriate with each culture.

Cultural diversity also affects the interpretation of findings based on the data collected. Stakeholders involved in the health program who come from different backgrounds and cultures will often hold different values and ideas. Their culturally based interpretations may be quite different from the interpretations of health professionals, who have their own professional culture.

Culture influences how meaning is attributed to findings and how data are collected for program evaluation. For example, a violence prevention program measured the program's effectiveness in terms of the lack of gang tags spray-painted on walls in a neighborhood that was next to a city park. When residents of the neighborhood were presented with the findings, they interpreted the findings in a skeptical manner. They explained that for them the lack of gang tags did not mean the lack of gangs, just that they no longer knew where the gang boundaries were and, therefore, where it was safe to go, including whether it was safe to go the park for exercise. This actual example exemplifies both the powerful influences of culture on interpreting data and the value of involving stakeholders in any data interpretation.

INTERVENTIONS

Program *interventions* are the actions done intentionally to have a direct effect on program participants or recipients. The interventions used in health programs must be tailored to the target audience if the program is to be successful in achieving the desired health effects. The choice of interventions and manner of intervention delivery ought to be based on both the sociocultural diversity of the target audience and the biological diversity within the target audience. Three approaches are evident in how culture is addressed during the development of program interventions. In addition, the diversity of the health professionals and health sectors plays a role in the effectiveness of program interventions.

Influences of Sociocultural Diversity on Interventions

Fisher, Burnet, Huang, Chin, and Cagney (2007) conducted a literature review of interventions focused on culture as means of improving health. They argue that *cultural leverage* is a strategy used to improve the "health of racial and ethnic communities by using their cultural practices, products, philosophies, or environments as vehicles that facilitate behavior change" (p. 245) of individuals and healthcare providers. Cultural leverage, therefore, encompasses culturally tailoring interventions to specific ethnic or cultural groups as well as culturally targeting specific ethnic or cultural groups. In addition, the interventions developed for cultural leverage are culturally competent (as discussed later in this chapter). The key point is that there is increasing emphasis on, and more sophisticated approaches to, addressing culture in ways that are appropriate and beneficial to improving health and decreasing health disparities.

Understanding how to tailor the program given cultural differences begins with having or collecting information about differences across and within cultural groups. Hsu and colleagues (2007), for example, found differences in hepatitis B knowledge and infection rates among different Asian American communities. Navarro, Wilson, Berger, and Taylor (1997), in providing Native American students with a program to prevent alcohol and substance abuse, found that tribal differences and conflicting religious themes among tribes were important to individuals participating in the program. This is not surprising given that more than 500 Native American languages exist, each associated with a different tribal culture. Among low-income, urban, African American women, Beckjord and Klassen (2008) found variations in cultural values such that the women with more traditional values were less likely to seek and receive breast cancer screening.

Studies such as these highlight the inadequacy of broad cultural classifications when developing a program for specific cultural or ethnic groups. The specificity with which a cultural group is defined makes a difference in the delivery strategies and interventions chosen. The health program interventions must be congruent with the values, norms, and expectations of the cultural group.

A current trend is to incorporate faith into health programs and to design programs that are church or parish based. In a review of the literature on church-based health promotion programs, Campbell et al. (2007) found that this approach is effective for African Americans. The practice of collaborating with spiritual leaders and basing health programs in places of worship is likely to continue as an approach to reducing disparities. Developing faith-based programs may or may not require first understanding the health disparity in terms of religion, but it certainly does require understanding ways to effectively collaborate with church leadership and members for the delivery of a health program.

Interventions may result in immediate or permanent changes, but most health behavior interventions are intended to change behaviors that must be sustained over time. Culture can affect whether behaviors are sustained. Potentially, one type of culturally tailored intervention might be needed to initiate change and another type of culturally appropriate and tailed intervention might be needed to maintain the change or program effects. Also, program outcome objectives need to be culturally appropriate, with correspondingly appropriate target levels.

Sociocultural influences on intervention may emerge in unanticipated ways, such as through program participants themselves. For example, program participants bring their culture to the program in ways that can affect the intervention and its effectiveness. Higginson (1998) studied adolescent mothers in a high school program to examine their competitive culture, concluding that it was shaped by the mothers' social class, age, and race. Their competitive culture also pervaded the beliefs and norms of the health program in which they participated. These adolescents socialized new program participants into the competitive culture, thereby creating a "program culture."

Kohn and Bryan (1998) argued that one way to understand the culture of a program is to analyze the ceremonies and rituals associated with it. They also suggested intentionally building ceremonies and rituals into programs for high-risk groups whose members need the sense of belonging that comes with having a program culture, so as to retain them as active program participants. These are some examples of how diversity can affect program interventions.

Influences of Biological Diversity on Interventions

For some health conditions, physiological responses may vary by race, gender, or age, which in turn affects decisions about the type and intensity of interventions used in the health program. Generational differences in values, norms, beliefs, and health problems all contribute to diversity. From the perspective of health program planning, age distribution is an important factor in reaching the intended audiences of a program. Gender and sexual orientation are other dimensions of physical diversity that have ramifications for program development. Disability—whether physical, mental, or developmental—is another dimension of diversity but is less often mentioned. Nonetheless, it may be extremely relevant for some health programs.

The distribution of physical characteristics within a population or community influences decisions during health program planning and later during program evaluation. Take age as an example. Imagine that the Bowe County Board wants to increase the physical activity of all county residents. The age distribution across the community and within its towns will affect the nature and content of the countywide media messages. Messages that relate to the physical abilities of the elderly will need to be quite different from messages that address the physical abilities of adolescents. Similar considerations would be needed for the other types of physical diversity.

Approaches to Developing Programs

Various perspectives exist in regard to explaining patterns of health behavioral differences by culture, ethnicity, and race. Kim, McLeod, and Shantzis (1992) suggest that three approaches are used in health-related programs: cultural content approaches, cultural integration approaches, and cultural conflict approaches.

In the cultural content approach, cultural backgrounds and norms are viewed as leading to behaviors and illnesses. For example, Kleinman (1980), a medical anthropologist, explains that illness is cultural in that sickness and symptoms are saturated with specific meaning and are given patterns of human behavior. The notion that illness is cultural, and not just biological, affects the degree to which individuals accept professional explanations of health and illness.

Cultural integration approaches to developing health programs focus on acculturation. *Acculturation,* the adoption and assimilation of another culture, affects behavior in that the less dominant group takes on behaviors of the dominant group. When planning programs, planners need to consider the degree of acculturation, because it affects health beliefs and behaviors. Behavior is also affected when individuals identify with more than one culture to varying degrees, such that bicultural individuals have health beliefs and behaviors that are a blend of the dominant and less dominant cultures. When targeting groups or individuals who identify with more than one culture, planners need to understand their health beliefs and behaviors as a "new" culture. This is particularly relevant for health programs targeting immigrants or first-generation U.S. citizens.

Cultural conflict approaches underscore conflict as the genesis of behaviors. Several areas of potential cultural conflict exist. One area stems from the generation gap, which leads to family conflict and unhealthy behaviors and illnesses. Differences between the role expectations of different cultures are another source of cultural conflict and unhealthy behaviors. Racism, oppression, and lack of political power lead to alienation and identity conflict, and subsequently to unhealthy behaviors and illnesses. From a psychological perspective, individuals who are experiencing these kinds of conflicts are more likely to be in some form of crisis and, therefore, have less attention and energy to engage in health-promoting behaviors or may be less receptive to making change. Thus an assessment of the target population ought to access the degree of cultural conflict. Program planners need to address the immediate causes of the cultural conflict if they are to develop appropriate interventions for the health program.

Profession and Provider Diversity

Health program planning and evaluation draw upon the expertise of individuals from a multitude of health disciplines, including medicine, nursing, pharmacy, social work, nutrition, physical therapy, and dentistry, as well as social science disciplines, including health education, health psychology, social demography, and medical sociology. Each discipline has its own specialized knowledge, values, and professional norms. Successful planning, implementation, and evaluation of health programs require working on teams that bring together the strengths of the various professions and that respect the different educational backgrounds of team members (Table 2.3). Each health discipline speaks a slightly different professional language, holds different beliefs about how to identify and address health problems, and adopts a different perspective on what constitutes a health outcome. To tap into the wealth of information and experience available through professional diversity requires that the team develop a common language and shared goals for the health program.

Health professionals do not reflect the diversity profile of the population of the United States in terms of cultural, racial, and ethnic diversity. For example, African Americans account for 3.2% of registered nurses, yet African Americans make up 12% of the overall population. Similarly, 1.2% of registered nurses are Hispanic, compared to 10% of the total population (U.S. Census Bureau, 2000; U.S. Department of Health and Human Services, 2006). This same pattern of under-representation of minorities is consistently evident across all health professions. The ensuing lack of racial and ethnic diversity among health professionals creates a cultural gap between professionals and patients, clients,

Table 2.3   Professional Diversity Among Health Professionals

Health Discipline	Average Education	Primary Focus	Licensure/ Certificate	Programmatic Contribution	Estimated Number in United States
Community health worker	High school or baccalaureate	Informal education, advocacy, assistance of community members	Varies by state for certification	Shares ethnic, linguistic, socioeconomic status, and life experiences with community members	86,000 in 2000[a]
Dentistry	Dental doctorate (3–4 years after baccalaureate)	Diagnosis and treatment of conditions of the teeth and gums	Licensure	Oral health knowledge	196,000[b]
Dietitian, nutritionist	Baccalaureate	Dietary and nutritional elements necessary for health	Licensure and certificate	Nutritional knowledge, influence of nutrition on health	96,000[b]
Health administration	Master's degree	Leadership and management of healthcare organizations	Certificate	Management and administration	N.A.[c]
Health education	Baccalaureate	Development and delivery of materials and curriculum designed to impart health knowledge and change behavior	Certificate	Social and behavioral knowledge	N.A.[c]
Medicine	Medical doctorate (4 years after baccalaureate), plus residency of 3–4 years	Differential diagnosis and treatment of illnesses	Licensure and certificate	Medical, pathology, and treatment knowledge	863,000[b]

Health Discipline	Average Education	Primary Focus	Licensure/ Certificate	Programmatic Contribution	Estimated Number in United States
Nursing	Baccalaureate (associate degree minimum requirement)	Promotion of health and well-being based on scientific knowledge	Licensure and certificate	Integration of behavioral and medical knowledge	2,529,000[a]
Physical therapy	Baccalaureate	Restoration and maintenance of body strength and flexibility for the purpose of maximizing physical capabilities	Licensure	Focus on enhancing capability within limitations	198,000[b]
Social work	Master's degree	Address basic needs; help people manage environmental forces that create problems in living	Licensure	Focus on family and psychological factors	698,000[b]

[a] Community Health Workers National Workforce Survey. Retrieved February 9, 2008, from http://bhpr.hrsa.gov/healthworkforce/chw/
[b] Bureau of Labor Statistics (BLS). (2006). *Current population survey*. Table 11: Employed persons by detailed occupation, sex, race, and Hispanic or Latino ethnicity. Retrieved February 9, 2008, from http://www.bls.gov/cps/cpsaat11.pdf
[c] Data not available on these health disciplines.

and program participants. The extent of the cultural gap between planners and a health program's target audience contributes to a reduced understanding of the target audience, a greater need to become informed about the target audience, and, potentially, tensions between the planners and advocates for or from the target audience. The more comprehensive the health program and the greater the cultural diversity of the target population, the greater the need to have parallel diversity among those planning, providing, and receiving the program.

The Three Health Provider Sectors

From an anthropological perspective, the effects of health provider diversity (or lack thereof) can be understood by considering the three sectors of the health–illness system from which individuals seek help when experiencing illness (Kleinman, 1980). Each sector has direct implications for planning, implementing, and evaluating health programs.

One sector consists of allopathic, naturopathic, and other formally trained health professionals who make up the medical healthcare system. Physicians, nurses, pharmacists, naturopathic physicians, chiropractors, and licensed massage therapists function within this sector. Professionals from this sector have legally sanctioned practice parameters. The insurance industry interacts and, to some extent, intersects with this sector. Although not the most widely used sector, it is the most expensive in societal terms. The notion of health program planning falls within this sector, as do the methods and knowledge about health program planning and evaluation. In addition, the preponderance of health programs are designed in accordance with theories and knowledge generated from this sector.

A second sector from which individuals might seek help is the folk healthcare sector, which comprises nonprofessional, secular, or sacred healers who have not received formal education but who are very likely to have received training through some type of apprenticeship. A wide variety of traditional healers makes up this sector—curanderos, espiritualistos, santerias, singers, shamans, and root-workers, among others. Some of these healers and their treatments are now collectively referred to as "complementary or alternative medicine." Evidence of the presence of folk healers can be found when visiting neighborhoods that are ethnically isolated or that maintain folkloric traditions. Individuals may consult healers from this sector while receiving more modern or Western health care. The theories of illnesses and diseases that are the basis of folk health practices can conflict with allopathic theories and thus may diminish the effectiveness of interventions based on an allopathic frame of reference. The role of folk healers in community health behaviors and in addressing health problems can be central for some health programs, especially those targeting individuals who have maintained "the old ways."

The third (and largest) sector of health providers is the popular or lay sector, consisting of family and friends. Undoubtedly, most of us talk to a family member or friend about our illness before seeking either professional or folk health care. This almost invisible sector is the most relied upon, from receiving the latest news disseminated through the mass media to getting a mother's recipe for chicken soup. Health information is spread through the lay sector through social networks, making it a powerful factor in influencing health knowledge and behavior. Health programs that seek to change social norms or population-level behaviors are essentially seeking to change the lay healthcare sector.

DIVERSITY WITHIN HEALTHCARE ORGANIZATIONS AND PROGRAMS

From a systems theory perspective, an organization that is internally diverse will be better able to respond to externally diverse needs and demands. This concept has been formalized into the concept of requisite variety (Weick, 1979). The concept of requisite variety suggests that healthcare organizations with a culturally diverse and culturally competent workforce are better suited to provide services that meet culturally diverse health needs. The need for requisite variety is a fundamental reason for having a culturally and ethnically diverse health professions sector. The need for a diverse workforce was recognized in a report to the Bureau of Health Professions, within the Health Resources and Services Administration (HRSA, 2006), especially to benefit underserved and minority populations.

Organizational Culture

Many different types of organizations offer health programs, including state or local health agencies, for-profit acute care networks, not-for-profit community-based agencies, and academic institutions. Each organization has a unique set of values, norms, and beliefs that are collectively held by its members and that are passed on to new employees; this constitutes the organizational culture (Deal & Kennedy, 1982; Schein, 1995). Organizational culture continues to be relevant, including in health care (Scott, Mannion, Davies, & Marshall, 2003). Well-known examples of organizational culture are the norms about starting meetings on time and the willingness to help other employees accomplish tasks.

Organizational culture is recognized as influencing the performance of health programs, as exemplified through studies of patient safety and rates of medical errors (e.g., Williams, Well, Konrad, & Linzer, 2007) and patient outcomes (Gershon et al., 2007). Sustaining new health programs has also been associated with better organizational cultures of mental health clinics (Glisson et al., 2008) and organizational climate with continued implementation of health promotion programs in schools (Parcel et al., 2003).

Program managers need to be sensitive to the degree of fit between the organizational culture and the goals of the health program. Not all good ideas for programs are good for the organization. A good match or fit between the organization's view of its mission and philosophy—in other words, its beliefs and values—and the purpose of the health program may be important to the success of the health program in terms of financial, personnel, and other organizational support. In a similar vein, the integration and sustainability of a program within an organization are affected by organizational culture. For example, Gager and Elias (1997) found that, for sustaining a mental health program in a school, a determinant factor was having the program become part of the school's culture.

Another implication of organizational culture for program managers is that staff with work experience hold some of the values and norms of their prior organizational culture. These values and norms can be shaped; in other words, new employees need to become acculturated into the new organization, a process that begins with their initial orientation. Cox (2001), an expert on multicultural organizations, defined diversity within an organization as the variation in the social and cultural identities of people existing together. For organizations, diversity provides value-added because it increases respect, improves problem solving, increases creativity and ideas, increases organizational flexibility, improves the quality of employees, and improves marketing strategies. Diversity within organizations does not just create benefits, however; it also poses challenges for managing and enhancing that diversity.

An essential element contributing to a healthcare organization's cultural competency is its ability to engage in self-assessment of its cultural competency. This endeavor requires having an understanding of the cultural competency continuum.

Cultural Competency Continuum

Accompanying the emphasis on diversity and health disparities is the emphasis on *cultural competency*, the extent to which individuals are able to live or work in a culture other than their own. Cultural competency, by its very nature, has shades of less and more that extend along a continuum (Orlandi, 1992; Table 2.4), an idea that has gained wide acceptance (Lewin Group, 2001). It is possible for health professionals and program staff to reside at different points along the continuum, depending on a variety of factors, such as the specific circumstances and the individuals' experiences with cultures other than their own. While the prevailing norm and politically correct stance is to be as culturally sensitive and as competent as possible, acceptance of different values and beliefs can be difficult, particularly those of cultures that are dramatically different from one's own.

Cultural Destructiveness.   At the least tolerant end of the continuum is cultural destructiveness (Orlandi, 1992), which includes a set of attitudes and practices that explicitly promote one culture over another based on the notion

Table 2.4 Cultural Continuum with Examples of the Distinguishing Features of Each Stage

	Cultural Destructiveness	Cultural Incapacity	Cultural Blindness	Cultural Openness	Cultural Competence	Cultural Proficiency
Attitude toward other cultures	Hostility	Dislike, separate but equal	Ambivalence, treat all alike	Curious, cultural awareness	Respect and tolerance, cultural sensitivity	Fully comfortable, cultural attunement
Knowledge of other cultures	Active avoidance of knowledge	None	Little or none	Some	Fair amount	Extensive
Degree of integration across cultures	None	None	None	Contemplation of potential benefits of integration	Some integration, some elements of multicultural integration	Extensive integration, fully multicultural, fusion of cultures
Implications for health program of participants at each stage	Programs address consequences of cultural destructiveness	Need to have programs provided to separate groups	If have multicultural elements, may need to justify and explain	Can provide program to participants from multiple cultures but will need to provide information and role modeling of competence	Can provide program to participants from multiple cultures with minimal adjustments	Can provide multilingual, multicultural interventions in one program

of one culture being superior to the other. The attitude of superiority of one's culture over the inferior culture stems from the notion of the other being different or distasteful. Often physical (visible) characteristics are used as the basis for cultural destructiveness, especially race, gender, sexual orientation, and age. While it is unlikely that the staff of a health program would be at this end of the continuum, health programs might be needed by and being planned for individuals who would reside at this end of the continuum. In fact, many of the global conflicts that lead to humanitarian crises and refugees have their roots in cultural destructiveness. Indeed, international health programs are likely to deal directly with the consequences of cultural destructiveness. For programs within the United States, program planners will need to have an

"insider" understanding of factors that would make the health program acceptable to culturally destructive groups.

Cultural Incapacity.   Individuals at the next stage, cultural incapacity, also
promote one culture over another, albeit more implicitly than individuals
at the cultural destructiveness stage. Cultural incapacity is manifested in the
doctrine of "separate but equal," with the accompanying segregation and dis-
crimination. In the United States, both cultural incapacity and cultural destructiveness have been made illegal through constitutional, federal, and various
state statutes.

Cultural Blindness.   Cultural blindness is a perspective of being unbiased,
such that people are viewed as being alike and, consequently, are treated alike.
At this stage, the definition of "alike" is based on the dominant culture, giving
cultural blindness ethnocentric overtones. Historically, health programs
sought and delivered universal solutions without regard to different communication patterns of different cultures (Airhihenbuwa, 1994). Treating everyone
in an unbiased manner would seem to be a reasonable premise for a health
program. Cultural blindness, however, does not lead to effective programs.

One explanation for this phenomenon, taken from educational psychology,
centers on the role of the dominant culture. Boekaerts (1998) suggests that
because culture affects self-constructs, it also affects key features of how individuals learn and process information. As a result, what may be an effective
learning environment for members of the dominant culture may not be effective for members of the less dominant culture, who are being treated like members of the dominant culture. This theory implies that health programs,
especially those with education or learning components that are based on a
cultural blindness perspective, are not likely to be effective for individuals not
from the dominant culture.

Another way of thinking about the consequences of cultural blindness is by
acknowledging its failure to recognize that ideas and concepts are not the
same across cultures, due to the differences in self-constructs and learning. From this perspective, the earlier discussion of the need to translate concepts used in questionnaires is another example of how to overcome cultural
blindness and its potential consequences for health program planning and
evaluation.

Cultural Openness.   Cultural openness is the attitude of being receptive to a
different culture and to active learning about other cultures. Although other
cultures are valued and some knowledge of other cultures exists, cultural
openness does not include any integration of cultures or cross-pollination of

cultural ideas. In this regard, cultural openness is similar to cultural aware-ness. Each culture is valued and understood as separate and distinct.

An example of being culturally open is someone from a dominant white cul-ture going to a local Native American powwow or to an inner-city Black Evange-list Church service simply to observe what happens. Cultural openness in health programs would be evident in having minority representation on community or advisory boards for the health program, using consultants with expertise in cul-tural awareness, and providing cultural sensitivity training for staff. Such cultur-ally open practices increase the likelihood that the health program will be culturally appropriate, but they do not ensure its appropriateness. To ensure that the health program is culturally appropriate requires actively seeking informa-tion and integrating that information into the design, delivery, and evaluation of the health program. This process requires cultural competence.

Cultural Competence. Cultural competence encompasses not only demon-strating respect for other cultures, but also actively seeking advice and consul-tation from members of the less dominant cultural group about what is culturally appropriate from their perspective. Acting in a culturally competent manner requires various skills that one needs to acquire intentionally. These skills are more specific than listening and being respectful. Continuing with the Native American example, if a tribal healer is consulted and included as a full member in the planning team for a health program intended for members of his tribe, then the health planning team is exhibiting culturally competent behaviors, especially if the hearler's approach to healing is included in the pro-gram. Generally, cultural competence is understood as an individual charac-teristic of providers. For example, in a study of medical clinics, Paez, Allen, Carson, and Cooper (2007) found that more culturally competent provider behavior was associated with the clinic having more nonwhite staff and more culturally adapted patient education materials.

One challenge to understanding what constitutes cultural competence is that other terms may be used to describe it, such as "cultural sensitivity" and "cultural attunement." Both sensitivity and attunement can be viewed as ele-ments of cultural competence. Hoskins (1999) has proposed five principles of cultural attunement: acknowledging the pain of oppression by the dominant cul-ture, engaging in acts of humility, acting with reverence, engaging in mutuality, and coming from a place of "not knowing." Hoskins's principles are notably developed for members of the dominant culture, with the implicit expectation that the member of the dominant culture needs to become culturally competent. In other words, it is incumbent upon the member of the dominant culture to strive for cultural competence. These principles also reveal that cultural compe-tence, as a set of behaviors, may be difficult to attain or maintain over time.

The Lewin Group (2001), writing in a report for HRSA on cultural competence, listed domains of cultural competence for healthcare organizations. One domain is the values and attitudes of mutual respect and regard, and acceptance of the role that values and beliefs play in health and illness. Another domain is a communication style of being sensitive and aware of cultural nonverbal language. Community and consumer involvement and participation in decision making constitute the third domain. The fourth domain is the cultural appropriateness of the physical environment, materials, and resources; use of posters and brochures with representatives from different races and ethnicities falls into this domain. The fifth domain encompasses policies and procedures of the organization that lead to hiring staff members who reflect the linguistic and cultural diversity of the community. Another domain is the self-awareness exhibited by the health professional in regard to his or her own beliefs, values, and knowledge about diversity. The final domain is the training and professional development provided to staff to ensure cultural competence across the organization.

This list of domains hints at the corresponding amount of work needed to achieve and maintain a culturally competent organization and workforce. These same domains clearly apply to programs.

Cultural Proficiency.   At the most culturally capable end of the cultural competency continuum is cultural proficiency, which involves proactively seeking knowledge and information about other cultures, as well as educating others about other cultures. Cultural proficiency, as with any end point on a continuum, is difficult to achieve and may not be sustained for a long period of time. Those rare individuals who can move seamlessly among cultures, be accepted in those cultures, and act as an ambassador of multiple cultures would be considered culturally proficient.

Being *multicultural*—that is, fully accepting and integrating two or more sets of cultural values and beliefs—is a manifestation of cultural proficiency. Multiculturalism in an organization or program (Cox, 1991) is the extent to which different cultures are fully integrated. It is manifested in programs that integrate folk or professional practitioners and treatment options, have predominantly bicultural staff, celebrate holidays important to cultural groups involved in the program, and synthesize different cultural beliefs into the program plan and implementation.

Enhancing Cultural Competency

Program managers can enhance cultural sensitivity, cultural awareness, and cultural competencies through several strategies other than hiring consultants or sending staff for cultural competency training. Cox (2001) has stressed that to have a diverse, friendly organization, workplace, or program requires making systemwide changes, affecting everything from hiring policies to the physical structure of the workplace, that are aligned with valuing and respecting the diversity of personnel.

For example, before making plans for organizational system changes, an organizational or program self-assessment of cultural competency is warranted. A variety of assessment tools serving this purpose have been developed and validated (i.e., Doorenbos, Schim, Benkert, & Borse, 2005). In addition, the National Center for Cultural Competence (Cohen & Goode, 1999) has developed a simple checklist (Exhibit 2.1) for use by program planners, as well as by other individuals who have roles in shaping policy at the federal, state, or local levels. Use of this checklist can help determine which areas are in need of attention (Goode, Jones, & Mason, 2002), with actions subsequently being taken to enhance the cultural competency of staff and the program as a whole.

Enhancing the cultural competency of health professionals begins with recruitment of minorities into the health disciplines, which remains a challenge (Pacquiao, 2007). During professional training, curricular attention to developing cultural competency also presents a challenge. Other problematic issues related to developing cultural competency curricula for health professionals are the need to overcome learner resistance and the need to avoid creating stereotypes (Boutin-Foster, Foster, & Konopasek, 2008), as well as the need for consensus on what ought to be taught and adequate preparation of faculty (Lipson & DeSantis, 2007). Katz, Conant, and Inui (2000), in a program to teach medical residents on a geriatric rotation, described the process used to build a dialogic relationship among participants from different generational cultures, as well as among lay and medical cultures. They learned that a special kind of listening was required that included a high degree of paying attention to the speaker. These findings suggest that specific efforts and skills are required to overcome the cultural differences between professionals and lay individuals.

One strategy to use with individual program staff is to make it acceptable to ask questions about cultural beliefs and practices and norms so that staff members can acquire the information necessary to become more culturally competent. Program personnel need to be able to express both their comfort and their discomfort with other cultures, as a step toward receiving whatever information or counseling is needed to overcome the discomfort. Out of respect, cultural labels ought to be avoided, using instead objective descriptors or names of individuals.

Not all staff members will be equally accepting and competent with all other cultures, depending on their cultural background. Some cultures are

Exhibit 2.1   Checklist to Facilitate Development of Cultural and Linguistic Competence Within Healthcare Organizations

Does the healthcare organization, primary healthcare system, or program have

☐ A mission statement that articulates its principles, rationale, and values for culturally and linguistically competent healthcare service delivery?

☐ Policies and procedures that support a practice model that incorporates culture into the delivery of services to racially, ethnically, culturally, and linguistically diverse groups?

☐ Structures to ensure consumer and community participation in the planning, delivery, and evaluation of its services?

☐ Processes to review policy and procedures systematically to assess their relevance for the delivery of culturally competent services?

☐ Policies and procedures for staff recruitment, hiring, and retention that will achieve the goal of a diverse and culturally competent workforce?

☐ Policies and resources to support ongoing professional development and in-service training (at all levels) for culturally competent healthcare values, principles, and practices?

☐ Policies to ensure that new staff are provided with training, technical assistance, and other supports necessary to work within culturally and linguistically diverse communities?

☐ Position descriptions and personnel performance measures that include skill sets related to cultural competence?

☐ Fiscal support and incentives for the improvement of cultural competence at the board, agency, program, and staff levels?

☐ Methods to identify and acquire knowledge about health beliefs and practices of emergent or new populations in service delivery areas?

☐ Policies and allocated resources for the provision of translation and interpretation services?

☐ Requirements for contracting procedures, announcement of funding resources, and/or development of requests for proposals that include culturally and linguistically competent practices?

☐ Policies for and procedures to review periodically the current and emergent demographic trends for the geographic area it serves?

☐ Policies and resources that support community outreach initiatives for limited-English-proficient and/or nonliterate populations?

Source: Excerpted from National Center for Cultural Competence, Georgetown University. (n.d.). *Policy brief 2: Linguistic competence in primary health care delivery systems: Implications for policy makers.* Retrieved February 23, 2008, from http://www11.georgetown.edu/research/gucchd/nccc/documents/Policy%20Brief%202%20Checklist.pdf

more accepting and seeking of new experiences than others. Being alert to cultural differences within program staff is an important step toward developing and ensuring organizational and program cultural competency. Ignoring the difficulties inherent in having diversity can lead to further problems; therefore, the challenges inherent in moving an organization, a program, or an individual toward cultural competency need to be acknowledged and addressed in a forthright, yet sensitive manner.

Another strategy for enhancing the cultural competency of program personnel is to make diversity visible. This effort might include displaying posters or cultural artifacts. It may also include making available to staff members professional journals with a health and culture focus, such as *American Indian Culture and Research Journal, Ethnicity and Disease, International Journal of Intercultural Relations, Journal of Black Psychology, Journal of Cross-Cultural Psychology, Journal of Health Care for the Poor and Underserved,* and *Journal of Multicultural Counseling and Development.* The high visibility of diversity in the workplace becomes a symbol that reflects the organizational culture of valuing and respecting cultural diversity.

Fong and Gibbs (1995) identified three factors that influence the process of increasing the cultural competency of staff: limits on staffing patterns, fit between staff and the organization, and barriers to organizational change. Limits on staffing patterns include having sufficient coverage so that staff members have time to receive the education necessary to increase their cultural competency. Staffing pattern also includes having a diverse workforce as a venue for staff to learn from each culture—that is, from other staff members. The beliefs, values, and goals of individual staff members need to be congruent with those of the organization, which results in the second factor, fit. Fit between an individual and the organization is well accepted as an appropriate criterion for hiring decisions (Cable & Judge, 1997; McCulloch & Turban, 2007) and may entail sensitive hiring decisions. Taking actions to become a culturally competent organization and program may involve fundamental changes for the organization or program. Naturally, there will be barriers to making changes that address cultural issues. Fong and Gibbs (1995) suggested that a key strategy for overcoming these barriers is developing shared goals for staff. In other words, the program personnel must believe in achieving cultural competency for all program staff, not just themselves or other staff.

Lientz and Rea (2002) offer realistic suggestions for addressing cultural issues in the workplace. They recommended avoiding open conflicts over cultural issues, especially given that no one "right way" exists. They also recommend working through informal communication channels when cultural issues need to be addressed or to achieve changes in organizational culture. Another realistic suggestion is for managers to focus on reinforcing those new behaviors that promote cultural competency and sensitivity. Finally, acknowledging that individuals have personalities, rotating staff members to other work units or programs may be the best approach in some situations. The positive aspect of this last suggestion recognizes a hard truth: When a fit between the program and staff does not exist, both parties may benefit from a change in the relationship. The trick to addressing this type of situation in a culturally and legally competent manner is for both parties to understand the issue as one of fit and not as a personal judgment.

In summary, efforts are needed to extend cultural competency across the healthcare organization and workforce. Betancourt, Green, Carrillo, and Ananeh-Firempong (2003) have identified sociocultural barriers to care at three levels: organizational, structural, and clinical. At each of these levels, a variety of approaches are available that might enhance cultural competency, which would then reduce the barriers to care and health programs. Cultural competency at the organizational level, for example, entails ensuring a diverse workforce. Structural aspects, such as the lack of translator, also need to be addressed. Lastly, clinicians and others who have direct contact with patients and clients need interpersonal cultural competency as a foundation for improving health.

STAKEHOLDERS AND COALITIONS

Another key approach to achieving requisite variety is through the inclusion of diverse stakeholders in the process of planning and evaluating the health program, which is often accomplished through the development of coalitions. Several federal agencies, such as the Office of Minority Health and the Centers for Disease Control and Prevention (CDC), and private foundations, such as the W. K. Kellogg Foundation and the Robert Wood Johnson Foundation, have funding priorities related to health disparities that require programs to engage in coalition development, often in the form of community engagement. The emphasis on developing coalitions parallels the emphasis on health disparities and diversity. Coalitions, partnerships, alliances, consortia, and collaborative linkages are some of the structural forms that result when stakeholders, interested parties, members of the target audience, and professionals with expertise agree to work together toward the common goals of community and health improvements for common constituents. The term "coalition" is used as the umbrella term for such agreements.

Coalitions, in whatever form, can be viewed as potentially having power and being power brokers (Braithwaite, Taylor, & Austin, 2000). Underlying the emphasis on coalition initiatives is growing evidence that collaboration among stakeholders is key to ensuring effective community involvement and to decreasing health disparities. For example, coalitions have proved effective in reducing the number of uninsured children (Stevens, Rice, & Cousineau, 2007). Coalitions for health programs may be developed for a variety of reasons, such as creating a power base from which to gain attention for the health problem or resources to address the problem or to achieve long-term sustainability of the health program. To achieve this purpose, of course, the coalition must be effective (i.e., successful). In a review of the literature, Zakocs and Edwards (2006) found some evidence that the following characteristics were associated with greater coalition effectiveness: use of formal rules and procedures, an inclusive leadership style, participation by members, a diverse membership, collaboration with agencies occurred, and group cohesion.

The process of forming a coalition follows commonsense, deceptively simple steps. At the core of a coalition is attention to group process, as the following discussion suggests. The initial step in forming a coalition is to identify potential coalition members who are either individual stakeholders or representatives of organizations with a potential stake in the healthcare program. Naturally, the potential members ought to reflect the diversity being addressed by the health program.

An early step is the task of articulating the common goal for the coalition. Coalitions are more likely to succeed if they have a defined goal with specific tasks that can be realistically accomplished with minimal expense. As coalition members change, funding priorities change, leadership changes, and time passes, the goal for which the coalition was established will need to be reiterated as a sounding board for decisions and directions. It is also worth noting that coalitions have a life cycle, which may begin with a programmatic focus but evolve to have a policy focus (Hill et al., 2007).

Also early in the formation of the coalition, it will be essential to build credibility and trust, both within the coalition and with stakeholders in its work. Relationships with these characteristics take time to build and are inevitably tested over time. Credibility and trust are extremely difficult to recover if lost. The credibility and trustworthiness of organizers are especially important considerations when working with culturally and ethnically diverse groups whose members have had negative experiences with coalitions or health programs in the past.

Rose (2000) suggested two strategies for building relationships in the coalition. One approach is to adopt issues of the coalition members as issues for the coalition. This strategy would be feasible when issues overlap—say, housing affordability and health programs for the homeless. The other strategy is to promote honest dialogue, in which members can be frank without feeling threatened by retribution for ideas. Complementing this strategy is the adoption of a policy of "agree to disagree." This ground rule for interactions tends to foster cooperation as well as trust. Rose reminded us that humor is a very effective tool for unifying members and for relieving tensions. It is always healthy to laugh at situations, to find the bright side, and to be amused. This need transcends cultures, despite cultural differences in what makes something humorous.

Throughout the process of forming and working with a coalition, attention to cultural competency is crucial. One aspect of being culturally competent involves conducting a self-assessment that assesses the values and principles that govern participation in coalitions. The National Center for Cultural Competence has developed a checklist that can be used to assess cultural competency in community engagement (Goode, 2001; Exhibit 2.2). The health program planners could use this tool—after substituting "program" for "organization"—as a means of gauging the cultural competency of the health program to engage the community in health program development.

ACROSS THE PYRAMID

At the direct services level of the public health pyramid, disparities are seen as affecting individuals and their health status. As individuals from diverse cultures, ethnicities, races, and SES backgrounds interact with health professionals and the health program staff, the training in cultural sensitivity and competency is put into practice. If the professionals and staff have not received or integrated this knowledge into their practice, the potential for continued healthcare disparities is present.

Health programs designed for the direct services level of the pyramid will need to verify that the interventions included in the program match the culture, language, and norms of the program recipients. It may also be necessary for the health program to be designed so that the intervention can be culturally, ethnically, and linguistically tailored "on the spot" to those participating in the program at the moment. In terms of measurement considerations at this level of the pyramid, the direct interaction with program participants allows for needs assessment, program process, and program effect data to be collected from individuals, through either quantitative questionnaires or qualitative interviews.

At the enabling services level of the pyramid, disparities are seen as they affect aggregates and families. Diversity is manifested in subcultures or enclave ethnicity, as well as in the larger cultural context. The interpersonal interaction between the program staff and the program recipients remains an essential element of services at this level. As a consequence, the cultural competency of individual members of the program staff continues to be important as they implement the program interventions.

Exhibit 2.2   Checklist to Facilitate Cultural Competence in Community Engagement

---

Does the healthcare organization, primary healthcare system, or program have:

☐ A mission that values communities as essential allies in achieving its overall goals?

☐ A policy and structures that delineate community and consumer participation in planning, implementing, and evaluating the delivery of services and supports?

☐ A policy that facilitates employment and the exchange of goods and services from local communities?

☐ A policy and structures that provide a mechanism for the provision of fiscal resources and in-kind contributions to community partners, agencies, or organizations?

☐ A position description and personnel performance measures that include areas of knowledge and skill sets related to community engagement?

☐ A policy, structure, and resources for in-service training, continuing education, and professional development that increase capacity for collaboration and partnerships within culturally and linguistically diverse communities?

☐ A policy that supports the use of diverse communication modalities and technologies for sharing information with communities?

☐ A policy and structures to periodically review current and emergent demographic trends to
 – Determine whether community partners are representative of the diverse population in the geographic or service area?
 – Identify new collaborators and potential opportunities for community engagement?

☐ A policy, structures, and resources to support community engagement in languages other than English?

Source: Excerpted from National Center for Cultural Competence, Georgetown University. *Policy brief 4: Engaging communities to realize the vision of one hundred percent access and zero health disparities: A culturally competent approach.* Retrieved February 23, 2008, from http://www11.georgetown.edu/research/gucchd/nccc/documents/Policy%20Brief%204%20Checklist.pdf.

The interventions provided as enabling services will need to be tailored to the specific sociocultural characteristics and preferences of the target aggregate. For example, an existing enabling service may be planned for a new target audience. This endeavor would result in fairly specific changes, modifications, or additions to the existing program in an effort to make it culturally and linguistically acceptable to the new target audience. In terms of measurement, data are likely to be collected from individuals, allowing for tailoring the data collection to the characteristics of the aggregate.

At the population-based services level of the public health pyramid, disparities within a population are revealed through the collection of data related to that population, such as vital statistics and healthcare utilization. For all practical purposes, disparities are most easily identified by examining differences within a population, although they can also be identified within large aggregates, such as schools. Because health programs designed for the population level of the pyramid are delivered or provided to the population, interpersonal interaction between program staff and program recipients will vary from minimal (e.g., in an immunization campaign) to none (e.g., in a media campaign). Thus issues of cultural competency for program staff are lessened.

The need for the intervention itself to reflect cultural competency remains at the population-based service level. Health programs targeted at populations face the challenge of deciding whether to make the program generically acceptable for most members of the population or whether to develop different versions of the intervention tailored to known, culturally distinct subpopulations or aggregates. This challenge, while similar to the need for flexibility in direct services programs, is complicated by the inability to tailor the intervention during a program encounter.

Finally, with regard to measurement, most data collected at the population-based services level of the public health pyramid will be on such a scale that simple, generic data collection methods will be needed. This will result in having data that offer less detail but cover more program recipients. Unlike programs at the direct services or enabling services levels, a population-based program may not be able to gather data on actual program recipients. This fact creates a situation in which program planners may need to work more closely with the organizations and agencies responsible for collecting population-level data to ensure that the measures employed are as relevant to the program as possible.

At the infrastructure level, personnel diversity, organizational culture, and program culture all play roles in program planning and delivery. Overall, diversity and disparities are visible through their effects on existing and new health policy and priorities and on organizational processes and culture. Interpersonal interactions among program planners, staff members, stakeholders, and policy makers are the focus of efforts to address health disparities and cultural issues. Programs at the infrastructure level aim to change the cultural competency of the workforce and the capacity of the workforce to address health disparities and cultural diversity.

As with programs for the other levels of the pyramid, interventions implemented at the infrastructure level need to be tailored to the sociocultural characteristics of the target audience within the infrastructure. In addition, they need to address the professional diversity that exists within the infrastructure, within specific healthcare organizations or agencies, and within the healthcare system as a whole.

With regard to measurement at the infrastructure level, the availability of individual data versus aggregate data will depend on the nature of the health program. Health programs provided to groups of workers, such as cultural competency training, make it possible to measure specific attributes of program participants. Health program interventions designed to change health policy are not amenable to direct data collection but would rely on population-level data, especially for program effects.

One other infrastructure issue that warrants mentioning is the legal implications of diversity. For example, the Americans with Disabilities Act of 1990 (ADA) requires that planning for programs take into account issues of accessibility for disabled persons. Another legal issue relates to antidiscrimination laws, which affect both the management of program personnel and the process by which program participants are recruited and accepted into the health program. State laws and local ordinances regarding same-sex marriage and civil unions may also affect reimbursement for programs, responses to survey questions about marriage, and recruitment of family members into programs. All of these factors influence the planning and evaluation of the health program and, therefore, fall within the purview of the infrastructure level of the public health pyramid.

DISCUSSION QUESTIONS

1. Discuss the ways in which the linguistic diversity of a target audience would affect programs being planned at each level of the public health pyramid.

2. Think of a specific health program provided by a specific healthcare organization with which you are familiar. Complete either of the cultural competency self-assessments included in this chapter (Exhibits 2.1 and 2.2). What surprised you about taking the self-assessment? Which recommendations would you make based on the results of the assessment?

3. Identify one health-related questionnaire that has been used with more than one cultural or linguistic group. Discuss the adequacy of the linguistic and conceptual translations of the questionnaire.

4. List four health programs in your community. Are they supported by coalitions? What is the composition of each coalition? Does there appear to be a relationship between coalition diversity and health program success?

INTERNET RESOURCES

Agency for Healthcare Research and Quality

The Agency for Healthcare Research and Quality's Minority Health Page (http://www.ahrq.gov/research/minorix.htm) offers an entire library of minority health resources, including information on health disparities and cultural competence.

Centers for Disease Control and Prevention

The Centers for Disease Control and Prevention's National Center for Health Statistics is a good resource for health statistics. It allows users to manipulate data on a specific health indicator by variables such as race or income. Find it at http://www.cdc.gov/nchs/Default.htm.

National Center on Cultural Competence

Georgetown University's National Center on Cultural Competence (NCCC) website (http://www11.georgetown.edu/research/gucchd/nccc/index.html) has a wealth of resources related to cultural competency. The mission of the NCCC is to increase the capacity of health and mental health programs to design, implement, and evaluate culturally and linguistically competent service delivery systems.

Bureau of Primary Health Care

The Bureau of Primary Health Care, which is part of the Health Resources and Services Administration (HRSA), has a website devoted to creating Centers of Excellence. The relevant document is called "Transforming the Face of Health Professions Through Cultural and Linguistic Competence Education: The Role of the HRSA Centers of Excellence"; it can be found at http://www.hrsa.gov/culturalcompetence/curriculumguide/executive.htm.

Public Health Services, Office of Minority Health

The document entitled "Cultural Competence Standards: Full Report" by the Public Health Services agency sets out the standards for linguistically appropriate health care can be found at http://www.omhresgov/CLAs/cultural1a.htm.

Medical Anthropology

This medical anthropology website includes a page of culture-specific syndromes, with some explanation and maps. Visit it at http://anthro.palomar.edu/medical/med_4.htm.

REFERENCES

Airhihenbuwa, C. O. (1994). Health promotion and the discourse on culture: Implications for empowerment. *Health Education Quarterly, 21*, 345–353.

Beckjord, E. B., & Klassen, A. C. (2008). Cultural values and secondary prevention of breast cancer in African American women. *Cancer Control, 15*, 63–71.

Betancourt, J. R., Green, A. R., Carrillo, J. E., & Ananeh-Firempong, O. (2003). Defining cultural competence: A practical framework for addressing racial/ethnic disparities in health and health care. *Public Health Reports, 118*, 293–302.

Bhopal, R. (2006). Race and ethnicity: Responsible use from epidemiological and public health perspectives. *Journal of Law, Medicine, and Ethics, 34*, 500–507.

Boekaerts, M. (1998). Do culturally rooted self-construals affect students' conceptualization of control over learning? *Educational Psychologist, 33*, 88–108.

Boutin-Foster, C., Foster, J. C., & Konopasek, L. (2008). Viewpoint: Physician, know thyself: The professional culture of medicine as a framework for teaching cultural competence. *Academic Medicine, 83*(1), 106–111.

Braithwaite, R. L., Taylor, S. E., & Austin, J. N. (2000). *Building health coalitions in the Black community.* Thousand Oaks, CA: Sage Publications.

Bureau of Health Professions, Health Resources and Services Administration (HRSA). (2006). The rationale for diversity in the health professions: A review of the evidence. Retrieved February 9, 2008, from http://bhpr.hrsa.gov/healthworkforce/reports/diversity/default.htm

Cable, D. M., & Judge, T. A. (1997). Interviewers' perceptions of person–organization fit and organizational selection. *Journal of Applied Psychology, 82*, 546–561.

Campbell, M. K., Hudson, M. A., Resnicow, K., Blakeney, N., Paxton, A., & Baskin, M. (2007). Church-based health promotion interventions: Evidence and lessons learned. *Annual Review of Public Health, 28*, 213–234.

Cohen, E., & Goode, T. (1999). *Policy brief 1: Rationale for cultural competence in primary health care.* Washington, DC: National Center for Cultural Competence, Georgetown University Child Development Center. Retrieved February 9, 2008, from http://www11.georgetown.edu/research/gucchd/nccc/documents/policy_brief_1_2003.pdf

Cotton, S., Zebracki, K., Rosenthal, S. L., Tsevat, J., & Drotar, D. (2006). Religion/spirituality and adolescent health outcomes: A review. *Journal of Adolescent Health, 38*, 472–480.

Cox, T. (1991). The multicultural organization. *Academy of Management Executive, 5*, 34–47.

Cox, T. (2001). *Creating the multicultural organization.* San Francisco: Jossey-Bass.

Deal, T. E., & Kennedy, A. A. (1982). *Corporate cultures: The rites and rituals of corporate life.* Reading, MA: Addison-Wesley.

Doorenbos, A. Z., Schim, S. M., Benkert, R., & Borse, N. N. (2005). Psychometric evaluation of the cultural competence assessment instrument among healthcare providers. *Nursing Research, 54*(5), 324–331.

Edwards, R. R., Moric, M., Husfeldt, B., Buvanendran, A., & Ivankovich, O. (2005). Ethnic similarities and differences in the chronic pain experience: A comparison of African American, Hispanic, and white patients. *Pain Medicine, 6*, 88–98.

Fisher, T. L., Burnet, D. L., Huang, E. S., Chin, M. H., & Cagney, K. A. (2007). Cultural leverage interventions using culture to narrow racial disparities in health care. *Medical Care Research and Review, 64*, 243s–282s.

Fong, L. G., & Gibbs, J. T. (1995). Facilitating services to multicultural communities in a dominant culture setting: An organizational perspective. *Administration in Social Work, 19*, 1–24.

Gager, P. J., & Elias, M. J. (1997). Implementing prevention programs in high risk environments: Application of the resiliency paradigm. *American Journal of Orthopsychiatry, 67*, 363–373.

Gershon, R. R., Stone, P. W., Zeltser, M., Faucett, J., MacDavitt, K., & Chou, S. S. (2007). Organizational climate and nurse health outcomes in the United States: A systematic review. *Industrial Health, 45*, 622–636.

Glisson, C., Schoenwald, S. K., Kelleher, K., Landsverk, J., Hoagwood, K. E., Mayberg, S., et al. (2008). Therapist turnover and new program sustainability in mental health clinics as a function of organizational culture, climate, and service structure. *Administration and Policy in Mental Health, 35*, 124–133.

Goode, T. (2001). *Policy brief 4: Engaging communities to realize the vision of one hundred percent access and zero health disparities: A culturally competent approach.* Washington, DC: National Center for Cultural Competence, Georgetown University Child Development Center. Retrieved February 9, 2008, from http://www11.georgetown.edu/research/gucchd/nccc/

Goode, T., Jones, W., & Mason, J. (2002). *A guide to planning and implementing cultural competence organization self-assessment.* Washington, DC: National Center for Cultural Competence, Georgetown University Child Development Center.

Hamilton, B. E., Martin, J. A., & Ventura, S. J. (2007). Births: Preliminary data for 2006. *National Vital Statistics Report, 56*(7).

Hamilton, B. E., Minino, A. M., Martin, J. A., Kochanek, K. D., Strobino, D. M., & Guyer, B. (2007). Annual summary of vital statistics: 2005. *Pediatrics, 119*, 345–360.

Hastie, B. A., Riley, J. L., & Fillingim, R. B. (2005). Ethnic differences and responses to pain in healthy young adults. *Pain Medicine, 6*, 61–71.

Herd, P., Goesling, B., & House, J. S. (2007). Socioeconomic position and health: The differential effects of education versus income on the onset versus progression of health problems. *Journal of Health and Social Behavior, 48*, 223–238.

Higginson, J. G. (1998). Competitive parenting: The culture of teen mothers. *Journal of Marriage and Family, 60*, 135–149.

Hill, A., De Zapien, J. G., Staten, L. K., McClelland, D. J., Garza, R., Moore-Monroy, M., et al. (2007). From program to policy: Expanding the role of community coalitions. *Preventing Chronic Disease, 4*, A103.

Hoskins, M. L. (1999). Worlds apart and lives together: Developing cultural attunement. *Child and Youth Care Forum, 28*, 73–84.

Hsu, C. E., Liu, L. C., Juon, H., Chiu, Y., Bawa, J., Tillman, U., et al. (2007). Reducing liver cancer disparities: A community-based hepatitis-B prevention program for Asian-American communities. *Journal of the National Medical Association, 99*, 900–907.

Hunter, D. J., Khoury, M. J., & Drazen, J. M. (2008). Letting the genome out of the bottle: Will we get our wish? *New England Journal of Medicine, 358*, 105–107.

Jefferys, K. (2007). U.S. legal permanent residents: 2006. *Annual Flow Report.* Washington, DC: United States Department of Homeland Security, Office of Immigration Statistics.

Katz, A. M., Conant, L., & Inui, T. S. (2000). A council of elders: Creating a multi-voiced dialogue in a community of care. *Social Science and Medicine, 50*, 851–860.

Kim, S., McLeod, J. H., & Shantzis, C. (1992). Cultural competence for evaluators working with Asian-American communities: Some practical considerations. In M. A. Orlandi, R. Weston, & L. G. Epstein (Eds.), *Cultural competence for evaluators: A guide for alcohol and other drug abuse prevention practitioners working with ethical/racial communities* (pp. 203–260). [DHHS Publication No. (ADM) 92–188]. Washington, DC: U.S. Government Printing Office.

Kleinman, A. (1980). *Patients and healers in the context of culture.* Berkeley: University of California Press.

Kohn, A., & Bryan, K. (1998). Ritual practice in a social model recovery home. *Contemporary Drug Problems, 25*, 711–739.

Kosa, J., & Zola, I. K. (1975). *Poverty and health: A sociological analysis* (rev. ed.). Cambridge, MA: Harvard University Press.

Lewin Group. (2001). Health Resources and Services Administration study on measuring cultural competence in health care delivery settings. Retrieved February 9, 2008, from http://www.hrsa.gov/culturalcompetence/measures/sectionii.htm

Lientz, B. P., & Rea, K. P. (2002). *Project management for the 21st century* (3rd ed.). San Diego, CA: Academic Press.

Lin, S. S., & Kelsey, J. L. (2000). Use of race and ethnicity in epidemiologic research: Concepts, methodological issues, and suggestions for research. *Epidemiology Review, 22*, 187–202.

Lipson, J. G., & DeSantis, L. A. (2007). Current approaches to integrating elements of cultural competence in nursing education. *Journal of Transcultural Nursing, 18*, 10S–20S.

Masters, K. S., & Spielmans, G. I. (2007). Prayer and health: Review, meta-analysis, and research agenda. *Journal of Behavioral Medicine, 30*, 329–338.

McCulloch, M. C., & Turban, D. B. (2007). Using person–organization fit to select employees for high-turnover jobs. *International Journal of Selection and Assessment, 15*, 63.

McDaniel, M., Paxson, C., & Waldfogel, J. (2006). Racial disparities in childhood asthma in the United States: Evidence from the National Health Interview Survey, 1997–2003. *Pediatrics, 117*(5), e868–e877.

Minino, A. M., Anderson R. N., Fingerhut, L. A., Boudreault, M., & Warner, M. (2005). Deaths: Injuries. 2002. *National Vital Statistics Reports, 54*(10). Hyattsville, MD: National Center for Health Statistics.

National Cancer Institute. (2007). *A snapshot of breast cancer.* Retrieved July 29, 2003, from http://planning.cancer.gov/disease/snapshots.shtml

National Diabetes Statistics. (2005). Retrieved January 23, 2008, from http://diabetes.niddk.nih.gov/dm/pubs/statistics/#10

Navarro, J., Wilson, S., Berger, L. R., & Taylor, T. (1997). Substance abuse and spirituality: A program for Native American students. *American Journal of Health Behavior, 21*, 3–11.

Orlandi, M. A. (1992). Defining cultural competence: An organizing framework. In M. A. Orlandi, R. Weston, & L. G. Epstein (Eds.), *Cultural competence for evaluators: A guide for alcohol and other drug abuse prevention practitioners working with ethical/racial communities* (pp. 293–299). [DHHS Publication. No. (ADM) 92–1884]. Washington, DC: U.S. Government Printing Office.

Pacquiao, D. (2007). The relationship between cultural competence education and increasing diversity in nursing schools and practice settings. *Journal of Transcultural Nursing, 18*(1), 28S–37S.

Paez, K. A., Allen, J. K., Carson, K. A., & Cooper, L. A. (2007). Provider and clinic cultural competence in a primary care setting. *Social Science and Medicine, 66, 1204–1216*.

Parcel, G. S., Perry, C. L., Kelder, S. H., Elder, J. P., Mitchell, P. D., Lytle, L. A., et al. (2003). School climate and the institutionalization of the CATCH program. *Health Education and Behavior, 30*, 489–502.

Park, C. L. (2007). Religiousness/spirituality and health: A meaning systems perspective. *Journal of Behavioral Medicine, 30*(4), 319–328.

Polednak, A. P. (1997). *Segregation, poverty, and mortality in urban African-Americans.* Oxford, UK: Oxford University Press.

Rose, F. (2000). *Coalitions across the class divide: Lessons from the labor, peace and environmental movements.* Ithaca, NY: Cornell University Press.

Schein, V. E. (1995). *Working from the margins: Voices of mothers in poverty.* Ithaca, NY: ILR Press, Cornell University Press.

Scott, T., Mannion, R., Davies, H., & Marshall, M. (2003). The quantitative measurement of organizational culture in health care: A review of the available instruments. *Health Services Research, 38*, 923–945.

Shakoor-Abdullah, B., Kotchen, J. M., Walker, W. E., Chelius, T. H., & Hoffman, R. G. (1997). Incorporating socio-economic and risk factor diversity into the development of an African-American community blood pressure control program. *Ethnicity and Disease, 7*, 175–183.

Smedley, B. D., Stith, A. Y., & Nelson, A. R. (2002). *Unequal treatment: Confronting racial and ethnic disparities in health care.* Washington, DC: National Academics Press.

Spector, R. E. (1991). *Cultural diversity in health and illness* (3rd ed.). Norwalk, CT: Appleton & Lang.

Stevens, G. D., Rice, K., & Cousineau, M. R. (2007). Children's health initiatives in California: The experiences of local coalitions pursuing universal coverage for children. *American Journal of Public Health, 97,* 738–743.

Su, C. T., & Parham, L. D. (2002). Generating a valid questionnaire translation for cross-cultural use. *American Journal of Occupational Therapy, 56,* 581–585.

Tseng, W. (2006). From peculiar psychiatric disorders through culture-bound syndromes to culture-related specific syndromes. *Transcultural Psychiatry, 43,* 554–576.

U.S. Census Bureau. (2000). Retrieved February 4, 2008, from http://www.census.gov/prod/1/pop/p25-1130/p251130b.pdf

U.S. Census Bureau. (2004). U.S. interim projections by age, sex, race, and Hispanic origin. Retrieved January 23, 2008, from http://www.census.gov/ipc/www/usinterimproj/

U.S. Department of Health and Human Services. (2006). *The registered nurse population: Findings from the 2004 national sample survey of registered nurses.* U.S. Department of Health and Human Services, Health Resources and Services Administration, Bureau of Health Profession, Division of Nursing. Retrieved February 4, 2008, from http://bhpr.hrsa.gov/healthworkforce/rnsurvey04/

Vlaar, A. P., ten Klooster, P. M., Taal, E., Gheith, R. E., El-Garf, A. K., Rasker, J. J., et al. (2007). A cross-cultural study of pain intensity in Egyptian and Dutch women with rheumatoid arthritis. *Journal of Pain, 8,* 730–736.

Weick, K. (1979). *Social psychology of organizing* (2nd ed.). Reading, MA: Addison-Wesley.

Williams, D. R. (1996). Race/ethnicity and socioeconomic status: Measurement and methodological issues. *International Journal of Health Services, 26,* 483–505.

Williams, E. S., Well, L. B. M., Konrad, T. R., & Linzer, M. (2007). The relationship of organizational culture, stress, satisfaction, and burnout with physician-reported error and suboptimal patient care: Results from the MEMO study. *Health Care Management Review, 31,* 203–212.

Willis, G., & Zahnd, E. (2007). Questionnaire design from a cross-cultural perspective: An empirical investigation of Koreans and non-Koreans. *Journal of Health Care for the Poor and Underserved, 18*(4S), 197–217.

Zakocs, R. C., & Edwards, E. M. (2006). What explains community coalition effectiveness? A review of the literature. *American Journal of Preventative Medicine, 30,* 351–361.

Defining the Health Problem

CHAPTER 3

Planning for Health Programs and Services

Planning is one of those undertakings that everyone thinks they can do. The reality is that planning is not a single task, and it can be time-intensive to do well. The term "planning" is also one of those words that has a plethora of implicit meanings.

Exploring the meaning and delineating the process of planning have a substantial history in public health. The pioneers of public health planning were primarily concerned with planning at the systems level—that is, with planning as it relates to the infrastructure of the healthcare or public health system. Planning with a global or national focus is different from planning for more discrete and specific health programs at a local level. Nonetheless, many of the concerns and processes used in planning for the health system as a whole are applicable and adaptable to planning of local health programs.

Tension will always exist between planning on a local level—say, within one small community organization or one county—and planning at a global level, such as through national health policy or the World Health Organization (WHO). At a minimum, local planning for health programs ought to be done with an awareness of the priorities and programs established through global and national planning. In addition, the local planning process for developing health programs can be enhanced by adapting the processes used at the systems level.

The purpose of this chapter is to draw upon and adapt approaches developed for systems for use in local program planning. To this end, it identifies tools and techniques currently used in planning public health programs or projects. The focus here is not on the type of strategic planning done by healthcare organizations or agencies, but rather on *tactical planning*, which is the set of planning activities carried out to implement a broader, more global strategy. Tactical planning is more time limited, is focused on meeting current needs and demands, incorporates current scientific knowledge in identifying

viable and feasible alternatives, and progresses in stages from problem definition to implementation. Although planning is generally described as a linear
process, program planning is a cyclical activity, with recursive events requiring additional or revised courses of action for the life of a health program.

DEFINITIONS OF PLANNING

A variety of definitions of "planning" have been suggested. Blum (1974)
defined planning as "the deliberate introduction of desired social change in
orderly and acceptable ways." Nutt (1984) identified several ways in which
planning is visible: as forecasting, as problem solving, as programming, as
design, as policy analysis, and as a response to a problem. He concluded that
planning involves synthesis in terms of putting together plans, policy, programs, or something else that is new. In this regard he viewed planning as creating change. Hoch (1994) described good planning as the popular adoption of
democratic reforms in the provision of public goods. Others have viewed planning as the effort to control social or collective uncertainty by taking action
now to secure the future (Marris, 1982, cited in Hoch, 1994).

All of these definitions share the elements of using a rational approach,
making change, and using a democratic or participatory process. In terms of
programs, *planning* is the set of activities in which key individuals define a set
of desired improvements, develop a strategy to achieve those desired improvements, and establish a means to measure the attainment of those desired
improvements.

HISTORICAL BACKGROUND ON PLANNING IN PUBLIC HEALTH

The planning of programs to address health problems essentially began as
public health planning. The history of public health planning began in antiquity
with the environmental planning of water and sewer systems in cities in the
West (Rosen, 1958) and civic planning in the East (Duhl, 2000). These early
forms of planning for the health and well-being of populations did not change
dramatically until the late twentieth century.

Population-based planning became necessary with the advent of immunizations, including the administration of the first polio vaccine. In public health,
Henrik Blum (1974) was among the scholars to formally consider what public
health planning is and how it ought to be done. He advocated the use of a rational approach to health planning, which included considering the problem and
systematically applying a solution. The rational approach to health planning was
further developed in Dever's work (1980), which extensively applied epidemiological techniques to the identification and prioritization of health problems.

Following more in the civic planning tradition, Duhl (1987) advocated for health planning from a social awareness perspective. In this sense, Duhl was building upon the work of LaLonde (1974), who is recognized as being the first public health scholar to articulate and emphasize the interaction of social conditions and well-being. The LaLonde report had a broad range of effects, including influencing Duhl to emphasize the involvement of community members in the betterment of their lives and environment. Duhl has continued to highlight the inseparable relationship between planning from a social framework and health.

During this period, considerable work was also being done in the organizational behavioral sciences on the issue of decision making and development of business strategies. This knowledge was eventually transferred into health care through the work of scholars such as Nutt (1979), who developed a model of the planning process that included stages and elements that were interactive and iterative. Nutt's model included not only activities, but also the central notion that a problem is real and that awareness of the problem is the stimulus of the planning activities. Nutt's work (1984) expanded on the model for organizational planning and focused on planning as done by healthcare organizations. Today, his field of study would be considered organizational strategic planning. The extent to which organizational strategic planning has influenced planning for population health and health programs is reflected in Dever's later work (1997), which drew more heavily on the strategic and organizational knowledge about planning.

These academic advances in health program planning have been paralleled by practitioner-focused advances. Beginning in the mid-1980s, the Centers for Disease Control and Prevention (CDC) began to develop and promote methodologies for systematic approaches to health planning for those working in public health. These models are important for their structured approach to planning health programs and for synthesizing the knowledge available at the time about health and program planning. Historical and current Internet resources related to each of the following programs are listed at the end of this chapter.

PATCH

The Planning Approach to Community Health (PATCH) was based on Green's PRECEDE (Predisposing, Reinforcing, and Enabling Factors in Community Education Development and Evaluation) model of health education planning (Green, Kreuter, Deeds, & Partridge, 1980). Built into the PATCH model of planning for public health was the notion that health promotion is a process that enables people to take greater control of their health and seek out ways to improve their health (U.S. Department of Health and Human Services [DHHS], n.d.). PATCH was implemented as the first national attempt to standardize public health planning and to provide technical assistance to local health agencies.

The PATCH model incorporated information on each of several elements viewed as key to the success of planning public health programs. One element was community participation in the process. Other elements were the use of data to drive the development of programs and a comprehensive health promotion strategy. The PATCH model also included the element of evaluation for program improvement and had as a long-term goal increasing community capacity for health promotion. These elements were to be achieved through steps outlined in the PATCH model: mobilize the community, collect data, choose health priorities, develop a comprehensive intervention plan, and evaluate the process. Although the CDC no longer provides training on using PATCH, PATCH materials are available online through the CDC website.

APEXPH

After working on the PATCH model, the CDC, in cooperation with the National Association of County and City Health Officials (NACCHO), developed and introduced the Assessment Protocol for Excellence in Public Health (APEXPH). Although development of APEXPH began in 1987, the manual for using the APEXPH approach was not released until 1999 (CDC PATCH, n.d.).

A key feature of the APEXPH approach is its addressing of the three core functions of public health: assessment, assurance, and policy development. These core functions were articulated in the Institute of Medicine's (1988) report on the future of public health and have since become pivotal in thinking about assuring the health of populations.

APEXPH differs from PATCH in that it provides a framework for assessing the organization and management of health departments, as well as a framework for working with community members in assessing the health of the community. The APEXPH workbook, which is available through the NACCHO website (NACCHO, n.d.), outlines planning in three parts: assessing internal organizational capacity, assessing and setting priorities for community health problems, and implementing the plans. In one study, 24 county health departments in the state of Washington used the APEXPH model to assess their strengths and weaknesses in each of these functional areas of assessment and implement (Pratt, McDonald, Libby, Oberle, & Liang, 1996). The results could then be used to identify specific areas that needed strengthening. To the extent that APEXPH addresses organizational capacity, it draws upon the strategic planning perspective of Nutt (1984) and others.

MAPP

More recently, the CDC and NACCHO have released the Mobilizing for Action through Planning and Partnership (MAPP) model. MAPP is a strategic planning tool that helps public health leaders facilitate community prioritization of public health issues and identify resources for addressing them. The first phase of MAPP is to mobilize community members and organizations under the leadership of public health agencies. The second phase is to generate a shared vision and common values that provide a framework for long-range planning. The third step of MAPP involves conducting four assessments of four areas: community strengths, the local public health system, community health status, and the forces of change. The final step is implementation. MAPP materials can be ordered from the MAPP website, which can be accessed through the NACCHO website (NACCHO, n.d.). Application of the MAPP process at a county level is possible and can result in a very user-friendly, public document outlining a long-term health improvement plan (e.g., http://www.bergenhealth.org/dept/resources/Chip_2006.pdf).

CHIP

The Community Health Improvement Process (CHIP), developed in 1997 (Durch, Bailey, & Stoto, 1997) is a less widely known tool for community health planning that incorporates organizational performance monitoring and community assets, followed by strategic planning, implementation, and evaluation. Like the other models, it involves two phases: (1) problem identification and prioritization and (2) implementation. CHIP was the first model that linked the community assessment and planning to the performance measures of *Healthy People 2000* and the *Healthy Communities 2000* model standards. The principles and recommended processes for conducting CHIP are similar to those of MAPP and APHEXPH—specifically, collection of data, involvement and engagement of the community, and priority setting. A variety of local governments have used CHIP by either explicitly or implicitly adopting its key elements.

PACE-EH

The Protocol for Assessing Community Excellence in Environmental Health (PACE-EH), developed by CDC and NACCHO, focuses the community assessment on evaluation of environmental health conditions (CDC, n.d.). Thus PACE-EH is a community environmental health assessment tool. The data gathered via this tool are then used to identify populations at risk and set priorities. A key feature of PACE-EH is the emphasis on health equity and social justice. As with the other public health planning models, PACE-EH focuses on building relationships with constituents and sharing the power and responsibilities with the community. PACE-EH has been used by county governments to improve the environment and, thereby, the health of their citizens.

In March 2006, a summit was held to address the barriers to the use of PACE-EH and the applications of this tool. The summary of the summit (NACCHO, 2006) highlighted the fact that more than 60 communities have used PACE-EH, primarily with a focus on improving air and water quality. Given the overall importance of air and water quality to individual and population health, using PACE-EH can be an effective approach to planning at local, county, and state levels.

In Summary

This brief overview of the models that have been used in planning public health programs highlights the ongoing evolution of thinking in this area. Evident in this evolution is the development of tools for designing health promotion programs, particularly those focused at the community or population level. Each model has a slightly different strength and emphasis (Table 3.1). Many of these materials are designed for public health agencies and leaders, as well as for use with community members. It is also worth noting that the content of the materials and the underlying philosophical perspectives are applicable to other types of health agencies that provide health programs to across the public health pyramid.

TRIGGERING THE PLANNING CYCLE

Common across the planning models that have been developed is the inclusion of various feedback loops among planning processes, implementation, evaluation, and the problem. Taken collectively, these feedback loops create a cycle (Figure 3.1).

One mechanism that initiates the planning cycle occurs when an influential individual's attention is caught. A wide variety of factors may act as the attention-getting event. New opportunities can stimulate planning for a health program, such as a grant announcement or the hiring of an enthusiastic, motivated, and knowledgeable employee who is passionate about a particular health problem. The trigger event might also be a mandated process, such as a five-year strategic planning process or a grant renewal. It might also be a less positive event, such as a news media exposé or legal action. For those seeking to initiate the planning process, getting the attention of influential

Table 3.1 Comparison of Models Developed for Public Health Planning

	PATCH	APEXPH	MAPP	CHIP	PACE-EH
Current practice	No	Yes	Yes, very widely used	Yes, but not widely used	Yes
Developers	CDC	CDC and NACCHO	CDC and NACCHO	NACCHO	CDC and NACCHO
Appropriate for which unit/level	City and county levels	Local health department, community assessments	Broadly community health at city, county, and state levels	Local health departments and county level	City, county, and state levels
Distinguishing emphasis	Health promotion programs and community capacity building	Emphasis on public health core functions of assessment, assurance, and policy development	Strategic planning, community involvement in planning process	Performance of local health departments, data used for planning	Environmental health, legal advocacy on environmental issues

individuals requires having access to them, packaging the message about the need for planning in ways that are immediately attractive, and demonstrating the salience of the issue. Thus, to get a specific health problem or issue "on the table," activists can use the salient events to get the attention of influential individuals. Although this may seem obvious, it is also a reminder that key individuals mentally sort through and choose among competing attention-getters.

As shown in Figure 3.1 by the arrows, there is also a link between the results of process and effect evaluations and program development. In other words, the indirect trigger for planning could be information generated from an evaluation that reveals either the failure of a health program, extraordinary success of the program, or the need for additional programs. Although information on developing and evaluating health programs is presented in subsequent chapters, the reality is that the multiple possible feedback paths throughout the planning cycle make the process far more iterative and fluid than can be adequately portrayed here.

Once the cycle has been triggered, the early stage of planning centers on how to progress from awareness of a need or opportunity to a formal assessment and program plan. During this formative stage, thinking about developing

Figure 3.1   The Planning and Evaluation Cycle

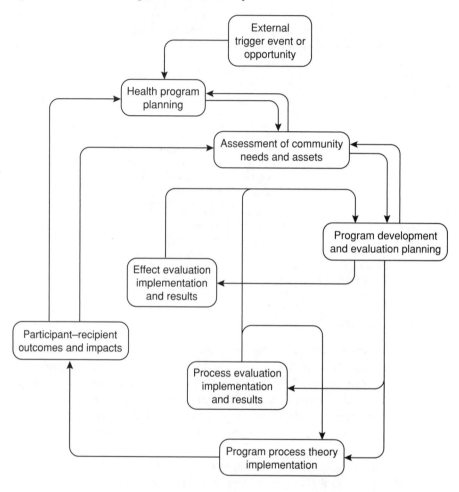

a program often generates a disorganized set of meetings and activities that eventually fall into a more organized pattern. One reason that the early planning stage is disorganized is that several paradoxes and assumptions about planning become apparent and must be addressed, or at least acknowledged.

THE FUZZY ASPECTS OF PLANNING

We like to think of planning as a rational, linear process, with few ambiguities and only the rare dispute. Unfortunately, this is not the reality of health program planning. There are many paradoxes inherent in planning, as well as implicit assumptions, ambiguities, and the potential for conflict. In addition, it is important to be familiar with the key ethical principles that underlie the decision making that is part of planning.

Paradoxes

Several paradoxes pervade health planning (Reinke & Hall, 1988), which may or may not be resolvable. Those involved also hold assumptions about planning that complicate the act of planning, whether for health systems or programs. Being aware of the paradoxes and assumptions can, however, help program planners understand possible sources of frustration.

One paradox is that planning is shaped by the same forces that created the problems planning is supposed to correct. Put simply, the healthcare, sociopolitical, and cultural factors that contributed to the health problem or condition are very likely to be same factors that affect the health planning process. In other words, the intertwined relationship of health and other aspects of life affects health planning. How can health be planned if the planning, particularly for public concerns, is limited to what occurs within the healthcare sector? For example, given that housing, employment, and social justice affect health, then health planning is automatically flawed to the extent that the context within which individuals live is not acknowledged or addressed in the health planning.

Another paradox is that the "good" of individuals and society experiencing the prosperity associated with health and well-being is "bad" to the extent that this prosperity also produces ill health. Prosperity in our modern world has its own associated health risks, such as higher cholesterol levels, increased stress, increased risk of cardiovascular disease, and increased levels of environmental pollutants. Also, as one group prospers, other groups often become disproportionately worse off. So, to the extent that health program planning promotes the prosperity of a society or a group of individuals, other health issues will arise that will require health program planning.

A third paradox is that what may be easier and more effective may be less acceptable. A good example of this paradox stems from decisions about active and passive protective interventions. Active protection and passive protection are both approaches to risk reduction and health promotion. *Active protection* requires that individuals actively participate in reducing their risks—for example, through diet changes or the use of motorcycle helmets. *Passive protection* occurs when individuals are protected by virtue of some factor other than their behavior—for example, water fluoridation and mandates for smoke-free workplaces. For many health programs, passive protection in the form of health policy or health regulations may be more effective and efficient. However, ethical and political issues can arise when the emphasis on passive protection, through laws and community-wide mandates, does not take into account cultural trends or preferences.

Another paradox is that planning of health programs ideally is triggered by those in need, rather than by health professionals. This paradox addresses the issue of who knows best and who has the best ideas for how to resolve the "real" problem. The perspective held by health professionals often does not reflect broader, more common health social values (Reinke & Hall, 1988), including the values possessed by those individuals with the "problem." Because persons in need of health programs are most likely to know what will work for them, community and stakeholder participation becomes not just crucial but, in many instances, is actually mandated by funding agencies. This paradox also calls into question the role of health professionals in developing health programs. Their normative perspective and scientific knowledge need to be weighed against individuals' choices that may have caused the health problem.

A corollary to the paradox dealing with the sources of the best ideas is the notion that politicians tend to prefer immediate and permanent cures, whereas health planners prefer long-term, strategic, and less visible interventions (Reinke & Hall, 1988). Generally, people want to be cured of existing problems, rather than to think probabilistically about preventing problems that may or may not occur in the future. As a consequence, the prevention and long-term solutions that seem obvious to public health practitioners can conflict with the solutions identified by those with the "problem."

One reason that the best solutions might come from those with the problem is that health professionals can be perceived as blaming those with the health problem for their problem. Blum (1982), for example, has identified the practice of "blaming the victim" as a threat to effective planning. When a woman who experiences domestic violence is said to be "asking for it," the victim is being blamed. During the planning process, blaming the victim can be implicitly and rather subtly manifested in group settings through interpretation of data about needs, thereby affecting decisions related to those needs. Having the attitude that "the victim is to blame" can also create conflict and tension among those involved in the planning process, especially if the "victims" are included as stakeholders. The activities for which the victim is being blamed need to be reframed in terms of the causes of those activities or behaviors.

Yet another paradox is the fact that planning is intended to be successful; no one plans to fail. Because of the bias throughout the program planning cycle in favor of succeeding, unanticipated consequences may not be investigated or recognized. The unanticipated consequences of one action can lead to the need for other health decisions that were in themselves unintended (Patrick & Erickson, 1993). To overcome this paradox, brainstorming and thinking creatively at key points in the planning process ought to be fostered and appreciated.

Assumptions

Assumptions also influence the effectiveness of planning. The first and primary assumption underlying all planning processes is that a solution, remedy, or appropriate intervention can be identified or developed and provided. Without this assumption, planning would be pointless. It is fundamentally an optimistic assumption about the capacity of the planners, the stakeholders, and the state of the science to address the health problem. The assumption of possibilities further presumes that the resources available, whether human or otherwise, are sufficient for the task and are suitable to address the health problem. The assumption of adequate capacity and knowledge is actually tested through the process of planning.

A companion assumption is that planning leads to the allocation of resources needed to address the health problem. This assumption is challenged by the reality that four groups of stakeholders have interests in the decision making regarding health resources (Sloan & Conover, 1996) and each group exists in all program planning. Those with the health problem and who are members of the target audience for the health program are one group. Another group of stakeholders is health payers, such as insurance companies and local, federal, and philanthropic funding agencies. The third group is individual healthcare providers and healthcare organizations and networks. Lastly, the general public is a stakeholder group because it is affected by how resources are allocated for health programs. This list of stakeholder groups highlights the variety of motives each group has for being involved in health program planning, such as personal gain, visibility for an organization, or acquisition of resources associated with the program.

Another assumption about those involved is that they share similar views on how to plan health programs. During the planning process, their points of view and cultural perspectives will likely come into contrast. Hoch (1994) suggested that planners need to know what is relevant and important for the problem at hand. Planners can believe in one set of community purposes and values, yet still recognize the validity and merit of competing purposes. He argues that effective planning requires tolerance, freedom, and fairness and that technical and political values are two bases from which to give planning advice. In other words, stakeholders involved in the planning process need to be guided into appreciating and perhaps applying a variety of perspectives about planning.

Each stakeholder group assumes that there are limited resources to be allocated for addressing the health problem and is receptive or responsive to a different set of strategies for allocating health resources. The resulting conflicts among the stakeholders for the limited resources apply whether they are allocating resources across the healthcare system or among programs for specific health problems. Limited resources, whether real or not, raise ethical questions of what to do when possible gains from needed health programs or policies are likely to be small, especially when the health program addresses serious health problems.

Interestingly, the assumption of limited resources parallels the paradox that planning occurs around what is limited rather than what is abundant. Rarely is there a discussion of the abundant or unlimited resources available for health planning. Particularly in the United States, there is an amazing abundance of volunteer hours and interest and of advocacy groups and energy. There is also an abundance of recently retired equipment that may be appropriate in some situations. Such resources, while not glamorous or constituting a substantial entry on a balance sheet, deserve to be acknowledged in the planning process.

Another assumption about the planning process is that it occurs in an orderly fashion and that a rational approach is best. To understand the implications of this assumption, one must first acknowledge that four key elements are inherent in planning: uncertainty, ambiguity, risk, and control. The presence of each of these elements contradicts the assumption of a rational approach, and each generates its own paradoxes.

Uncertainty, Ambiguity, Risk, and Control

Despite the orderly approach implied by use of the term "planning," this process is affected by both the limits of both scientific rationality and the usefulness of data to cope with the uncertainties, ambiguities, and risks being addressed by the planning process.

Uncertainty is the unknown likelihood of a possible outcome. Rice, O'Connor, and Pierantozzi (2008) have identified four types of uncertainty: types and amount of resources, technological, market receptivity to the product, and organizational. Each of these uncertainties will be present in planning health programs. *Ambiguity* is doubt about a course of action stemming from awareness that known and unknown factors exist that can decrease the possibility of certainty. In this sense, ambiguity results in uncertainty. Both uncertainty and ambiguity pervade the planning process because it is impossible to know and estimate the effect of all relevant factors—from all possible causes of the health problem, to all possible health effects from program interventions, to all possible acts and intentions of individuals. A rational approach to planning presumes that all relevant factors can be completely accounted for by anticipating the effect of a program, but our experiences as humans tell us otherwise.

Ambiguity is a feeling that tends to be both uncomfortable and undesirable. Change, or the possibility of change, is a likely source of ambiguity. This may explain why change is distasteful to those affected and subsequently influences the likelihood of successfully implementing programs (Reinke & Hall, 1988). So, generally, steps are taken either to deny the ambiguity, regardless of its source, or to eliminate it. Both of these actions have the potential to lead to conflict among stakeholders and planners, among planners and those with the health problem, and among those with various health problems vying for resources. The conflict, whether subtle and friendly or openly hostile, detracts from the planning process by requiring time and personnel resources to address and resolve the conflict. Nonetheless, to the extent that the conflict is open and constructive, it can lead to innovations in the program.

Risk is the perceived possibility or uncertain probability of an adverse outcome in a given situation. Health planners need to be aware of the community's perception and interpretation of probabilities as they relate to health and illness. Risk is not just about taking chances (such as bungee jumping or having unprotected sex), but is also about uncertainty and ambiguity (as is the case with estimates of cure rates and projections about future health conditions). Risk is pervasive and inherent throughout the planning process in terms of deciding who to involve and how, which planning approach to use, and which intervention to use, and in estimating which health problem deserves attention. The importance of understanding risk as an element both of the program planning process and of the target audience provides planners with a basis from which to be flexible and speculative.

Control, as in being in charge of or managing, is a natural reaction to the presence of ambiguity, conflict, and risk. It can take the form of directing attention and allocating resources or of exerting dominance over others. Although control has historically been a key element of management, advances in complexity theory highlight its detrimental effects in situations of uncertainty (McDaniel, 1997). In other words, addressing the ambiguity, uncertainty, and risk that might have been the trigger for the planning process requires less—not more—control. Those who preside over and influence the planning process are often thought of as having control over solutions to the health problem or condition. They do not. Instead, effective guidance of the planning process limits the amount of control exerted by any one stakeholder and addresses the anxiety that often accompanies the lack of control.

Ethics and Planning

Bioethics, or the application of ethical and philosophical principles to medical decision making, tends to focus on decision making within the context of acute care or end-of-life decisions. However, global concerns over the possibility of *pandemics*, the spread of a disease over a large portion or entire population, and the need for greater disaster preparedness have led to the application of ethical principles to population-focused health planning. Ethical principles, as derived from the philosophy of moral behavior and used as guides to health planning, determine the priority given to health problems and the approaches to deal with those problems. The choice of which ethical principles and frameworks to apply from among the variety that exists subsequently has consequences throughout the program planning and evaluation cycle.

For this reason, a brief overview of some of the frequently applied ethical frameworks and principles (Table 3.2) is in order. This overview is not intended to be comprehensive or thorough. Rather, the intent here is to introduce the major ethical principles that play crucial roles in health program planning.

Table 3.2   Ethical Frameworks and Principles for Planning Health Programs

Approach	Principle	Health Application	Examples in Health
Autonomy	Personal right to self-determination and choice	Individual choice takes priority, avoidance of coercion	Pro-life and pro-choice, living will
Criticality (contractarian)	The worst off benefit the most	Greatest problem, severest health risk	WIC, Medicaid, SCHIP
Egalitarian	All persons of equal value, minimize disparities	Hardest to reach, most marginalized, most in need	*Healthy People 2010* goals
Needs based	Equal opportunity to meet own needs, such as a healthy life	Future oriented, strategies to promote health and prevent diseases and illnesses	Early childhood intervention programs
Resource sensitive	Resources are scarce	Cost-effectiveness as the standard	Oregon Health Plan
Utilitarian	The greatest good for the greatest number; the ends justify the means	Collective benefits outweigh individual choices	Required immunization

Autonomy, as an ethical principle, is the right to make a decision on one's own behalf. Applied to health programs, autonomy is the decision that each potential participant makes whether to join the health program. It is such a basic ethical principle that it is often taken for granted as being an option. However, for some groups, such as those with intellectual disabilities, language deficits or persons in a coma, autonomy is compromised.

One ethical approach, *criticality*, is to focus on providing for those who have the greatest or severest health problem or risk. Under this ethical philosophy, persons with life-threatening illnesses would receive high priority, such as individuals at highest risk for exposure to air particulate pollution or in need of an organ transplant. Taking this approach is likely to be costly for the healthcare organization and for society.

In contrast, the *egalitarian* ethical approach would assert that the most neglected, hardest to reach, and most in need ought to receive the highest priority under the health program. This approach would lead to an emphasis on addressing the health problems of groups such as substance-abusing sex workers, isolated women suffering physical abuse, and illegal farm workers. The *Healthy People 2010* objectives operationalize an egalitarian ethic by directing attention, and thus efforts, toward those groups that are farthest from national target objective levels.

The *needs-based* approach directs attention to the future potential. From this perspective, efforts to prevent the development of unhealthy lifestyles, habits, and situations take priority. Also, high priority would be given to interventions intended to ensure healthy pregnancy, breastfeeding, and safe playgrounds because of their preventive aspects.

The *resource-sensitive* ethical approach emphasizes being cost-effective, such that the least resources are expended for the greatest amount of health gain. A cost-effectiveness ethic would target common health problems with inexpensive solutions, such as primary prevention.

Lastly, prioritization could be approached from a *utilitarian* philosophy, in which achieving the greatest good or benefit for the greatest number of persons is the guiding principle. The utilitarian ethic would give a high priority to the reduction in air pollutants and quarantine of individuals with highly contagious infectious disease. The vast majority of public health programs are predicated on the utilitarian principle, making it an integral element of public policy making. This also makes it appear to be a core value rather than an ethical principle.

There is growing global, national, and local awareness of the need for preparedness for disasters with both natural and human causes. Along with planning efforts geared toward being prepared to respond to disasters has come a parallel awareness that planning for disasters has profound ethical implications. Measures focusing on isolation via quarantine, degree of public health authority, and extent of response force all have the potential to conflict with individual autonomy and freedom. Thus, increasingly, public health disaster preparedness planning is including explicit statements of ethical principles to be followed during a response and used to guide the planning.

APPROACHES TO PLANNING

An awareness of the various approaches used to accomplish planning helps planners interpret events and guide others through the planning process. Each of the approaches provides a basis for assessing possible points of contention or agreement regarding health and program priorities. Six different perspectives on planning are offered here as different lenses through which the program planning process can be viewed, understood, and used to address the health problem. These perspectives are based on the processes identified by Beneviste (1989), whose international work on planning includes a broader set of approaches than those described by Blum (1974) or Nutt (1984). Each approach is typified by various planning activities (Table 3.3). None of the approaches is inherently better or worse than any of the others. Rather, the purpose of becoming aware of all six approaches is to select an approach that matches the situation and to use the strengths of the approaches to arrive at an optimal process for developing a health program and its evaluation.

Incremental Approach

The incremental approach to planning does not attempt to address the problem in any context or across any time span. Instead, the approach is one of addressing immediate concerns and, to some extent, having faith that the small, rather disconnected plans and actions will have a cumulative effect on the problem. Incrementalism, by its very nature, focuses only on the immediate, without attempting to see the "big picture" or implement a long-term plan.

In the very early days of the HIV/AIDS epidemic, before the causative virus had been identified or named, the only health planning options were incremental: shut down bath houses, use infectious disease precautions, and seek funding to study the health problem. These actions were isolated, disjointed efforts, but under the circumstances, the incremental approach was the only available option. Advocates for infected individuals had not yet emerged, nor was there a scientific basis for making rational, apolitical decisions.

As this example points out, incrementalism, while not the most effective planning approach, may be the only option in some circumstances. In addition, when resources are limited, incrementalism can lead to small gains related to

Table 3.3   Summary of the Six Approaches to Planning, with Public Health Examples

Approach	Underlying Assumptions	Consequences of Use	Public Health Application
Incremental	Not feasible to do more than small portions at a time; the parts are greater than the whole	Can be done quickly; results in plans that may be redundant or leave gaps; no guarantee that the parts will build on one another	Specific programs implemented that reflect discrete, categorical funding, despite potential overlap or existing similar programs
Apolitical	Options are known; technicalizes the problem; the means to the ends are known; can anticipate all caveats	Plans may fail because of unforeseen or unaccounted-for factors	Evidence-based practice
Advocacy	An external expert can accurately speak for those with less power	Experts may not accurately speak for others; media attention is likely to focus on the spokesperson rather than the issue	Activists for marginalized groups and environmental issues
Communication action	Language is powerful; those with the problem have the capability to enact a solution	An increased sense of confidence and an increased ability to solve one's own problems; potential for conflict	Community coalitions that take on a program or become not-for-profit organizations
Comprehensive rational	System feedback loops are contextual and can be known; rational choices are preferred	Takes considerable time and effort to implement; likely to have more dissent to overcome; results in an encompassing, intertwined set of actions	Community-focused initiatives
Strategic planning	Can anticipate and predict the future; stability is more pervasive than change	Lacks flexibility to respond to emerging issues; a costly process to arrive at a plan	*Healthy People* series; states' two- to five-year plans; Title V two-year plans

immediate problems. The major disadvantage of incrementalism is that the myriad small planning efforts may lead to conflicting plans, confusing programs, programs or services that are not integrated, or personnel redundancy or mismatch with the "new" program.

Apolitical Approach

The apolitical approach to planning relies solely on technical knowledge to arrive at a solution and assumes that technical knowledge makes it possible to achieve compromises among those involved in the health problem and the planning process. In a sense, the apolitical approach is fundamentally a problem-solving approach that relies on current knowledge about the problem and known alternatives to address the problem. The name of this approach reflects the fact that its focus on the technical aspects ignores the political aspects inherent in any problem. This approach is implicitly a gold standard of planning, particularly when those involved in the planning process are more technically inclined and focused.

To the extent that the apolitical approach relies on objective information for decision making, the application of evidence-based medicine (EBM) and evidence-based practice (EBP) guidelines can be viewed as essentially apolitical approaches to planning. In *EBP*, guidelines for practice by individual practitioners and complex health promotion programs are developed solely based on the best available scientific knowledge, without consideration of the context of the practice or the preferences of those experiencing the health problem. When planners use EBP guidelines as the basis for health program planning without taking other factors into account, they are engaged in apolitical planning.

One criticism of the apolitical problem-solving approach is that it does not account for interpersonal dynamics and possible struggles for control (Forester, 1993). This approach also neglects cultural issues involving the potential program participants and program staff, which can be substantial stumbling blocks in applying the health programs. Nonetheless, the apolitical approach has the advantage of being—or at least providing—the appearance of being logical and rational and of specifying solutions with the documented highest efficacy.

Advocacy Approach

The advocacy perspective on planning focuses on the client and mandates citizen participation in planning activities. Beneviste (1989) described advocacy planning as a bottom-up form of comprehensive rational planning. Planners using the advocacy approach, however, would be likely to speak for or on behalf of those with the health problem.

For example, experts in environmental hazards may testify before city or county elected officials to plead the case for people living in areas where hazardous waste is generated or stored. When those who live in the area are unaware of a problem but an expert is nevertheless safeguarding their best interest, advocacy planning is occurring. Another example of the advocacy approach is the trend for many federal granting agencies, such as the CDC, to mandate participation of community members in health planning activities. These federal agencies now regularly require that, during a year of program planning, representatives from the community be included in the development of the priorities and the action plan for addressing those health priorities. In this instance, the federal agencies are advocating for the communities that will be affected by the grant they are about to fund.

As Guerin, Allotey, Elmi, and Bho (2006) discovered, advocacy is personal because of the intense involvement between the advocate and those receiving advocacy. They also see political advocacy as a final stage of community-based participatory research. This perception is similar to the findings of Hill and colleagues (2007), who noted that community planning groups that begin with a focus on program development often evolve into policy planning and advocacy. These reports suggest that an advocacy approach to planning is more likely when the group has been established long enough to acquire an in-depth understanding of the health problem and a deep appreciation that an advocacy planning approach is needed to further address the health problem.

The advantages of the advocacy approach are most readily evident in situations in which clients or citizens are, for whatever reasons, not empowered to convey their own preferences or concerns. In such situations, having an advocate may be the only option for planning a needed health program. The disadvantages are that the clients or citizens may not agree with the opinions or views of the advocate. In fact, their "advocate" may not even be representing those he or she claims to speak for, because this individual implicitly holds a normative view of the needs of the clients or citizens. The advocacy approach also implicitly entails some degree of conflict or confrontation, which may have negative repercussions over the long term. Social irresponsibility arises when the solution ignores important social or cultural factors (Blum, 1982). Strong advocates and users of the apolitical approach to planning may be prone to this pitfall simply because a scientific basis may not take into account social realities and needs.

Communication Action Approach

Communication action, or critical planning theory, is concerned with the distribution of power and communication. From this perspective, those involved in the planning make efforts to empower those with the problem through sharing of information. Whereas the advocacy approach does not enable those with the problem to participate as equals with the "experts" in the planning process, the critical or communication action approach is predicated on making those with the problem equals in the planning process. According to Forester (1993), this perspective leads planners to think of planning as shaping attention, changing beliefs, gaining consent, and engendering trust and understanding among those involved. This approach to planning, which is now called community-based participatory research (CBPR; see Minkler, Wallerstein, & Hall, 2003), has gained such wide acceptance that basic knowledge about CBPR and skills in CBPR are included in the competencies for public health professionals (Institute of Medicine, 2003).

One of the many examples of this approach to planning is evident in mental health. The National Alliance on Mental Illness (NAMI) is a not-for-profit organization whose purpose is to support those with mental illness, and it is run by individuals with mental illness. Individuals with mental health problems are taught and guided in the process of developing small-scale, community-based programs and services for those with mental illnesses. This approach exemplifies the communication action approach.

A major advantage of the communication action approach is that members of the target audience gain skills, knowledge, and confidence in addressing their own problems. However, the health planner who is involved in critical planning needs to have a different set of skills from those needed to do rational or incremental planning. Also, because time and effort are needed to enable those with the problem to participate fully in the planning process, planning may proceed more slowly. The time needed to implement communication action lengthens the planning timeline such that it is not useful in emergencies.

Comprehensive Rational Approach

The comprehensive rational perspective on planning is fundamentally a systems approach. It involves analyzing the problem by drawing upon ideas from systems theory—namely, feedback loops, input and output, systems, and subsystems. The systematic, logical sequence of thought processes and actions employed explains why this approach is termed "rational." Assumptions are made that the factors affecting the problem (the elements of the systems that contribute to the goals) are knowable and that virtually all contingencies can be anticipated. In this sense, this perspective is rational and logical. The approach is comprehensive in the sense that planners can take into account those contingencies and peripheral influences.

In the comprehensive rational approach, the planners set goals, identify alternatives, implement programs, and monitor results. This approach is clearly the dominant perspective of this textbook and of most courses in planning and evaluation. Health program planning—particularly of national initiatives—often reflects the effort to use a comprehensive rational approach. In fact, one of the planning principles outlined by Reinke and Hall (1988) is to be as objective as possible, given the context, and to use rationality rather than status or position as much as possible as a basis for power.

One benefit of this approach is that it facilitates obtaining information from stakeholders who might otherwise be reluctant to share information, because it diffuses authority in favor of an information and rational base. The comprehensive rational approach allows planners to address issues faced by the entire system rather than just by subsystems; in this respect it resembles quality improvement methodologies. Another benefit of the comprehensive rational approach is that it yields more information for decision making than does an incremental approach.

The comprehensive rational approach is not without its flaws. Forester (1993), for example, critiqued the cybernetic (systems) perspective that underlies this approach for its failure to take into account the norms and values of individuals either involved in the planning process or affected by the planning process. Beneviste (1989) acknowledged that the comprehensive rational approach separates planners from the political realities of the health situation.

Forester (1993) also pointed out that this approach assumes that the means and the ends are known, which may not be the case. Claims of professional expertise about the relationship of means to ends may be dysfunctional when the claims cannot be substantiated, according to Forester. The claim that means and ends are understood leads to a choice that also takes into account other system constraints. When planners choose an option that satisfies the need—in other words, when they take the path of least effort that will meet the minimum requirements—*satisficing* has occurred. Although satisficing is certainly rational and often observed in the real world, a satisficing decision inherently includes the assumption that the decision is rational and based on a comprehensive understanding of the consequences—which may not be true. Finally, the idea that planners know best, in terms of which means are optimal, reveals a normative perspective on planning that may be unacceptable to stakeholders with less expertise.

Strategic Planning Approach

The strategic planning perspective focuses on the organization and its ability to accomplish its mission in a fiscally responsible manner. While this approach is rarely used to address specific health conditions, it is particularly applicable to the infrastructure level of the public health pyramid. Through strategic planning, resources needed to address the health problem are identified and considered in terms of the mission of the organization. This widely used approach often affects program choices, as in healthcare organizations whose services center on one disease entity, such as Planned Parenthood or the March of Dimes, or on one aggregate, such as the Boys and Girls Club or the American Association of Retired Persons. To some extent, the national goals and objectives set forth in *Healthy People 2010* are also an example of strategic planning.

This approach, when used by one member of a planning team, can affect the planning of the whole team. For example, the CDC awarded a large city a grant for a one-year planning phase of a major community-based health promotion initiative. The funded agency involved numerous local community agencies in the planning process. At one planning meeting, the chief executive officer of one of the community health agencies asked what his organization could do, what was being asked of his organization, and how his organization would benefit from participating in the health programs that would result from the planning process. His questions reflect implicit thinking about how to strategically place his organization within the field of contenders for grant money. His participation in the planning process also implied that his organization's mission was compatible with the general direction being taken to address the health problem.

The strategic planning approach has some clear advantages: It takes into account the context, whether competition or policy, and it has a slightly longer-term focus. Most strategic planning scholars recommend a time frame of approximately five years when planning, because it typically takes that long to make strategic changes in programs and services. Because strategic planning is a rational model or systematic approach to decision making, decision points can be quantified, weighted, and sequenced, although programmed into computer software that then shows which option is the "best."

Despite the capability to quantify mathematically the decision-making process, identifying the best option does not guarantee that the best decision option, or program plan will be adopted. Human beings are irrational (March, 1988), with biases in how they think about probabilities and possibilities (Tversky & Kahneman, 1974). These human characteristics are usually not quantified in the decision models, but they are powerful forces in interpreting information and then shaping the actions taken. This irrationality can lead to situations in which the broad goals developed during the planning process are not, in fact, acted upon. Another disadvantage of the strategic planning approach is its lack of flexibility to respond to newly emerging environmental opportunities or threats (Egger, 1999). In addition, strategic planning, if properly done, is time and resource intensive.

Summary of Approaches

To some extent, all of the approaches to health planning discussed in this section are likely to occur during the planning phase of addressing a health problem. One example is the efforts to increase adult immunization in Bowe County. The need to track immunizations necessitated the involvement of both state health officials and representatives from large health maintenance organizations (HMOs) in the planning process. A lobbyist used advocacy to gain passage of state legislation supportive of financing immunizations across all age groups, particularly for underinsured individuals from minority groups. The choice of vaccines was an apolitical decision, based on research indicating which combinations were likely to result in the highest levels of protection for the population. Senior citizens were involved as informed consumers in shaping policy and tracking procedures, so communication action was also part of the planning process.

It is quite unlikely that all of the individuals involved in the immunization planning efforts recognized the mixture of approaches being used in this community-based effort. Had they been aware of the approaches being used by various constituents, additional strategies could have been developed that would have made the planning process more effective, efficient, and palatable to parents, providers, and policy makers alike. Undeniably, a blend of approaches is typically needed, particularly in health program planning that aims to address more recalcitrant or population-based health problems.

Each of the six approaches to health planning represents a way to identify a problem, identify options, and make a choice—the classic definition of decision making. In other words, planning is decision making (Veany & Kaluzny, 1998). From the perspective of an organization or agency engaged in health planning, health planning activities can be framed in terms of managerial and organizational decision making. This fact is important when assessing (constraints for implementing the health program) and developing the organizational resources.

PLANNING STEPS AND STAGES

The steps or sequence of considerations commonly encountered across the planning models are essentially a form of problem solving, with a mixture of empowerment. Planning rarely occurs in a step-by-step, linear fashion; rather, it is an iterative process, particularly when it responds to data gathered from community needs assessments and previous program evaluations, as shown by the feedback arrows in Figure 3.1. For the sake of simplicity, the diagram shows only the key planning steps. These steps are inevitably revised, expanded, and adapted to the particular situation, using the community needs assessment data and resulting in a priority given to a health problem. To the extent that cost considerations are included in the steps, they can apply to making decisions about health resource allocation (Patrick & Erickson, 1993).

Planning also tends to evolve as a process though stages that are common to workgroups, beginning with their formation. The formation and team development stage ought to be viewed as the groundwork that lays out the processes and oversees the cycle, from assessment through program and evaluation development to implementation and evaluation.

Team Formation and Development

Planning is a collective activity. The individuals involved at the various stages of the planning cycle easily influence the directions and decisions made. A key strategy for achieving successful planning is to have a visible, powerful sponsor. Given that politics of one form or another are inherently a part of the planning process, having a backer who is recognized, respected, and influential becomes an essential element to successfully planning and implementing a health program.

Selection of the planning team members is influenced by legal considerations (such as antidiscrimination laws and municipal mandates for advisory boards), the reasons for wanting to participate, the level and type of expertise that an individual can contribute to the process, the amount and type of resources that an individual can contribute to the process, the person's status as a current or potential user or client of the health program, and the person's role as an advocate for a group likely to be affected by the health program. Group size is another consideration, with groups of 10 to 15 being acceptable for the planning process, recognizing that an optimal size for a task force or workgroup is 5 to 7 persons.

One "law" of groups points out the challenges in working collectively: There will always be one person who is not a team player. Given this likelihood, it is crucial to know the strengths and weaknesses of the individuals involved and to understand why each individual has been selected as a member. Having such information helps ensure that a planning group possesses a balance of strengths that will contribute to an efficient and effectively functioning group. Attention to the composition of the planning group also ensures that a breadth of knowledge and concerns are represented, while eliminating disruptive individuals. Reinke and Hall (1988) also remind us that it is critical to have trained, skilled, and knowledgeable planning staff. Similarly, a growing consensus suggests that successful planning processes begin with developing the planning group's awareness, concern, and skills to address the problem at hand.

Different types of public health planning groups exist, but the most common type is a consortium. A *consortium* is a quasi-temporary body that is formed for a specific programmatic purpose and that has an independent sponsor, broad representation, and experts as members. Consortia are popular means to increase involvement of community members and to address (implicitly) the paradox of professionals not having the "right" solution.

Formation of a planning board is one way to ensure that both professionals and those affected by the planning become involved in the planning process. Research has shown that participation of those affected by a decision in the actual decision-making process tends to enhance the strategic ability of organizations (Issel & Anderson, 2001). It follows, then, that involving stakeholders in decisions inherent in program planning will lead to a better plan for the program. Participation in the decision-making process by those who will do the work also has a notable benefit: It increases worker satisfaction (Coopman, 2001; Wagner, 1994). Similarly, involving the future program employees, if possible, will increase their commitment to the program.

Overall, the literature on participation in decision making reveals a pattern in favor of involving those affected by the decision in the decision-making process. For this reason, the involvement of stakeholders throughout the planning, implementation, and evaluation cycle is highly recommended. It is also important to educate those involved in the planning process, using a communication action approach (as discussed earlier in this chapter). When those individuals who will be affected by the decision are involved in making it, their resistance to the change is likely to be diminished and they will begin to "own" the program or plan, although participation does not guarantee ownership (Goodman, Steckler, Hoover, & Schwartz, 1993).

The last consideration in the team development stage is the selection of a leader for the planning group. Duhl (2000) argues that many types of leaders may be necessary for an effective planning process. A leader can emerge or be appointed based on his or her capability to function as an educator, a doer, or even a social entrepreneur. At any point in the planning process, or even during oversight of the program implementation, different individuals may be better suited to play a leadership role. Recognizing the fluidity of the leadership situation and acting on that recognition are both healthy and useful.

What may be less fully articulated, especially during the earliest stages, is the degree of formalization of leader selection. In other words, the planning group needs an acknowledged and standard process for designating a legitimate leader. This process can and does vary, ranging from the ad hoc emergence of a natural leader to the election of an individual from a slate of candidates according to formalized bylaws. Regardless of where along that continuum the group wants to be, the key will be to have an articulated and accepted process that facilitates the planning process, rather than hindering team members' creativity and commitment. Ideally, each member of the planning group needs to be actively involved in ensuring that the process is open and agreed upon.

Creation of a Vision

The first step in planning, according to the American Planning Association, is to create a vision. Development of a vision is also one of the first steps in the CHIP and MAPP models of assessment.

Specific elements of the mission statement appear to have a bearing on the success of healthcare organizations (Bart, 1999). For example, *Healthy People 2010* outlines a national vision of eliminating racial and ethnic disparities in health and increasing the quality of life. Whatever the trigger event, health program planners must create a vision with which existing and future stakeholders can identify and to which they can devote attention and energy. Patrick and Erickson (1993), in their discussion of health resource planning, suggested that this effort begin by specifying the health decision. A vision frames information for the stakeholders and helps identify economic assumptions that may affect the overall health program.

Part of the process of creating a vision of the final "product" is reaching a consensus on how to arrive at that final ideal. In this regard, one element of creating a vision is deciding on a system for prioritizing both problems and possible solutions to the highest-priority problems. How decisions are made—whether by voting, consensus, or complex algorithm—should be one of the first decisions of the planning group.

Investigation

During the investigation phase of planning, data are gathered that will be used to first prioritize health problems and then prioritize possible programmatic solutions. Generally, data relevant to planning health programs come from community assessment, population preferences, previous program evaluations, and research on possible interventions. The importance and possible scope of data collection carried out through community assessment is such critical factor that the next chapter is entirely devoted to community assessment.

Two elements of the nonlinear nature of health program planning are worth introducing during this stage of planning. One is the need to focus on future considerations—specifically, interventions—even before the program direction has been decided. The other is the need to be aware of the willingness of key individuals to support the planning and program process and to understand the quantification of health problems in terms of quality of life.

Interventions are actions that are done intentionally to have a direct effect on the health problem or condition. This broad definition of intervention includes medical treatments, pharmacological treatments, behavioral treatments, and health policy development, as well as education and skill enhancement, social support, and financial aid. In the healthcare realm, research resulting in EBM and EBP can be used to determine the effectiveness of potential interventions. Of particular concern are the sensitivity of the health problem to the intervention and the specificity of the intervention with regard to the health problem it addresses. Another consideration in determining the effectiveness of an intervention is the theoretical or conceptual logic underlying the way in which the intervention alters the health problem or condition. Chapter 6 discusses this issue in more detail.

Solutions, whether programmatic interventions or other ideas, often exist even before the problem is formally identified. Proponents of the solution might, for example, be waiting for a window of opportunity for "their" idea to be applied. Although having ready-made solutions available can certainly be helpful, too many individuals are inclined to jump on a particular solution bandwagon before the planning process has fully explicated the problem and all of its potential solutions. To the extent that any intervention or solution is well suited to a clearly defined problem, the planning process is effective.

One factor that adversely affects planning is wishful thinking, according to Blum (1982). In other words, solutions are sometimes based on idealistic and overly optimistic hopes rather than on scientific knowledge. This factor leads to the failure to examine the range of possible effective interventions or solutions to the problem. A key to avoiding this pitfall is the use of EBM and EBP, even though facts may not convince individuals with strongly held beliefs about what is scientifically the right thing to do.

An additional benefit of focusing on interventions is that this tactic helps avoid an undue emphasis on needs assessment and data collection. Goodman et al., (1993) found that planning groups have a tendency to "frontload" the planning cycle, by devoting considerable time and effort to collecting risk and health problem data and conducting data analysis. Focusing on identifying realistic interventions balances the early planning stages with the later stages of implementation.

Prioritization

During the prioritization stage, data and information gathered during the community health assessment (Chapter 4), along with the information on preferences and interventions, are integrated into a decision about what to address and how. During the establishment of priorities, the planning group is likely to face conflicts stemming from the group members' different philosophies about how to establish priorities. As discussed earlier with regard to ethics, no single ethical approach to prioritizing issues is inherently right or wrong. Thus, centering the team's debates on what ought to be the guiding philosophical and ethical framework for making prioritization decisions can be an important step toward building consensus, trust, and mutual respect among stakeholders. Once these underlying principles have been agreed upon, a systematic, quantitative approach can be applied to determine health priorities. These established priority-establishing techniques are covered in more detail in Chapter 5.

Decision

Inevitably, the priority ranking of health problems will not be acceptable to some stakeholders. As a consequence, the rankings may need to be revised by seeking stakeholder input or until a consensus is gained. Such an activity reflects the reality of blending the rational and political approaches to program planning. These decisions regarding which health problems to address serve as the starting point for program development and then implementation.

Decisions about which health problems to address can fail for two major reasons. First, the organizational norms and institutionalized objectives may support conflicting priorities regarding health problems, limiting which interventions are acceptable. For this reason, the organizational assessment discussed in Chapter 4 is critical. Second, the experts conducting the community health needs assessment may be biased, which will shape their findings. In other words, data from the community health assessment that are made available for planning may reflect the views of those who conducted the assessment, rather than revealing the full scope of what exists as both strengths and problems in the community.

Once a health problem or condition has been chosen as the focus of a health program or service, a detailed implementation plan needs to be developed, along with a plan for conducting the evaluation. Planners should be aware that once a health problem has been identified, the composition of the planning group is likely to change. Members with vested interests will remain part of the team, while those with little expertise or interest in the chosen priority will fade away. At this point in the cycle, it may be important to revisit the group's composition and address why potential key stakeholders should become involved.

Implementation and Continuation

The planning cycle is complete after one full iteration until the program is implemented, monitored to determine the extent of the implementation, and assessed for its effectiveness. For some health programs, implementation includes a termination phase or phase-out period, as happens with health programs funded for a limited time. Evaluation, whether of immediate effects or long-term outcomes, provides a basis for further program planning and completes one cycle.

Throughout the planning process, multiple foci are useful as evaluation end points: an epidemiological focus on the characteristics of the health problem; a scientific focus on identifying the best possible, feasible programmatic interventions; and a managerial focus on the planning cycle and program implementation. If these foci are maintained, then feedback loops will develop more quickly, new triggers to additional planning activities will be perceived, and the evolution of involvement of stakeholders will be more rapid.

ACROSS THE PYRAMID

At the direct services level of the public health pyramid, planning focuses on individual health problems and the most prevalent or most costly health problems addressed by direct services. Planning, therefore, can be rather clinical in nature, involving only those individuals affected by the clinical decision. It can also address issues affecting small aggregates, such that the planning results in the development of health educational offerings to patients who visit a certain clinic, for example.

At the enabling services level of the public health pyramid, planning focuses more on aggregates and prioritizing among available or potentially available enabling services. It may also target the creation of enabling services to address high-priority problems. In contrast to direct services planning, which might occur within the boundaries of a clinic, planning at the enabling services level requires the involvement of a wider body of constituents. This broader scope reflects the fact that the nature of the health problems addressed at the enabling services level is likely to lead to plans that require a broader base of support and cooperation. For example, if health planning includes a focus on accessibility of primary health care and transportation emerges as an element in the planning process, the transportation authority needs to be included in the planning activities.

At the population-based services level, health planning is most evident in state health plans, although health systems and networks have begun to use a

DISCUSSION QUESTIONS

1. Given the many different ways that planning bodies can accomplish their tasks and the diverse backgrounds of those involved, planners assume different roles in various situations. For example, planners can act as facilitators and educators. What other roles might planners take on to be effective at planning?
2. In what ways, if any, would you modify the planning steps for developing programs at each level of the public health pyramid?
3. Consider the strengths of and the differences among the MAPP, PACE-EH, and CHIP models. Under which circumstances would you choose which approach? Access the websites for these programs (see the Internet Resources list), and compare the planning models in terms of how they demonstrate the planning approaches identified by Forester (1993).
4. Being effective in participation in program planning often means being comfortable with using different approaches in different situations. Choose a planning approach and describe an ideal situation and a least ideal situation for its use.

population-focused approach as well. State health agencies regularly conduct assessment and planning activities whose outcomes serve as the basis for developing state-supported or state-implemented health programs. As with planning for enabling services, planning of population-based services is likely to require the involvement of a wider array of stakeholders.

At the infrastructure level, planning is an activity of the infrastructure. Given this point, the issues of resource allocation, planning for the planning, and collection of the planning data are relevant. For example, one area that is likely to be addressed through health planning at the infrastructure level is determination of the qualifications and number of health personnel needed to implement the plan. Health personnel and resource planning (Blum, 1982; Reinke & Hall, 1988) are appropriate planning foci and are needed to sustain the infrastructure.

INTERNET RESOURCES

Heidi Deutsch, "Performance Improvement Processes: Survey of Tools and Approaches"

This PowerPoint presentation gives a nice comparison of the major models for doing an assessment. Retrieved January 28, 2008, from http://www.Phf.org/infrastructure/resources/assessmentpresentation.ppt.

Centers for Disease Control and Prevention: PATCH

CDC's link to PATCH is found at http://www.cdc.gov/nccdphp/publications/PATCH/index.htm.

National Association of City and County Health Officers: PACE-EH

NACCHO's webpage has links to PACE-EH resources and support: http://www.naccho.org/topics/environmental/CEHA.cfm.

Other PACE-EH Sources

You can look at the tool box developed by New Mexico at this site: http://www.health.state.nm.us/eheb/rep/Community/Community%20Env.%20Health%20Ass.pdf. At the county level, Multnomah, Oregon, has created a nice website describing its efforts: http://www.pace-eh.org/index.shtml; find its publication at http://www.pace-eh.org/documents/pilot_nne.pdf. Another example of PACE-EH being used by a county government is available at http://www.co.burlington.nj.us/departments/health/information/pace_eh/index.htm.

Disaster Preparedness

Examples of ethics in disaster preparedness planning in Canada can be found at http://www.waterlooregionpandemic.ca/en/planning/resources/Chapter3.pdf and http://www.utoronto.ca/jcb/home/documents/pandemic.pdf.

World Health Organization: Ethics

The WHO has prepared a paper on ethics that is relevant to planning: http://www.who.int/eth/ethics/PI_Ethics_draft_paper_WG2_6_Oct_06.pdf.

REFERENCES

Bart, C. K. (1999). Mission statement content and hospital performance in the Canadian not-for-profit health care sector. *Health Care Management Review, 24*(3), 18–29.

Beneviste, G. (1989). *Mastering the politics of planning: Crafting credible plans and policies that make a difference.* San Francisco: Jossey-Bass.

Blum, H. L. (1974). *Planning for health.* New York: Human Sciences Press.

Blum, H. L. (1982). Social perspective on risk reduction. In M. M. Faber & A. M. Reinhart (Eds.), *Promoting health through risk reduction* (pp. 19–36). New York: Macmillan.

Centers for Disease Control and Prevention (CDC). (n.d.). Retrieved February 13, 2007, from http://www.cdc.gov/nceh/ehs/PIB/PACE.htm

Centers for Disease Control and Prevention (CDC) PATCH. (n.d.). Retrieved March 5, 2008, from http://www.cdc.gov/nccdphp/publications/PATCH/index.htm

Coopman, S. J. (2001). Democracy, performance, and outcomes in interdisciplinary health care teams. *Journal of Business Communication, 38*(3), 261–284.

Dever, G. E. (1980). *Community health analysis: A holistic approach.* Germantown, MD: Aspen Systems.

Dever, G. E. (1997). *Improving outcomes in public health practice: Strategy and methods.* Gaithersburg, MD: Aspen.

Duhl, L. S. (1987). *Health planning and social change.* New York: Human Science Press.

Duhl, L. S. (2000). A short history and some acknowledgements. *Public Health Reports, 115*, 116–117.

Durch, J. S., Bailey, L. A., & Stoto, M. A. (Eds.). (1997). *Improving health in the community: A role for performance monitoring IOM.* NAP. Retrieved February 13, 2008, from http://www.nap.edu/readingroom/books/improving/

Egger, E. (1999). Old ways of planning, thinking won't work in today's volatile health care industry. *Health Care Strategic Management, 17*(9), 18–19.

Forester, J. (1993). *Critical theory, public policy and planning practice: Toward a critical pragmatism.* New York: State University of New York Press.

Goodman, R. M., Steckler, A., Hoover, S., & Schwartz, R. (1993). A critique of contemporary community health promotion approaches: Based on a qualitative review of six programs in Maine. *American Journal of Health Promotion, 7,* 208–220.

Green, L. W., Kreuter, M. W., Deeds, S. G., & Partridge, K. B. (1980). *Health education planning: A diagnostic approach.* Palo Alto, CA: Mayfield.

Guerin, P. B., Allotey, P., Elmi, F. H., & Bho, S. (2006). Advocacy as a means to an end: Assisting refugee women to take control of their reproductive health needs. *Women and Health, 43,* 7–25.

Hill, A., De Zapien, J. G., Staten, L. K., McClelland, D. J., Moore-Monroy, M., Meister, J. S., et al. (2007). From program to policy: Expanding the role of community coalitions. *Preventing Chronic Disease: Public Health Research, Practice, and Policy, 4.* Retrieved February 13, 2008, from http://www.cdc.gov/ped/issues/2007/oct/07_0112.htm

Hoch, C. (1994). *What planners do: Power, politics and persuasion.* Chicago: Planners Press.

Institute of Medicine. (1988). *The future of public health.* Washington, DC: National Academies Press.

Institute of Medicine. (2003). *The future of the public's health in the 21st century.* Washington, DC: National Academies Press.

Issel, L. M., & Anderson, R. A. (2001). Intensity of case managers' participation in organizational decision making. *Research in Nursing and Health, 24,* 361–372.

LaLonde, M. (1974). *A new perspective on the health of Canadians.* (Ottawa Catalog No H311–374.) Ottawa, Canada: Government of Canada.

March, J. G. (1988). *Decisions and organizations.* New York: Basil Blackwell.

Marris, P. (1982). *Community planning and conceptions of change.* New York: Routledge and Kegan Paul.

McDaniel, R. R. (1997). Strategic leadership: A new view from quantum and chaos theory. *Health Care Management Review, 22*(1), 21–37.

Minkler, M., Wallerstein, N., & Hall, B. (2003). *Community-based participatory research for health.* San Francisco: Jossey-Bass.

National Association of City and County Health Officers (NACCHO). (2006). PACE EH National Summit Proceedings, March 28–29, 2006. Retrieved February 13, 2008, from http://www .naccho.org/topics/environmental/documents/PACEEHSummitProceedings-final.pdf

National Association of County and City Health Officials (NACCHO). (n.d.). Retrieved March 5, 2008, from http://www.naccho.org/topics/infrastructure/apexph.cfm

Nutt, P. C. (1979). Calling out and calling off the dogs: Managerial diagnosis in public service organizations. *Academy of Management Review, 4,* 203–214.

Nutt, P. C. (1984). *Planning methods for health and related organizations.* New York: John Wiley.

Patrick, D. L., & Erickson, P. (1993). *Health status and health policy: Allocating resources to health care.* Oxford, UK: Oxford University Press.

Pratt, M., McDonald, S., Libby, P., Oberle, M., & Liang, A. (1996). Local health departments in Washington State use APEX to assess capacity. *Public Health Reports, 111,* 87–91.

Reinke, W. A., & Hall, T. L. (1988). Political aspects of planning. In W. A. Reinke (Ed.), *Health planning for effective management* (pp. 75–85). New York: Oxford University Press.

Rice, M. P., O'Connor, G. C., & Pierantozzi, R. (2008). Implementing a learning plan to counter project uncertainty. *Sloan Management Review, 29*(2), 54–62.

Rosen, G. (1958). *A history of public health.* Baltimore: Johns Hopkins University Press.

Sloan, F. A., & Conover, C. J. (1996). The use of cost-effectiveness/cost–benefit analysis in actual decision making: Current status and prospects. In F. A. Sloan (Ed.), *Valuing health care: Costs, benefits, and effectiveness of pharmaceuticals and other medical technologies* (pp. 207–232). Cambridge, UK: Cambridge University Press.

Tversky, A., & Kahneman, D. (1974). Judgment under uncertainty: Heuristics and biases. *Science, 18*(4157), 1124–1131.

U.S. Department of Health and Human Services (DHHS). (n.d.). *Planned approach to community health: Guide for the local coordinator.* Atlanta, GA: U.S. Department of Health and Human Services, Department of Health and Human Services, Centers for Disease Control and Prevention National Center for Chronic Disease Prevention and Health Promotion. Retrieved February 13, 2008, from http://www.cdc.gov/nccdphp/publications/PATCH/pdf/PATCHCh4.pdf

Veany, J. E., & Kaluzny, A. D. (1998). *Evaluation and decision making for health services.* Chicago: Health Administration Press.

Wagner, J. A. (1994). Participation's effects on performance and satisfaction: A reconsideration of research evidence. *Academy of Management Review, 19,* 312–330.

CHAPTER 4

Community Health Assessment for Program Planning

This chapter begins with a definition of community. It then provides an overview of needs assessment with full acknowledgment that, as with many aspects of program planning and evaluation, this field is an area of specialization. The various models that underlie an assessment are reviewed, as are the prototypical types of assessment. The distinctions made among the models and the types of assessment do become blurred in practice. Nonetheless, having a clear sense of what could be involved allows for more thoughtful and intentional decisions on how best to design and carry out the community health assessment.

DEFINING COMMUNITY

The use of the ecological model and the public health pyramid leads naturally to considering community and its role in health program planning and evaluation. Community is a concept that has been the subject of debate and deliberation by sociologists, beginning with Tonnies in 1897 (Bell & Newby, 1971). The term "community" is increasingly used to refer to almost any group of people, which results in a lack of conceptual clarity. This ambiguity, in turn, can lead to conflicts and confusion during program planning. To minimize the ambiguity and confusion, it is worth considering what is and is not a community, as a prelude to clarify thinking and as a foundation for better planning of health programs.

A *community* encompasses people and some form of proximity or place that enables interaction, and that interaction leads to shared values or culture (Bell & Newby, 1971; Table 4.1). A defining characteristic of a community is people with the potential for interaction. Without the potential for interaction, the sharing of values and norms is not possible. In today's world of electronic communication, interactions can be virtual as well as taking the more traditional person-to-person approach. To the extent that a large number of interacting individuals share values and culture, a community can exist even in the electronic sphere. Of course, virtual communities that exist via electronic media extend the traditional, anthropological notions of community that grew from the study of tribes and villages.

Another defining characteristic of a community is that its members have shared values and norms of behavior. The prerequisite that a community have commonly held values precludes in many instances a census tract, a ZIP code, a telephone area code, a consortium of health agencies, or a catchment area for a health service from being a community in the more pure sense. In contrast, active members of a church or residents of a small and homogeneous neighborhood might be a community.

This distinction between a convenient geographic designation and an actual community is important for planning how to have participation by community members in the planning process. Nilsen (2006) reminds us that the major problem with defining a community based on geographic location is that the geography does not ensure that a sense of community exists. Shared values form the basis for the cultural unity of a community, which in turn is the basis for the perception of being connected and belonging to a community. From that sense of belonging stems the subsequent behaviors that might be attributed to members of a particular community.

The concept of a "sense of community" has been studied and found to include aspects of membership, influence over what occurs within the community, shared values and needs fulfillment, and a shared emotional connection. Perhaps not surprisingly, given the breadth of this list of the elements fostering a sense of community, community and its associated emotional and cultural components create challenges for health program planning and

Table 4.1   Three Elements of Community, with Examples

Elements	Examples of the Community Elements
People	Values, beliefs, behaviors, size, membership, demographic characteristics, social and economic status, sense of power or influence, sense of belonging
Place	Geography, boundaries, housing, industry, air, water, land, virtual presence
Interaction	Communication, familial, education, religious based, political, recreational, virtual

evaluation. Interestingly, individuals' sense of community varies according to their race/ethnicity and income (Belue, Taylor-Richardson, Lin, McClellan, & Hargreaves, 2006). This lack of homogeneity suggests that disparities exist in more than health statistics. Thus, to achieve participatory planning, it may first be necessary to understand the local variations in sense of community. Regardless of the size of the population, the sense of community can be a key factor in gaining support for the program and for maximizing the health effects of some programs.

Community as Context and Recipient

Distinguishing one community from another, while perhaps necessary from the perspective of a health planner, may lead to artificial demarcations. Program planners must clarify the purpose for which "the community" is being delineated. A community, as a unit of individuals with some degree of cultural cohesion, can be both the target of a health program and the context in which a health program is provided and evaluated.

When a community is the target of a health program, some or all of the community members are the intended recipients of the health program. Thus, to establish the size of the health problem, planners must delineate the community boundaries. In this sense, a community is akin to a population. Community assessments or community needs assessments are processes by which planners seek to more fully understand and describe the health problem. The word "community" is used irrespective of whether a community or a population is being assessed. However, if an actual community—in contrast to a population or an aggregate—is the focus, planners must clarify the boundaries of the community membership if they are to truly understand the specific health and social conditions within that community.

The community may be viewed as the context of the program in two different ways. First, the notion of community embodies a myriad of sociopolitical and economic factors that can influence the program plan and implementation. It may be possible only to acknowledge, articulate, and take into account these influences as contextual to the program (if resources will address these influences directly). Second, from a different perspective, community members who are invited to participate in the planning process become an immediate, intimate context of the program intervention.

The concepts of community as target and community as context are not mutually exclusive. An example helps demonstrate their interactive nature. At a university health promotion program, students, faculty, and university staff were involved in planning the program, and they also received the wellness program (Reger, Williams, Kolar, Smith, & Douglas, 2002). They were a community as target to the extent that all those individuals working and going to school on campus were the intended recipients of the wellness program and were assessed as a unit to identify health problems. They were community as context to the extent that their values, norms, social structure, and university bureaucracy were influences on the program.

In this case, to address the contextual influences, the program initiators included and promoted participation by members of the university community in planning the wellness program. In so doing, they overcame institutional barriers and mobilized resources for the program. The synergies achieved by involving community members became possible because the university community was understood not as a single thing or a simple geographic location, but rather as a group of individuals. In other words, to involve "the community" in program planning requires having influential, energetic, devoted actual individuals who serve as representatives of or from that group actively participate in planning activities.

Collaboration between health program planners and formal or informal leaders from a community, and the participation of those community leaders in the development and evaluation of a health program, are increasingly valued. In fact, such collaboration is increasingly mandated by funding agencies as a prerequisite to being considered for funding. Collaboration creates interaction, which can intensify the sense of community and promote synergy among the community representatives, the agency sponsoring the health program, and the program staff (Figure 4.1). These interactions and influences move in two directions, with ideas and energy flowing toward the health program and results and respect flowing from the health program.

Defining Terms: Based, Focused, and Driven

Three terms related to community need to be defined in any discussion of community health planning: community based, community focused, and community driven.

Community based is an adjective describing where a program or service is provided. A health program is community based if it is delivered at locations considered within the boundaries of the community, rather than at a centralized location outside the community boundaries. Generally, this understanding translates into a program being delivered in local churches, schools, recreation centers, local clinics, or libraries.

Community focused refers to the way in which the program is designed. Health programs that seek to affect the community as a whole, as a unit, are best described as community focused. A community-focused program may seek to change the norms or behaviors of the members of a community that

Figure 4.1 Connections among Program, Agency, and Community

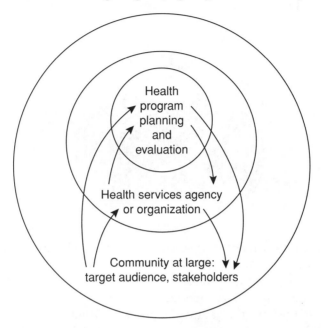

contribute to the health problem, or it may seek to reach all members of the community.

In contrast, if a health program is the result of the involvement of community members and is based on their preferences and needs, it is referred to as *community driven*. A community-driven program has its genesis—that is, its design and implementation—in the involvement, persistence, and passion of key representatives or members from the community.

Three points are worth noting about these qualifiers. First, the terms "based," "focused," and "driven" are not mutually exclusive (Figure 4.2). In other words, a program can be a combination of being based in, focused on, and driven by a community.

Second, the degree to which a program is community based, community focused, or community driven can vary. For example, it is easy to imagine a city health clinic that is very community based, moderately community focused, and not at all community driven.

Third, the designations of "based," "focused," and "driven" can also apply to families, populations, or other aggregates. Thus family-based programs might be provided to individuals but within the theoretical or physical

Figure 4.2   Venn Diagram of Community Based, Community Focused, and Community Driven

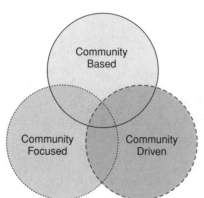

presence of families, family-focused programs would be designed to enhance the family as a unit, and family-driven programs would be the result of a group of families advocating for or demanding the programs.

These distinctions can be important in terms of describing health programs and of conceptualizing the nature of a program. Whether a health program is based or focused on a unit ought to flow from an understanding of the health problem and the best strategy for addressing it.

COMMUNITY NEEDS ASSESSMENT: TYPES OF NEEDS

Four types of needs (Bradshaw, 1972) ought to be considered in a needs assessment. Understanding the characteristics of each type of need as it relates to the population of interest is critical to successful health program planning.

Expressed need is the problem revealed through healthcare-seeking behavior. In other words, expressed need is manifested as the demand for services and the market behavior of the target audience. It is measured in terms of the number of people who request services, the types of services sought, and in utilization rates.

Normative need is a lack, deficit, or inadequacy as defined by experts and health professionals, usually based on a scientific notion of what ought to be or what the ideal is from a health perspective. A norm or normal value is used as the gauge for determining if a need exists. Given that the health professional is an outside observer, normative need can be viewed as similar to an *etic* perspective—that is, the view through the eyes of an observer.

The third type of need is the *perceived need*, which is the felt lack as experienced by the target audience. Perceived needs are demonstrated in what members of the target audience say they say they want, and in their stated deficits and inadequacies. Perceived need is similar to an *emic* perspective—that is, the view through the eyes of the person having the experience.

Finally, the comparative or *relative need* is the identified gap or deficit as identified through a comparison between advantaged and disadvantaged groups. Relative need entails a comparison that demonstrates a difference that is interpreted as one group having a need relative to the other group. Most of the health disparities are stated as relative need. Either health professionals or community members can choose the point of comparison, but are likely to choose different points of comparison. Thus the relative needs would also be different.

The ways in which the interaction of these needs plays out in day-to-day situations can be seen in the experiences of a group of health planners who conducted a community needs assessment in the fictitious town called Layetteville. In conducting their assessment, they identified a neighborhood as having a relative need. The planners found that the neighborhood had higher rates of adolescent pregnancy, deaths due to gunshot injuries, birth defects, and diabetes than other neighborhoods in the city, and that these rates were two to three times higher than those set out in the *Healthy People 2010* objectives. When the group explored the healthcare utilization patterns of the residents of the neighborhood, they found that the residents rarely used a primary healthcare clinic; instead, they used the local emergency department.

Confident in their understanding of what was needed to improve the health of the neighborhood, the group of planners approached the residents with a plan to establish a primary care clinic in the neighborhood that would provide prenatal care and diabetes management. Bluntly, the residents indicated that they were not interested: They wanted a community swimming pool in their neighborhood. They felt a strong need for recreation, a community meeting place, and an equal opportunity to engage in the healthy behavior of swimming as an alternative to the gang activities that were contributing to the shootings. Only after those conducting the assessment agreed to address the community's perceived need for a community swimming pool did the residents then consider how to address the normative, comparative, and relative needs that had been identified.

PERSPECTIVES ON ASSESSMENT

The goal of a needs assessment is to guide and inform decisions related to program prioritization and development. Basically, a needs assessment is a procedure used to collect data that describe the needs and strengths of a specific group, community, or population. To simplify the language, *needs assessment* is the term used in this chapter to broadly encompass both the deficit and the asset perspectives. Also, the term *target audience* is used as a way to denote those for whom a program is intended. Only if the program is targeted at a true population is the term *target population* used. The intended audiences can be a group (a relatively small set of individuals who interact), a community, a neighborhood, an *aggregate* (a set of individuals who share one characteristic in common, such as a school or a health condition), or a complete population. One of the first tasks in planning and conducting a needs assessment is to determine who is likely to make up the target audience or target population and in what larger unit they are situated.

Five types of models exist for conducting a needs assessment: the epidemiological model, the public health model, the social model and the asset model. Each model has its own intellectual perspective, as well as both advantages and disadvantages (Table 4.2). Nonetheless, each model has a role in a health needs assessment.

Epidemiological Model

The epidemiological model of needs assessment focuses on quantifying health problems, using national data sets and applying epidemiological methods and statistics. This model seeks to answer questions with an epidemiological focus, such as "What is the magnitude of the problem?" or "What illness and disease trends are evident?" or "What patterns of selectivity are exhibited in the distribution of the problem?" Other questions stemming from this perspective would be "Is the problem preventable?," "How treatable is the problem?," and "What is currently being done?" As these questions suggest, epidemiological models often include a focus on identifying hazards, risks, and precursors to the health problem.

Examples of tools used in the epidemiological model are disease and death registries and national probability sample surveys such as the National Health Information Survey (NHIS) and the National Health and Nutrition Examination Survey (NHANES). An advantage of epidemiological models is that they provide data for assigning relative weights to the seriousness of a health problem, the importance of that health problem, and its prevalence. However, these models do not provide a breadth of data that might also be key in prioritizing health problems.

Table 4.3 is a summary of commonly used epidemiological rates, with their corresponding numerators and denominators. As the entries in the table suggest, the epidemiological model relies heavily on having accurate counts that can be used in the denominators and numerators. To the extent that data are

Table 4.2 A Comparison of the Five Dominant Models of Community Needs Assessment

	Epidemiological Model	Public Health Model	Social Model	Asset Model	Rapid Model
Population assessed	Populations	State and communities	Populations, selected aggregates	Community, neighborhoods	Community, neighborhoods
Data sources	Registries, national probability sample surveys, existing national databases	State and local agencies, vital records	Individual surveys, national surveys	Rosters of agencies, focus groups, maps	Windshield surveys, existing data, interviews
Examples	National Health Interview Survey (NHIS), Healthcare Cost Utilization Profile (HCUP)	MAPP, CHIP, PATCH	U.S. Census	Assets-Based Community Development Institute	Rapid Assessment and Response (RAR), Rapid Assessment and Response and Evaluation (RARE)
Types of needs assessed	Normative, expressed, and relative needs can be estimated	Normative and relative needs can be estimated	Relative needs can be estimated, perceived needs are directly determined	Perceived needs, perceived strengths	Normative and perceived needs
Advantages	Statistically sound and generalizable findings	Administratively sound; includes focus on constituent concerns	Statistically sound; provides information on factors contributing to health problem	Existing resources are identified	Quickly completed and provides basic information
Disadvantages	No information on perceived needs; local variations may not be captured or described	Relies on other data sources; perceived needs are not directly determined	Does not directly measure the extent of the health problem	Does not measure the extent of the health problem	Does not measure the extent of the health problem; may miss problems or causes

Table 4.3   Numerators and Denominators for Selected Epidemiological Rates Commonly Used in Community Health Assessments

Rate	Numerator	Denominator	Per
Crude death rate	Total number of deaths in a given time period	Total population	1000
Cause-specific death rate	Number of deaths due to a specific cause in a given time period	Total population	100,000
Birth rate	Number of live births in a given time period	Total population	1000
Fetal death rate	Number of fetal deaths of 28 weeks' gestation or more that occur in a given time period	Number of fetal deaths of 28 weeks', gestation or more plus number of live births that occur in a given time period	1000
Neonatal death rate	Number of deaths of infants 28 days old or less that occur in a given time period	Number of live births that occur in a given time period	1000
Infant mortality rate	Number of infants (age birth to 1 year of age) who died in a year	Number of births in a year	1000

available, key elements of the epidemiological model are incorporated into most community health assessments.

Public Health Model

Public health models focus on quantifying health problems for the purpose of prioritizing the identified health problems being addressed with limited resources. These models seek to answer the questions that reflect an interest in the health of a population. Needs assessment questions from this perspective might be "What is the seriousness of the problem?" or "What is the distribution of the problem?" Other questions relate to the prioritization aspect, such as "What is the perceived importance of the problem?" or "What resources are available to address the problem?"

Public health approaches to needs assessment typically rely on existing data and epidemiological data. Specific tools or models are used in the public health approach to needs assessment, such as PATCH and MAPP. These models, which were described in Chapter 3, provide a framework for determining which types of data ought to be collected as part of the needs assessment. There is considerable overlap between public health models and the epidemiological approach to needs assessment. Although these models are fairly comprehensive, they are somewhat weak in terms of their ability to account for the sociocultural aspects of health.

Social Model

The social model of needs assessment focuses on quantifying characteristics that contribute to the socioeconomic and political context that may affect the health of individuals. This model seeks to answer questions focused on societal trends. For example, using the social model is appropriate if the question is "What is the relationship among health problems and social characteristics?" or "Which social trends are evident?" Other questions appropriate for this model are "What is the relationship between the use of social and health resources and the problem?" and "How have social and health policies affected the magnitude, distribution, or trends of the problem?" Key characteristics of a social model needs assessment are a focus on collecting data regarding social characteristics, such as income, and on collecting data from specific aggregates about specific social and economic topics. Specific information is collected through national household surveys, such as the U.S. Census.

The value of the social model approach has been demonstrated in a variety of studies. For example, Sorensen and colleagues (2007) used a social context model to guide their evaluation of two randomized controlled trials of health behavior change. They found that variables measuring the social context, such as supportive social norms and more social ties, were associated with increased fruit and vegetable consumption. Such studies reinforce the value of including data on social indicators as part of a needs assessment.

In health care, reliance on social indicators alone as a sole basis for program planning is not considered acceptable. Without the health indicators, the community needs assessment is incomplete. Nevertheless, social models of assessment do generate crucial information that might help identify antecedents or prior conditions leading to the health problems.

Asset Model

A fourth perspective on needs assessment is based on asset models, which focus on the strengths, assets, abilities, and resources that exist and are available, rather than focusing on the needs, deficits, lacks, and gaps between the healthy and ill. These models seek to answer the questions such as "Which social and health resources exist within the community experiencing the health problem?"or "What do community members view as strengths and resources within their community?" Another question might be "To what extent are the resources mobilized or able to be mobilized to address health problems?"

Asset-based community development (ABCD) has been recognized as potentially useful for creating healthy communities for children (Pan, Littlefield, Valladolid, Taping, & West, 2005). Indeed, asset models represent an important counterbalance to deficit models (Morgan & Ziglio, 2007) in efforts to overcome barriers to improving community health. Inherent in the asset perspective is a focus on the collective resources of individuals, particularly in the form of their social networks. In this regard, the asset perspective is aligned with the current emphasis on social capital. An asset model assessment could reasonably include an inventory of the social capital within the community being assessed for health problems.

Taking the social context into account in understanding a health problem stemmed from the older view of health in which the environment was seen as one of four forces either fostering health or leading to illnesses (Blum, 1981; Dever, 1980): environment, genetics, medical care system, and lifestyle. Blum (1982), in discussing considerations related to risk reduction, introduced the "force field" perspective, suggesting that both forces that lead to risk conditions and forces that lead to risk minimization need to be considered. This perspective, he suggested, could be used to organize areas to be assessed.

Asset models also incorporate another concept with a long history: community competence (Cottrell, 1976; Goeppinger, Lassiter, & Wilcox, 1982). *Community competence* is the process whereby a community is able to identify problems and take actions to address those problems, and it is increased by community organizing (Denham, Quinn, & Gamble, 1998). Greater community competence has been associated with both better health of the community and larger amounts of social capital (Lochner, Kawachi, & Kennedy, 1999).

The asset perspective on community assessment seeks to identify and then build on the capabilities of a community so as to resolve health issues. Although the asset models have some appeal, especially to community stakeholders, gathering asset data can be challenging. No generally accepted set of asset indicators exists. Likewise, rarely does asset information exist at the time of the assessment, making data collection necessary. These disadvantages contribute to asset models being less widely used as a sole approach to needs assessment, and they are poorly integrated into the more widely used models of needs assessment.

TYPES OF ASSESSMENTS

Before initiating a full-scale needs assessment, planners and planning groups need to be familiar with assessment as a process. This process begins by studying available data in order to gain a working knowledge of the community and the prevalent health problems. The familiarization assessment, as it is called, is a starting point from which to consider whether more data are needed and whether to proceed with conducting a larger-scale needs assessment. It is possible that a local agency has already done a needs assessment that might be adequate for the task at hand. Thus, becoming familiar with the community, the health problem, and existing assessments can save time and effort during the planning process. If it appears that an assessment is needed, six types of assessments may need to be performed.

Organizational Assessment

An organizational assessment determines the strengths, weaknesses, opportunities, and threats to the organization providing the health program. While an organizational assessment can be thought of as part of the logistics planning for a health program, it is critical to have a good sense of the organizational willingness and capabilities to provide a program to address the health problem under consideration *before* planning proceeds. In the PRECEDE-PROCEED model (Green & Kreuter, 2005), which is widely used by health educators, an organizational assessment is viewed as a key component in planning health educational interventions. The organizational assessment seeks to answer the key question "What is the capability and willingness of the organization to provide the health program?"

Data for an organizational assessment are gathered from members of the organization as well as from existing organizational records and documents. These data help determine the organizational feasibility of providing the health program—that is, whether adequate and appropriate resources are available and whether the health program fits with the organization's mission and goals. One key aspect of the organizational assessment is the assessment of human resources within the organization, with particular attention being paid to their ability to meet the needs identified in the community needs assessment. This type of assessment can also identify changes needed within the organization as a prerequisite to providing the health program. In this way, the organizational assessment provides critical information for developing internal strategies to ensure the success of the health program.

The extent to which an organizational assessment is critical to the success of a health program is reflected in the organizational capacity study carried out by Roberts-Gray, Gingiss, and Boerm (2007). These authors developed a valid and reliable tool to assess the capacity of schools to implement a smoking prevention program funded by the Texas Department of State Health Services. Ultimately, their measures of organizational capacity predicted both the quantity of implementation activities and the quality of the implementation of the schoolwide intervention geared toward smoking prevention.

A case study is another potential source of data for an organizational assessment. Case studies involve multiple sources and types of data that are descriptive of one or more specifically selected cases, whether the case is a clinic, a program, or an individual. Although they are time intensive, case studies about health agencies, communities, or community action groups may be constructed as a part of a community health assessment. The advantage is that these studies provide comprehensive information, although it may not be generalizable to the current situation. Case study methodology is discussed in greater detail in Chapter 15.

Marketing Assessment

Just as understanding the needs and assets of a target audience is key in program planning, it is equally important to understand the extent to which the target audience would be interested in the health program. Although market assessment is usually considered a part of actual program planning, the data for such an assessment can be collected at the same time as the needs assessment data are gathered. This type of assessment seeks to answer the key question of "What will draw the target audience into the program?"

Typical market analyses, such as those conducted in businesses, differ from marketing assessments for health programs in several ways. As discussed in Chapter 8, in health programs, marketing concepts are adapted to reflect the programs' social and behavioral intervention focus. In addition, the price and packaging aspects that are addressed in marketing assessments play different roles in health programs.

The key data to be collected in a marketing assessment deal with competitive programs (available community resources) and overall interest in the intended program. Incorporating the marketing assessment into any early assessment activities minimizes lost opportunities to collect key data and helps to provide a more complete assessment of the conditions that might affect both services utilization and health outcomes.

Needs Assessment

A needs assessment, in the more narrowly defined, traditional sense, is a means by which to determine the gaps, lacks, and wants relative to a defined population and to define a specific health problem. Data from a needs assessment are used to identify health problems or conditions that can be addressed by a health program. In this way, the assessment serves as a starting point for planning, implementing, and evaluating a program (Scriven & Roth, 1990).

A needs assessment provides health-related information that enables planners to gauge the priorities to be given to specific health problems, and it helps identify the trade-offs that inevitably arise in addressing one health problem rather than another. Often a needs assessment is done to answer the question "What health problems exist, and to what extent?"

Findings from the needs assessment help identify health problems or conditions that should be addressed in future health programs. In other words, this effort provides data necessary for program development—specifically, regarding which health interventions are needed, where, and with which target audience. A needs assessment helps make decisions more defendable and acceptable to the stakeholders. Ideally, it results in the flow of money and effort to meet the needs of the target audience.

Typically a needs assessment is problem oriented; thus it tends to begin with a stated health problem about which more information is wanted or needed. Another facet of needs assessment is the delineation of the community as a subsystem deserving of specific assessment. Sometimes more detailed information is needed about one aspect of a community, and a needs assessment focused on the community can provide such information.

Community Health Assessment

A community health assessment is used to establish the magnitude of selected health problems in a selected community, neighborhood, or other designated locality relative to the strengths and resources within that community, and to determine the priority the community gives to addressing the health problem. A community health assessment casts a broad net, encompassing all aspects of the community. It examines health and human service resources and assets, as well as the health problem and other community weaknesses. This type of assessment seeks to answer the question "What are the health problems, and which resources are available to address those health problems?" In this sense, a community health assessment encompasses and integrates each of the four assessment models described previously. From this integrative perspective, the chapter provides details on conducting a community health assessment.

Rapid Assessment

In some circumstances, expediency is needed or desirable when conducting an assessment. Over the past 20 years, a consensus has emerged that a rigorous, reliable approach to rapidly assessing the health of a population or community is both possible and of value. Essentially, the rapid assessment approach uses multiple methods—such as focus groups, existing data, interviews, and mapping—to involve the community in rapidly developing and implementing needed health interventions. A rapid assessment seeks to answer the key question "What are the most immediate and pressing needs that can be addressed with readily available resources?" As this question implies, the focus is on obtaining a quick response rather than ensuring the depth or breadth of the assessment.

Various terms are used as names for this type of assessment: rapid assessment and response (RAR) and rapid assessment and response and evaluation (RARE). These names denote the process by which an assessment is rapidly conducted and used to develop interventions. The RARE model consists of community participation, use of multiple methods and triangulation, and evaluation of both short- and long-term outcomes (McNall & Foster-Fishman, 2007; Needle et al., 2003). These basic steps are also part of the RAR model, which has been used as part of the response to natural disasters, such as Hurricane Katrina (Rogers, Guerra, Suchdev, & Chapman, 2006). Stimson, Fitch, and Don Des Poznyak (2006), in a review of RAR studies conducted in several countries, found that RAR was effective in linking the assessment findings to the development and implementation of new or modified interventions.

Workforce Assessment

A workforce assessment is not commonly thought of as part of a community health assessment. However, at the infrastructure level of the public health pyramid, workforce assessments are particularly germane. A workforce assessment seeks to answer the question "Which human resources exist at which level of expertise to address the health needs?" A workforce assessment examines the current competencies among the workforce, trends and drivers of change related to the quantity and quality of the workforce, and building scenarios to understand the potential size of the gap between projected needs and projected available workforce.

Across the health professions, workforce assessments conducted by scholars as rigorous research projects have revealed a dire situation for health care. In the foreseeable future, there are predictions of shortages of personnel in the fields of nursing (Buerhaus, Donelan, Ulrich, DesRoches, & Dittus, 2007; Hinshaw, 2008), occupational health (Powell, Kanny, & Coil, 2008), environmental health (EPA, 1999), medicine (Salsberg & Grover, 2006), and public health (ASPH, 2008). These predictions make it necessary that before undertaking the development of any health program, a local assessment be conducted to identify the current and future workforces that will be tapped into to support the anticipated program. After all, there is no point in developing a great program on paper if it will not be possible to hire health professionals with the qualifications needed to make the program a success in the real world. Just as the organizational assessment is critical to determining the support of potential programs, so the workforce assessment is critical to determining the feasibility of having program personnel.

STEPS IN CONDUCTING THE ASSESSMENT

There is no one way and no one right way to conduct a community health assessment. Nevertheless, certain basic steps are incorporated into any approach to community health assessment. The first step is to involve community members in the development and execution of the community assessment. The next step is to define the community or population to be assessed, followed by making decisions about which data to collect regarding the nature of the health problem, such as the magnitude of the problem, precursors to the health problem, and demographic and behavioral characteristics. The next step is to collect these data, using a variety of data sources and approaches. Once the data have been collected, the assessment and planning team must analyze the data using statistical procedures to arrive at statistical statements about the health problems in the population. Based on these data and the statistics obtained via their analysis, the final step seeks to develop a summary statement of the need or the problem that ties together the antecedent and causal factors of the health problem, along with the asset factors that counter the existence of the health problem.

Involve Community Members

Ideally, before starting a community health assessment, the planners will devote time to developing a strategy for involving members of the community to be assessed. The rationale behind involvement of those likely to be targeted by a program stems from a philosophy of empowerment as well as a practical concern with stakeholder and consumer reactions to the data. From the philosophical perspective of empowerment, involvement by community members enhances both their capacity to assist in the assessment and their ownership of the data gathered and results produced by the assessment. This theme of involvement is carried throughout the phases of planning and evaluating a health program.

From a practical perspective, involving those likely to be affected by the assessment has immediate and direct consequences for how the community health assessment evolves. The involvement of community members can even shape the questions addressed by the needs assessment, as reported by Teufel-Shone, Siyuja, Watahomigie, and Irwin (2006). Of course, the strong views and bias of any one group can also become evident during the planning of the assessment. Program planners can use these revelations to begin to anticipate how those views might influence the interpretation of the data. By involving community stakeholder groups in the community health assessment, planners can uncover, acknowledge, and, hopefully, address their concerns.

Involving community members is rarely an easy venture. Numerous barriers to their involvement must be overcome: time constraints on busy individuals, competing interests for available time, parking problems, limited accessibility of the meeting location, lack of awareness of the opportunity for involvement, feelings of inadequacy or insecurity about being involved, lack of day care for members' children. There is no one best way to increase involvement of community members. Instead, multiple strategies are needed, and the ones used are likely to evolve as the community health assessment proceeds. In addition to strategies that specifically address barriers to community participation, other strategies to increase involvement can include obtaining names of key individuals from agency personnel, providing food as an incentive, providing informal training or skills related to being involved, having specific tasks in which individuals can be involved, or having regularly scheduled meeting dates and times.

Sometimes, however, it may not be wise to focus on involving community members: when severe time constraints on completing the community health assessment exist, when severe fiscal constraints limit the scope of the assessment, when profound allegiances might affect the quality of interactions among community members, or when insufficient leadership skills exist to initiate and sustain community involvement. At other times, community members simply must be involved in the community health assessment: when there is a mandate from a funding agency for community involvement, when doing so will reduce the perception of being excluded, when insiders' connections and perceptions are needed to ensure a complete community health assessment, or when the goal is to have the community take responsibility for sustained implementation of the health program.

Define the Population

Delineating who is to be assessed is an important early step in conducting a community health assessment. The question of who to assess is often influenced by who is doing the assessment. That "who" can be defined geographically, enabling the population of interest to be delineated by a site, such as workplace, location of residence, or school. Using locality as the defining characteristic is common, such that ZIP code areas, census tracts, community areas, or legal boundaries are often used to define who is assessed. A state health department or a state health program will focus on the state population, whereas a small, local, not-for-profit agency is likely to focus only on individuals who are potential customers. For example, the Traditional Indian Alliance in Tucson serves only Tucson's Native American population. Not surprisingly, its needs assessment was very limited in terms of both geography and population segment (Evaneshko, 1999). In contrast, a United Way organization in a large metropolitan area will assess the health and social needs of the population in its catchment area.

Using highly specific parameters to define "who" allows the assessment to be more encompassing and detailed. For example, work-site needs assessments, like the one carried out by Phillips and Belcher (1999), tend to yield data on a range of employee risk factors for health conditions, some of which are not related to the workplace. The data from these authors' work-site assessment enabled them to develop work-site health promotion programs that addressed both work-site and other health risks. This example shows that defining "who" based on a narrowly defined location may be a convenient means to access an aggregate, obtain detailed information, and very specifically tailor a health program.

In program planning and evaluation, the term *target audience* refers to those for whom the program or intervention is designed and intended—in other words, those who are targeted by the program. The term *target population* is used if the program is intended for an entire population, rather than a subpopulation. Put simply, the target audience includes all potential participants. Those who actually receive the program or intervention are referred to as the *recipient audience*. Thinking about this distinction between targets and recipients helps clarify who ought to be included in the community health assessment: Basically, both groups should be included, and the target audience encompasses the potential recipients.

The parameters used to distinguish individuals for whom the program or intervention is intended from individuals for whom it is not intended become the boundaries of the target population. The target audience is usually some portion of the *population at risk*—that is, those individuals who have some social, physical, or other condition that increases their likelihood of an undesirable health problem or state. The term *at high risk* is usually reserved for those individuals with the highest probability of having an undesirable health state or outcome.

When conducting a community health assessment, planners must recognize that the boundaries of the target audience are likely to change with the collection and analysis of the data. For example, imagine that when a community health assessment is begun, an entire neighborhood or community area is viewed as the target audience. As epidemiological data and asset data are analyzed and interpreted, the planners may realize that only the black elderly residents, or white adolescent residents, or working mothers are at high risk for a health problem that can be addressed by the organization. This evolution of "who" from the broad boundaries to a more refined definition of the target audience is what ought to occur as a result of the community health assessment.

Define the Problem to Be Assessed

Just as the "who" of a community health assessment evolves with the collection of data and synthesis into information, so the "what" is also likely to evolve as the assessment process unfolds.

Community health assessments are undertaken to address a purpose—and that purpose is never an altruistic desire to identify the breadth of the health problems that exist within a community. More likely, the community health assessment will be performed in response to a specific mandate. For example, the federal Maternal and Child Health Bureau mandates that all states conduct a statewide needs assessment every five years as part of the states' application for Title V block grant funding. Similarly, local jurisdictions may request a needs assessment as part of a strategic plan to be more responsive to changing health and social needs of their constituents and to address challenges created by budgetary constraints. If township or county officials face pressure to address the health or social problems of a particular group, such as adolescents, immigrants, or disabled, those officials may request a community assessment to substantiate or discredit the needs of the group. This may be one way that the political aspect of program planning is played out.

For larger health agencies, organizations, or jurisdictions, a community health assessment might be conducted in response to calls for grant proposals that specify health problems or conditions as a high priority for being addressed. For example, the Centers for Disease Control and Prevention (CDC) has funded health promotion programs designed to reduce racial and ethnic disparities with regard to diabetes, cardiovascular diseases, infant mortality, HIV/AIDS, and immunizations. An agency wishing to compete for these CDC funds needed to identify within its community the specific racial or ethnic disparities as well as needs and assets relative to one of those five health problems.

ANTICIPATE DATA-RELATED AND METHODOLOGICAL ISSUES

Data-related issues associated with conducting a needs assessment are well recognized and documented (Altschuld & Witkin, 2000; Lee, Altschuld, &

White, 2007). Such issues must be addressed to enhance the quality of the data collected, thereby improving the accuracy of the community health assessment. Several types of methodological issues are discussed here in the context of conducting a community health assessment, rather than within the more typical research framework.

First, when one is attempting to uncover what is occurring, there is a temptation to ask those experiencing the problem to provide information about the problem. As mentioned earlier, the trouble with this approach is that those receiving services may be systematically different from those not receiving services. Also, this approach is unlikely to uncover latent needs, meaning that some needs may not be manifested in an easily recognizable form. Going back to the earlier example of the community that wanted a swimming pool, a latent need was to have an inequity addressed as manifested in community members' perceived need for recreational opportunities.

Another methodological problem is that asking potential consumers of the program about their needs has the potential to bias the answer. In other words, when asked about their needs, community members may take the opportunity to express all kinds of frustrations, wants, and needs. In addition, asking about needs, problems, and deficits does not allow for understanding the community's assets, strengths, potential, resources, and capabilities. Thus data collection methods are best designed to enable the collection of data that would fall on both sides of the equation.

Community health assessments can take as long as a year to accomplish, particularly if the assessment is comprehensive in scope and involves community members in the process. Unfortunately, time constraints are a reality that can heavily influence both the quality and the quantity of data collected as part of the assessment. Realistic strategies and designs for collecting data must match the timelines; otherwise, only partial data will be collected and will most likely be imbalanced in nature, leading to faulty conclusions.

In addition, the measures used to collect data must adhere to scientifically rigorous standards. Most importantly, the instruments used must have both validity and reliability. *Validity* is the degree to which that instrument measures what it is intended to measure. *Reliability* is the degree to which the instrument will yield the same results with different samples. Epidemiological measures, such as mortality, have high validity; death is rarely misdiagnosed. By contrast, the underlying causes of death as reported on death certificates are prone to both validity and reliability problems. The validity problems stem from conceptual issues of whether the cause of death ought to be the immediate cause or the underlying cause. The reliability problems relate to how each death certificate is completed and coded. Similarly, other epidemiological measures, such as adequacy of prenatal care, have been questioned with regard to validity and reliability. In terms of conducting a community health assessment, the point being made here is that no data are perfect, and these imperfections can lead to inaccurate numbers and hence faulty program planning decisions. Given this potential for error, planners should openly discuss the limits of the data and take reasonable scientific steps to obtain the best data possible.

The issue of determining from whom to collect the community health assessment data will always be important. This is a sampling problem. Sampling is a science, with numerous sampling strategies (presented in detail in Chapter 13) being possible. In terms of conducting a needs assessment, the sampling decision will depend on the degree to which individuals providing community health assessment data must be representative of the entire target population. The epidemiological and social approaches to assessment would favor strategies that include individuals who look as much as possible like the target audience. However, if primary data are being collected, developing and employing strategies to achieve representativeness of the sample can be very difficult and costly. This issue is especially critical with hard-to-reach populations, such intravenous drug users, emotionally abused spouses, or women who have experienced a perinatal loss. Less expensive, but also less scientifically rigorous, sampling strategies are certainly possible. The key decision to be made is how important it is to describe the population with a high degree of accuracy, based on data from less than the entire target population or target audience.

An overarching concern is the cultural appropriateness of the data collection methods and the cultural competence of the data collectors and interpreters. As discussed in Chapter 2, culture, language, and ethnicity may all influence the responses of individuals to survey questions. The match between measurement approaches and the conceptualization of the neighborhood, for example, has subsequent implications for program intervention development (Nicotera, 2007).

Another key issue is the need to have community-level indicators—that is, data about the community, rather than data about individuals that are then aggregated by community. For example, daily intake of fat is an individual-level indicator, and an average of percentage of daily intake of fat based on sampling of all residents in the community is still an individual-level indicator. The percentage of grocery store shelf space allocated to low-fat foods, by contrast, is a community-level indicator. Similarly, the percentage of workers at a work site who smoke is an individual-level indicator, but the number of antismoking posters or announcements at the work site is a work-site-level measure.

Very few ready sources of community-level measures or indicators of aggregates such as work sites or communities are available. Rather, it takes creativity, working with the community members, and careful consideration to develop community-level indicators and then to reliably collect data. But this extra work is worth the effort: For many of the health problems targeted by health promotion or disease prevention programs, what exists in the community will be extremely important as a component of assessing the antecedents and causal factors to the health problems.

After analyzing community-level data, planners can develop community-level interventions. In addition, community-level interventions may sometimes be necessary when interventions at the individual level need to be reinforced with community-level changes. For example, Fikree, Khan, Kadir, Sagan, and Rahbar (2001) have suggested that to increase the use of family planning methods, community-level interventions are needed, such as engaging religious leaders in family planning programs and encouraging outreach efforts by community-based workers. Only by collecting community-level data as part of the community health assessment can planners identify community-level interventions that are truly relevant in addressing the health problem.

In summary, there are five "principles" of collecting data for a community health assessment. One, collect data from more than one source. In other words, use multiple methods and multiple sources, and be multicultural. Two, involve members of the community in the design, collection, and interpretation of the community health data: Be inclusive and be empowering. Three, give full disclosure and then get informed consent from individuals from whom data are being collected: Be forthright, be honest, and be safe. Four, go beyond the available and collect data from unlikely but enlightening sources: Be creative, be inventive, and be open. Finally, be as scientifically rigorous as time and other resources allow: Be scholarly, be interdisciplinary, and be systematic.

ACROSS THE PYRAMID

At the direct services level of the public health pyramid, health problems and conditions are viewed as individual problems that are best addressed by individual practitioners. Thus, at this level, assessments are of a focused type. A needs assessment is likely to concentrate on describing the magnitude of a specific medical problem. In addition, such an assessment would describe a subsystem of the community—namely, the diagnostic and treatment capabilities of the direct services providers within that community.

At the enabling services level of the public health pyramid, health problems and conditions are viewed as individual problems that are the direct results of non-individual factors and that require community-based or social services interventions. Thus assessments at this level would focus on describing the social context of those individuals with the health problem or condition, as well as the community subsystem in terms of local infrastructure capabilities and human services agencies.

At the population services level of the public health pyramid, health problems are viewed across a population. As a consequence, assessments at this level are likely to be epidemiological in approach, with attention being paid to describing the magnitude of various health problems or conditions. At the same time, social sciences approaches to assessment, using population data on social indicators, may provide valuable information about contributing and antecedent factors to the health problems and conditions.

At the infrastructure level of the public health pyramid, the concerns relate to the capabilities of the organization or the health delivery system to address the health problems or conditions at the direct, enabling, and population services levels of the pyramid. In the more ideal sense, the community health assessment is most appropriate for this level because it encompasses understanding the health problems and conditions within the social context of the target population as well as identifying the assets that are available to address those health problems and conditions. In addition, the organizational assessment fits at this pyramid level because it focuses on identifying the resources, capabilities, and mission currently available. The findings of the organizational assessment, when considered in conjunction with the findings of the community health assessment, ought to establish a solid foundation for garnering resources and planning health programs at the corresponding optimal level of the pyramid.

DISCUSSION QUESTIONS

1. Select one of the perspectives on assessment. In what way does that perspective change, alter, or influence each step in the process of performing a needs assessment?
2. Why is each type of assessment relevant to health program planning?
3. Do a search on Internet sites about community assessments. One suggestion is to begin with state health departments or the Community Tool Box. Which perspective on assessment is reflected in the context of the Internet site? Which of the steps described in this chapter received more or less emphasis by the authors of the Internet site? What implications does that shift in emphasis have for the problem statement?
4. Discuss the relevance of each perspective for developing programs at each level of the public health pyramid. What effect might choosing

one perspective have on the level of the program subsequently developed based on its assessment results?

5. A health program planning committee wants to address various health problems by developing programs for each health problem at all four levels of the public health pyramid. What would be some implications of this perspective on setting priorities and on the nature of the subsequent community health assessment?

INTERNET RESOURCES

Community Tool Box

The Community Tool Box, found at http://ctb.ku.edu/, has gained wide recognition for its information on community building, community assessment, and program evaluation (evaluation framework, funders, developing evaluation plan, and more).

Group Dynamics and Community Building

This website offers a different perspective on thinking about communities, with a wealth of links to resources on community and team building. Find it at http://www.community4me .com.

National Center for Health Statistics

The NCHS website (http://www.cdc.gov/nchs/about.htm) has information on accessing and using existing national data sets.

Institute for Policy Research: ABCD

For information on the ABCD approach, check out the website http://www.northwestern.edu/ ipr/abcd.html, maintained by the Institute for Policy Research at Northwestern University.

PRECEDE-PROCEED Model

The PRECEDE-PROCEED model can be viewed at the personal webpage of Lawrence Green, its author: http://www.lgreen.net/precede.htm.

Environmental Protection Agency

The EPA has conducted a workforce assessment that led to a strategic plan. The report found at http://www.epa.gov/epahrist/workforce/wap.pdf shows the importance of attending to the workforce in planning for future programs.

Maternal and Child Health Bureau

The Maternal and Child Health Bureau has published a guide on conducting a needs assessment that can be found at http://mchb.hrsa.gov/programs/womeninfants/naguide.htm. Although the focus is on maternal and child health needs, the process is applicable across populations.

REFERENCES

Altschuld, J. W., & Witkin, B. R. (2000). *From needs assessment to action: Translating needs into solution strategies.* Thousand Oaks, CA: Sage Publications.

Association of Schools of Public Health (ASPH). (2008). *Confronting the public health workforce crisis: ASPH statement on the public health workforce.* Retrieved March 6, 2008, from http://www.asph.org/UserFiles/PHWFShortage0208.pdf

Bell, C., & Newby, H. (1971). *Community studies: An introduction to the sociology of the local community.* London: George Allen & Unwin.

Belue, R., Taylor-Richardson, K. D., Lin, J. M., McClellan, L., & Hargreaves, M. K. (2006). Racial disparities in sense of community and health status: Implications in community-based participatory interventions targeting chronic disease in African-Americans. *Journal of Ambulatory Care Management, 29,* 112–124.

Blum, H. L. (1981). *Planning for health: Generics for the eighties* (2nd ed.). New York: Human Sciences Press.

Blum, H. L. (1982). Social perspective on risk reduction. In M. M. Farber & A. M. Reinhart (Eds.), *Promoting health through risk reduction* (pp. 19–36). New York: Macmillan.

Bradshaw, J. (1972). The concept of social need. *New Society, 30,* 640–643.

Buerhaus, P. I., Donelan, K., Ulrich, B. T., DesRoches, C., & Dittus, R. (2007). Trends in the experiences of hospital-employed registered nurses: Results from three national surveys. *Nursing Economic$, 25,* 69–79.

Cottrell, L. S. (1976). The competent community. In B. H. Kaplan, Leighton, A., & Wilson, R. (Eds.), *Further explorations in social psychiatry* (pp. 195–209). New York: Basic Books.

Denham, A., Quinn, S. C., & Gamble, D. (1998). Community organizing for health promotion in the rural South: An exploration of community competence. *Family and Community Health, 21,* 1–21.

Dever, G. E. (1980). *Community health assessment.* Germantown, MD: Aspen Systems.

Environmental Protection Agency (EPA). (1999). *Workforce assessment project: Executive summary and tasks 1–4 final reports.* Office of Administration and Resources Management. Retrieved March 6, 2008, from http://www.epa.gov/epahrist/workforce/wap.pdf

Evaneshko, V. (1999). Mental health needs assessment of Tucson's urban Native American population. *American Indian and Alaska Native Mental Health Research, 8*(3), 41–61.

Fikree, F. F., Khan, A., Kadir, M. M., Sagan, F., & Rahbar, M. H. (2001). What influences contraceptive use among young women in urban squatter settlements in Karachi, Pakistan? *International Family Planning Perspectives, 27,* 130–136.

Goeppinger, J., Lassiter, P. G., & Wilcox, B. (1982). Community health is community competence. *Nursing Outlook, 30,* 464–467.

Green, L. W., & Kreuter, M. W. (2005). *Health promotion planning: An educational and environmental approach* (4th ed.) New York: McGraw-Hill.

Hinshaw, A. S. (2008). Navigating the perfect storm: Balancing a culture of safety with workforce challenges. *Nursing Research, 57*(1 suppl), S4–S10.

Lee, Y., Altschuld, J. W., & White, J. L. (2007). Problems in needs assessment data: Discrepancy analysis. *Evaluation and Program Planning, 30,* 258–266.

Lochner, K., Kawachi, I., & Kennedy, B. P. (1999). Social capital: A guide to its measurement. *Health and Place, 5,* 259–270.

McNall, M., & Foster-Fishman, P. G. (2007). Methods of rapid evaluation, assessment, and appraisal. *American Journal of Evaluation, 28,* 151–168.

Morgan, A., & Ziglio, E. (2007). Revitalising the evidence base for public health: An assets model. *Promotion and Education, 2*(Suppl.), 17–22.

Needle, R. H., Trotter, R. T., Singer, M., Bates, C., Page, J. B., Metzger, D. (2003). Rapid assessment of the HIV/AIDS crisis in racial and ethnic minority communities: An approach for timely community interventions. *American Journal of Public Health, 93*, 970–979.

Nicotera, N. (2007). Measuring neighborhood: A conundrum for human services researchers and practitioners. *American Journal of Community Psychology, 40*, 26–51.

Nilsen, P. (2006). The theory of community based health and safety programs: A critical examination. *Injury Prevention, 12*, 140–145.

Pan, R. J., Littlefield, D., Valladolid, S. G., Taping, P. J., & West, D. C. (2005). Building healthier communities for children and families: Applying asset based community development to community pediatrics. *Pediatrics, 115*, 1185–1187.

Phillips, J. M., & Belcher, A. E. (1999). Integrating cancer risk assessment into a community health nursing course. *Journal of Cancer Education, 14*, 47–51.

Powell, J. M., Kanny, E. M., & Coil, M. A. (2008). State of the occupational therapy workforce: Results of a national study. *American Journal of Occupational Therapy, 62*(1), 97–105

Reger, B., Williams, K., Kolar, M., Smith, H., & Douglas, J. W. (2002). Implementing university-based wellness: A participatory planning approach. *Health Promotion Practice, 3*, 507–514.

Roberts-Gray, C., Gingiss, P. M., & Boerm, M. (2007). Evaluating school capacity to implement new programs. *Evaluation and Program Planning, 30*, 247–257.

Rogers, N., Guerra, F., Suchdev, P. S., & Chapman, A. S. (2006). Rapid assessment of health needs and resettlement plans among Hurricane Katrina Evacuees—San Antonio, Texas. *Morbidity and Mortality Weekly Report, 55*, 242–244.

Salsberg, E., & Grover, A. (2006). Physician workforce shortages: Implications and issues for academic health centers and policymakers. *Academic Medicine, 81*, 782–787.

Scriven, M., & Roth, J. (1990). Special feature: Needs assessment. *Evaluation Practice, 11*, 135–144.

Sorensen, G., Stoddard, A. M., Dubowitz, T., Barbeau, E. M., Bigby, J. A., Emmons, K. M., et al. (2007). The influence of social context on changes in fruit and vegetable consumption: Results of the Healthy Directions studies. *American Journal of Public Health, 97*, 1216–1227.

Stimson, G. V., Fitch, C. J., & Don Des Poznyak, V. (2006). Rapid assessment and response studies of injection drug use: Knowledge gain, capacity building, and intervention development in a multisite study. *American Journal of Public Health, 96*, 288–295.

Teufel-Shone, N. I., Siyuja, T., Watahomigie, H. J., & Irwin, S. (2006). Community-based participatory research: Conducting a formative assessment of factors that influence youth wellness in the Hualapai Community. *American Journal of Public Health, 96*(9), 1623–1628.

CHAPTER 5

Characterizing and Defining the Health Problem

In this chapter, the focus on the community health assessment phase of the planning cycle continues with a review of data collection options. This is followed by a discussion of the basic epidemiological analyses often used in community health assessment. After program planners have identified health problems through the assessment process, those health problems need to be summarized into statements and diagrams that facilitate both prioritization and the subsequent detailed program planning. A statement of the health problem can be developed in many ways and take a variety of forms. This chapter introduces an approach to developing a health problem statement which is then used throughout this textbook as a means of linking the elements of the planning and evaluation cycle. The last phase of the assessment process is to prioritize the problems, preferably through a systematic and intentional process.

COLLECTING DATA FROM MULTIPLE SOURCES

Numerous types and sources of data are used in a community health assessment. Each has the potential to contribute to an understanding of the parameters of the health problem or condition. However, each has limitations and caveats that need to be considered.

Archival Data

Archival data, as existing but not current, include medical records and other types of agency records. On a local level, clinics, agencies, and not-for-profit organizations may have data appropriate for a community health assessment they may be conducting. Archival data can provide information about the demand or need for a source as well as the characteristics of program participants. The types and uses of archival data are discussed more fully in Chapter

11. One limitation to archival data is that the data may not include key information that is sought or may not be complete. Another potential problem with archival data is that the extent to which the data were initially collected accurately is unknown. These factors will influence the data's overall usefulness and trustworthiness.

Public Data

Public data include national surveys, vital statistics, and census social indicators. These data include data gathered through the national surveys administered by the National Center for Health Statistics (NCHS) of the Centers for Disease Control and Prevention (CDC), such as the National Health and Nutrition Examination Survey (NHANES) and the National Health Interview Survey (NHIS). Secondary analyses of these public data sets can be used to extend data available for the community health assessment. Such national data have been helpful in making decisions about specific health problems, targeting populations, identifying barriers, and influencing health policy. They can also be used to create synthetic estimates, as explained later in this chapter.

Proprietary Data

Another possible source of data is proprietary data sources—specifically, data that are owned by an organization and that can be purchased for use. For example, the American Hospital Association, the American Medical Association, and health insurance companies own databases about their members that can contain information needed for a comprehensive community health assessment. Like archival data, the information that can be gained from proprietary data is limited to what has already been collected.

Primary Data

Primary data are often specifically collected to illuminate a need of interest. A wide variety of methods can be used to collect primary data, including interviews, surveys, community forums, focus groups, and interviews with key informants and service providers. These data collection methods are discussed more fully in Chapters 11 and 14.

There are three key points to keep in mind when collecting primary data for a community health assessment. One, data from participants in a program are rarely used as the sole source of data for a community health assessment. Although the program participants can provide valuable insights into the perceived needs of the target audience, that information must be considered in light of the fact that the participants are already in the program. This fact alone makes them potentially dissimilar to those persons targeted by the program. Two, rigor is required to obtain valid, reliable, trustworthy data. In most cases, only minor modifications to rigorous designs are needed for conducting a community health assessment. Three, primary data can, of course, be collected from members of the target audience, but providers can also provide valuable insights into the needs of the target population. Although data from providers are useful in identifying specific service needs of the target population, this information must be viewed as revealing the normative needs only. That is, providers are notorious for holding views of what is needed that differ from the views held by their clients. Naturally occurring discrepancies between providers' normative assessment of a problem and the clients' perceived needs can pose a particular challenge for the health program planning. Making program development decisions based only on provider data is likely to result in programs that are not attractive to the intended audience.

Observational Data

Unobtrusive (Webb, Campbell, Schwartz, & Sechrest, 2000) or nonreactive (Webb, Campbell, Schwartz, Sechrest, & Grove, 1981) measures are also sources of data and are particularly relevant to community characteristics. For example, walking around a neighborhood and observing how many blocks contain abandoned buildings or storefront churches is an unobtrusive measure. Going through the garbage to count the number of liquor bottles, counting the number of billboard advertisements for unhealthy behaviors, estimating the ratio of bars and pubs to banks, watching the interactions among residents in a local bakery, and collecting local community newspapers are all examples of data collection of the least invasive nature. Each of these examples provides some clues to the character, strengths, and problems in the community as a whole. The use of unobtrusive measures is inexpensive and can provide interesting clues about what the health problem is and what may be contributing to that problem.

Published Literature

The published literature is an excellent source of information, particularly for determining relative and normative needs. In other words, information may be available that allows for comparative statements about the health status either in reference to other groups or to professional health standards. This inexpensive, reliable source of information ought not be overlooked in a community needs assessment.

Other Data Sources

Lastly, it can be important to collect data from sources that are not readily available. This practice is called "going beyond the street lamp," which derives its name from a little story.

One night, a man lost his keys. He began to look for them, crawling around on his hands and knees beneath a street lamp. Before long, a stranger stopped and asked the man what he was doing on his hands and knees. He replied that he was looking for his keys. The stranger offered to help and asked where he had lost his keys. The man replied, "Over there," pointing to a dark area down the block just outside the bar. So the stranger asked, "Then why are you looking over here?" To which the man replied, "Because there is more light over here."

The point of this story is that the information you need may not be the same as the data to which you already have access: You need to go beyond the street lamp. Some of the sources of data just described are available under the street lamp, whereas others are not readily available and will require primary data collection. What determines the extent to which data need to be collected from beyond the street lamp are factors such as time constraints, fiscal resources, level of expertise, and endorsement or expectations of those who will be using the community health assessment.

COLLECTING DESCRIPTIVE DATA

To understand the health problem and formulate a definition of the health problem or condition, it is necessary to collect data. Baker and Reinke (1988) suggest that from an epidemiological perspective, four categories of information need to be collected as a prelude to health planning: the magnitude of the problem, the precursors of the problem, population characteristics, and attitudes and behaviors. These four categories provide a useful framework for organizing a community health assessment, especially when they are expanded to include elements from the public health, social, and asset perspectives.

Magnitude of the Problem

One category of information needed is the magnitude of the problem. The magnitude can be described in terms of the extent of the disease or health condition, the acute or chronic nature of the problem, and the intensity of the problem.

The extent of the health problem is described in terms of incidence and prevalence. The *incidence* is the rate at which new cases occur. The *prevalence* is the extent to which cases currently exist in a population. Incidence and prevalence, although typically used in reference to disease conditions, can be used to think about behaviors as well. For example, the number of new smokers among a defined group of adolescents (incidence) and the percentage of that same adolescent population that is currently smoking (prevalence) provide information that can be used to determine whether smoking is a problem of sufficient magnitude to warrant attention in the program planning effort.

The magnitude of a problem is also conveyed through measures such as rates and proportions. In epidemiological terms, these measures are a matter of numerators and denominators. The *denominator* is generally the total number in the population or the total number in the population that is potentially at risk. The *numerator* is generally the number of individuals who have the health problem or condition or who are actually found to be at risk. Using these basic numbers, a wide variety of commonly defined rates and proportions can be developed related to health, a few of which are given in Table 4.3. Increasingly, the rates and proportions for various health problems are available online at the websites for local and state health departments and federal agencies, such as the National Center for Health Statistics, which is housed within the CDC.

The ability to obtain accurate rates and proportions depends, in part, on the quality of the tests used to identify cases. Ideal tests have both high *sensitivity* (the extent to which there are no false negatives) and high *specificity* (the extent to which there are no false positives). Sensitivity and specificity are often used in reference to medical tests, such as occult blood tests, mammography, or urine tests for cocaine use, but they are also important characteristics of psychological and behavioral measures, such as the CES-D, which measures the level of depression in an individual (Radloff, 1977), and the SF-36, which measures overall health and functioning (Ware, 2000; Ware, et al., 1995). The sensitivity and specificity of medical tests and of psychological or behavioral measures determine the extent to which a condition is accurately identified, which in turn influences the estimated incidence or prevalence rates for a given condition or behavior. In this way, sensitivity and specificity affect the accuracy of an estimated magnitude of a health problem or condition within a population.

Dynamics Leading to the Problem

Another category of data is information about the precursors of the health problem or condition. As the community health assessment progresses, the planning group uses the data collected to generate lists of factors, conditions, situations, and events that in some way contribute to the health problem coming into existence and being observable. All of these factors are precursors or antecedents to the health problem. In addition, those factors, conditions, situations, and events that mediate, potentiate, or suppress the expression of the health problem may be uncovered during an assessment. While much may be known about a health problem from the scientific literature, the community health assessment is done to elucidate specific precursors that are unique to a locality, whether a neighborhood or a state, or to a target population. Such information is necessary in order to later tailor interventions to the specific precursors of the health problem.

From an epidemiological perspective, the precursors to a health problem are understood in terms of agent, host, and environment. Baker and Haddon (1974), in studying childhood injuries, developed a model of factors associated to a health problem—namely, the human, physical, environmental, and socio-cultural factors. Table 5.1 is based on this model, albeit with the addition of the healthcare system as another element in analyzing the health problem or condition. Each cell in the table contains a definition of what might go into that cell, along with a few examples. For any single health problem that is the focus of a needs assessment, data can be placed into the cells in Table 5.1, thereby giving an overview and a preliminary analysis of precursors to the health problem or condition. This format is especially useful for infectious diseases and injuries. The Haddon (1972) model reveals the complexity of data that might need to be analyzed to fully understand the health problem or condition.

Population Characteristics

Population characteristics data, the third category, relate mainly to the social model of needs assessments. Obtaining this information involves collecting data on characteristics, such as distribution of age categories, income levels, educational levels, and occupation distribution within a community. If the "who" has been narrowly defined in terms of location, the population characteristics uncovered through this effort can be very specific. For example, if the assessment focuses on prison inmates, then their characteristics—such as types of crime committed, length of time incarcerated, or race—can become part of the population characteristics data collected for the community (prison) health assessment.

Attitudes and Behaviors

The fourth category of information concerns the attitudes and behaviors of the population being assessed, with particular attention being paid to the attitudes and behaviors of the target audience. Data about attitudes and behaviors help complete or flesh out the description of the factors related to a health problem.

Table 5.1 Haddon's Typology for Analyzing an Event, Modified for Use in Developing Health Promotion and Prevention Programs

	Agent Factors	Human Factors	Physical Environment	Sociocultural Environment	Health System Environment
Pre-event	Latency	Genetic makeup, motivation, knowledge	Proximity, transportation, availability of agent (e.g., alcohol or drugs)	Norms, policy and laws, cultural beliefs about causes, family dynamics	Accessibility, availability, acceptability
Event (behavior)	Virulence, addictiveness, difficulty of behavior	Susceptibility, vulnerability, hardiness, reaction	Force	Peer pressure	Iatrogenic factors, treatments
Post-event	Resistance to treatment	Motivation, resilience, time for recovery	Proximity, availability of agent (e.g., alcohol or drugs)	Meaning of event, attribution of causality, sick role	Resources and services, treatment options, emergency response

Source: Adapted from Haddon, W., Jr. (1972). A logical framework for categorizing highway safety phenomena and activity. *Journal of Trauma, 12,* 193–207. Cited in Grossman, D. C. (2000). The history of injury control and the epidemiology of child and adolescent injuries. *Future of Children, 10*(1), 23–52.

Some attitudes and behaviors may be antecedents to health problems or conditions. For example, culturally held beliefs about illnesses, illness prevention, and treatments, as well as beliefs concerning appropriate health behaviors and the sick role, may all be important to understanding the health problem. Other lifestyle behaviors contribute to the existence of health problems. For example, secondhand smoke contributes to childhood asthma, whereas regular aerobic exercise contributes to reduced numbers of health problems. Still, other attitudes and behaviors have a more direct, causal relationship with health problems. Distrust in medical providers and a failure to obtain preventive health services lead directly to severe morbidity conditions in some populations. Accordingly, attitudes toward health promotion and disease prevention behaviors as well as attitudes toward healthcare services and providers must be considered in order to have a comprehensive data set for a community health assessment.

Years of Life and Quality of Life

A number of measures have been developed to account not only for deaths, but also the quality of years lived with an illness and the number of those years. Table 5.2 summarizes these measures, whose definitions are drawn from a variety of sources. These measures are widely used to make international comparisons, not only by the World Health Organization (WHO), but also by researchers such as Lopez and colleagues (Lopez, Mathers, Ezzati, Jamison, & Murray, 2006). These burden of disease measures can also be used as part of a community needs assessment, albeit only if the population being assessed is sufficiently large to have stable statistics. Thus measures of burden of disease might be used for larger states within the United States or regions of the United States. In the United States, national surveys, surveillance registries, and hospital discharge data are major sources that can be used to calculate burden of disease measures (McKenna, Michaud, Murray, & Marks, 2005). These measures also are used in the economic evaluations of programs, particularly in cost–benefit analyses (see Chapter 16). Data on the negative consequences of health problems, beyond the familiar mortality rates, can be quite influential during the problem prioritization processes.

Definitions of quality of life include the notions of a perceived overall state of well-being across various domains such as sociocultural relationships and physical functioning or in relation to goals and expectations. Often quality of life is measured as pertains to a particular illness or disease process—usually a chronic disease such as asthma or arthritis. Although each person has a sense of what constitutes quality of life, its measurement is complex; hence the plethora of quality-of-life measures that are available (Dijkers, 1999). An

Table 5.2   Quality-of-Life Acronyms and Definitions

Acronym	Spelled-Out Form	Definition
QALYs	Quality-adjusted life-years	Number of years of life expected at a given level of health and well-being.
DALYs	Disability-adjusted life-years	Number of years of life lost from living with a level of morbidity or disability.
YLL	Years of life lost	Number of years a person is estimated to have remained alive if the disease experienced had not occurred.
YPLL	Years of potential life lost	A measure of the impact of disease or injury in a population that calculates years of life lost before a specific age (often age 65 or age 75). This approach assigns additional value to deaths that occur at earlier ages.
HYE	Healthy years equivalent	Number of years in perfect health that are considered equivalent to a particular health state or health profile.
YHL	Years of healthy life	Number of healthy years of life lived or achieved, adjusted for level of health status.

issue with quality-of-life measures, as Kaplan (1996) stressed, is that quality of life is multidimensional, so the measures must address the relative importance of the many dimensions of quality of life. The choice of which measure to use in health program planning will depend on the resources available for the assessment phase, the sophistication of the planning team, and the role played by the rational approach in the planning process.

The length of life is as important as its quality. Because individuals may live with the same health condition for varying lengths of time, the length of life as affected by that health condition is what becomes important. In other words, the assessment must take into consideration the quality of the life as lived with the health condition. The measures known as quality-adjusted life-years (QALYs) and disability-adjusted life-years (DALYs) were developed specifically to give a numeric value to the quality of years of life (Table 5.2). These composite scores are used with populations and, therefore, have the advantage of being indifferent to individual preferences. However, because the number of years for which quality can be adjusted is naturally shorter for older persons, QALYs and DALYs mathematically discriminate against the elderly. Nonetheless, the use of DALYs reveals the extent to which diseases affect the years of life (Table 5.3).

For example, in the United States based on 1996 data, McKenna and colleagues (2005) reported that for males and females, ischemic heart disease was the number one cause of DALYs, followed by road traffic injuries for males and unipolar depression for females. They also reported the leading cause of DALYs by race: ischemic heart disease for whites and Asians, HIV/AIDS for blacks, and alcohol use for Native Americans. As these data reveal, having data available that can be separated out by gender and race can lead to very different impressions and priorities.

A slightly different perspective is based on the number of years of life that are lost due to a health condition. *Years of life lost* (YLL) reveals the number of years lost at the end of life because of a health condition. The shortened life-span could be due to acute or chronic health problems, chronic environmental conditions, or injuries. *Years of potential life lost* (YPLL) is a similar measure but indicates the number of years of life lost at the beginning of life, such as the shortening of life caused by neonatal sepsis or childhood drowning.

All of these quality-of-life and life-year measures are particularly useful in public health assessments. They assist program planners in deciding which health condition warrants health promotion or disease prevention programs, particularly when resources are severely limited. Unfortunately, these measures are difficult to calculate and exist for nations or very specific populations. Therefore, it is challenging to use these measures in local community assessments.

STATISTICS FOR DESCRIBING HEALTH PROBLEMS

Data collected from the community health assessment need to be analyzed and interpreted, particularly the primary data that were collected. For example, if surveys were conducted or if data were abstracted from medical records, those data need to be analyzed. This section briefly reviews statistical approaches, with particular attention to epidemiological considerations relevant to community health assessment. More details about quantitative data analysis are provided in Chapter 14 as well as in statistical textbooks. The intention of this section is to relate what is learned in statistics and epidemiology to the community health assessment.

Given that most community health assessments involve some population-based data, it is worth reviewing basic epidemiological techniques here. More

Table 5.3   Global Leading Causes of Disability-Adjusted Life-Years (DALYs) and Years of Life Lost (YLL)

Rank	DALY Causes	DALY	Percentage
1	Neuropsychiatric conditions	193,278,495	13.0%
2	Cardiovascular diseases	148,190,083	9.9%
3	Unintentional injuries	133,111,628	8.9%
4	Perinatal conditions	97,335,086	6.5%
5	Respiratory infections	94,603,349	6.3%
6	HIV/AIDS	84,457,784	5.7%
7	Malignant neoplasms	75,544,632	5.1%
8	Sense organ diseases	69,380,870	4.7%
9	Diarrheal diseases	61,966,183	4.2%
10	Respiratory diseases	55,153,199	3.7%
	Total for top 10 causes	**1,013,021,309**	**68.0%**
	Total for all causes of DALY	**1,490,125,643**	
Rank	YLL Causes	YLL	Percentage
1	Cardiovascular diseases	125,998,313	13.7%
2	Respiratory infections	88,455,607	9.6%
3	Perinatal conditions	82,189,042	8.9%
4	Unintentional injuries	82,022,787	8.9%
5	Malignant neoplasms	71,603,522	7.8%
6	Diarrheal diseases	56,132,786	6.1%
7	Childhood-cluster diseases	38,626,775	4.2%
8	Intentional injuries	38,296,385	4.2%
9	Tuberculosis	29,681,283	3.2%
10	Respiratory diseases	28,317,733	3.1%
	Total for top 10 causes	**450,269,271**	**69.5%**
	Total for all causes of YLL	**922,476,312**	

Sources: World Health Organization. (2004). Revised global burden of disease (GBD) 2002 estimates: Years of life lost (YLL). Geneva, Switzerland: Author. Retrieved June 17, 2008, from http://www.who.int/healthinfo/statistics/gbdwhoregiony ll2002.xls

World Health Organization (2004). Revised global burden of disease (GBD) 2002 estimates: Disability adjusted life years (DALY). Geneva, Switzerland: Author. Retrieved June 17, 2008, from http://www.who.int/healthinfo/statistics/gbd whoregiondaly2002.xls

complete and in-depth presentations are available in traditional epidemiology textbooks, such as the one by Mausner and Baum (1974). For a direct application of epidemiology to community health assessment, Dever's (1980) book is a classic. However, the more recent publications by Dever (1997) and by Fos and Fine (2000) also cover basic epidemiological techniques, but from the point of view of healthcare executives planning for population health. Health program planners would do well to have at least one of these texts on their bookshelves for quick reference. With the widespread availability of computer spreadsheet and database programs, the calculation of most statistics is less a matter of doing the math and more a matter of understanding which numbers to use and how to make sense of the numbers generated by the software.

Descriptive Statistics

Descriptive statistics—the fundamentals of statistics—are a family of statistics that portray the distribution of values for a single variable. These statistics provide an amazing wealth of information but are often underappreciated for their ability to communicate important information simply.

The simplest descriptive statistic is the frequency, or count of occurrences. Based on the frequency, two other very informative descriptive statistics can be calculated. Mean is a measure of central tendency, whereas variance and standard deviation are measures of dispersion. The standard deviation is related to the range of values in the data and thus indicates the dispersion of the data. Remember that 68.3% of data are contained within one standard deviation, 95.5% within two standard deviations, and 99.7% within three standard deviations.

Descriptive statistics are easy to calculate with a hand calculator or spreadsheet software, such as Excel. They are often presented in the form of graphical displays of frequency such as bar graphs. A bar graph of frequencies provides a rough picture of the distribution, thereby visually revealing whether the data approximate the normal curve.

Odds Ratio and Relative Risk

Two statistical tests that help estimate the likelihood of having or getting a given health problem are the *odds ratio* (OR) and the *relative risk* (RR). The odds ratio is calculated as the odds of having the health problem if exposed divided by the odds of having the problem if not exposed. The relative risk is calculated as the cumulative incidence in the exposed population divided by the cumulative incidence in the unexposed population. In conducting a community health assessment, planners mostly obtain the odds ratio and relative risk from published studies because having data on exposure usually requires epidemiological research.

Relative risk ranges from 0.0 to infinity: The larger the relative risk, the greater the chance of developing the health problem with exposure. Similarly, the odds ratio ranges from 0.0 to infinity. Odds ratios from 0.0 to 1.0 indicate a protective effect, whereas odd ratios greater than 1 indicate an increased likelihood of having the health problem. The larger the odds ratio, the more likely one is to have the health problem. Although the odds ratio can range to infinity, in practice it rarely exceeds 10. Relative risk compares two cumulative incidences, thereby providing a direct comparison of the probabilities. This makes the relative risk measure preferable to the odds ratio (Handler, Rosenberg, Kennelly, & Monahan, 1998). The odds ratio does not use the population in the denominator, making it less accurate than the relative risk. However, when the health problem is rare, the odds ratio begins to approximate the relative risk.

Both the relative risk and the odds ratio are used widely in epidemiology and thus are likely available for use in community health assessments. Both convey information about the comparative influence of factors or "exposure" variables on health outcomes. Having this information available then allows planners to prioritize which causal or exposure factors to address in a health program.

Population Parameters

The *confidence interval* (CI) indicates the upper and lower range of values between which the value for the true population is likely to fall. It helps to understand the likelihood that the score or mean value for a health condition derived from a sample is similar to the value in the true population. Confidence intervals, like standard deviations, provide a level of assurance about whether the mean or score value for the variable reflects the value for the whole population. For example, if a score is within the CI, then the value falls within a range that is reflective of the larger population. However, if the value falls outside the CI, then that score can be viewed as being important because it is not different from the value in the general population.

Confidence intervals play a valuable role during the community health assessment by focusing attention on values that are unusual and thus merit attention. They also provide a clue as to relative need, in that values which fall outside the CI are "abnormal" relative to the population. Naturally, the reverse of this can also be true in terms of a value falling within the CI as being a cause for concern.

Tests of Significance

A test of significance is done to assess whether the probability is high or low that the statistical result can be accepted as being true. The test of significance is the same across the types of statistics used and the interpretation of significance is the same. The first step is to set the alpha level, which is the probability of rejecting a null hypothesis, when in fact it is true. Commonly, the alpha is set at 5% and the null hypothesis is stated as there will be no difference between groups. Using a table of critical values for the type of statistical test used, one can then determine whether the statistical result was above or below the cutoff for the alpha.

In analyzing community health assessment data, a critical issue for program planners might be to determine whether the difference between two communities or two groups is just a random variation or whether the difference is sufficiently large to suggest something else is contributing to their difference. If the two groups are compared, the p-value gives the probability of falsely claiming that the groups are different. For example, if a test of significance is reported as $p < .05$ for a comparison of two groups, then there is less than a 5% chance that the two groups were actually the same.

Synthetic Estimates

In reviewing available data, program planners may find that data for a specific group or location are lacking, yet it may be important to have some estimate of the magnitude of a health problem for that group. *Synthetic estimation* is a technique that converts rates or means of a known group into frequencies (counts), which can then be used to calculate an approximate number (count) for the other group (Dever, 1980).

As an example, suppose the percentages of whites and blacks with diabetes are known for a state as a whole, but not for the neighborhood included in the community assessment. To estimate the number of whites with diabetes in the neighborhood, planners would multiply the percentage of whites statewide with diabetes by the number of whites in the neighborhood. Next, they would multiply the percentage of blacks in the state with diabetes by the number of blacks in the neighborhood. These two synthetic estimates yield the approximate number of blacks and whites in the local neighborhood with diabetes. The same calculation steps would then be repeated for each health problem and each group of individuals for whom synthetic estimates are needed.

Synthetic estimates have been shown to be useful at a state level (Dietz, Adams, Spitz, Morris, & Johnson, 1998), but they do have some notable deficiencies. First, there is no way to know how accurate these estimates are. Second, they do not take into account local environmental or social factors that can affect the health problem or condition. Third, synthetic estimates based on a total population are affected by differences within the population characteristics, such as age and race. Nonetheless, in some instances a synthetic estimate hints at whether a health problem or condition might warrant further assessment, as well as the relative needs of the groups.

Geographic Information Systems: Mapping

Historically, an element of the epidemiological assessment model has been the geographic mapping of health problems or population characteristics. With the advent of mapping software, the usual map-based display of the distribution of health problems or conditions can be done at any level, such as by state, county, parish, census tract, ZIP code, or street address. Mapping at very specific levels of geography provides an extremely refined picture of what is where. The same geographic mapping technology can accommodate social data and asset data, thereby enabling a more rapid and potentially more interesting analysis of the intersection of needs or problems and resources. One example of using the visual representation of assets in conjunction with a health problem is the development of a map with hospitals overlaid on rates of chronic health conditions. Such a map would reveal that the highest rates of chronic health conditions are found in geographic areas with the lowest density of hospitals.

Mapping health problems and suspected factors in the causal path provides very engaging information and can be crucial in reaching a consensus or attracting the attention of key stakeholders. Mapping, however, does not provide "hard" information, as in statistical evidence of association, importance, or need. It does lend itself to creative thinking that can lead to additional searches for those "hard" data.

Small Numbers and Small Areas

Small numbers are a big problem, whether one is looking at epidemiological data or social data. In particular, those conducting the community assessment and health planners for rural areas face the issue of how to portray rates. The problem is a simple one: If a geographic area has a small population (denominator), then a small variation in the occurrence of a health problem (numerator) will inevitably lead to a large change in the rate or proportion of that health problem. This instability of the rate affects the conclusions that can logically be drawn from the data. The same statistical problem also occurs when the analysis focuses on a small geographic area, such as a parish, county, or legislative district.

Small numbers can also be a problem if the data collected are of a social or qualitative nature, as might be the case in an asset assessment. If the number of respondents to a community survey or the number of participants in a community focus group is small, then the information those individuals provide has a higher likelihood of not being representative of the range of views and opinions in the community. Once data are collected, those conducting the assessment rarely have an opportunity to go back and gather more data. Given this caveat, careful planning and execution of the data collection must be done to avoid having too few respondents.

Several statistical techniques exist for addressing the small numbers problem, utilizing counts, rates, or proportions (Dever, 1997) or pooling years of data (Cawley, Schroeder, & Simon, 2006). Additional techniques continue to be developed as well (Yu, Meng, Mendez-Luck, Jhawr, & Wallace, 2007). One set of techniques focuses on comparing the small area (population) with a larger area (population) or a standard. Another set of techniques is based on comparing two small areas. Yet another approach is to use data from multiple time periods, which may cumulatively produce a sufficient sample size to make comparisons either across time periods or with another small area using a similar time period.

One study of immunization rates (Jia et al., 2006) is illustrative of the challenge inherent in dealing with small numbers. Jia and colleagues color coded county data to reflect whether the county was more than two standard deviations above or below the state mean, between one and two standard deviations above or below the state mean, or less than one standard deviation above or below the state mean. Their choice of displays on a map of the United States demonstrates the creativity that may be needed to deal with small numbers and small area data.

STATING THE HEALTH PROBLEM

Data collected for the community health assessment can be organized in a variety of ways, such as a community profile, a wellness profile, a behavioral profile, a service profile (Paronen & Oje, 1998), or a community diagnosis (Muecke, 1984). Regardless of which format is chosen, the community health assessment ought to lead to some statement of what was found, phrased in such a way that stakeholders, constituents, community members, and multidisciplinary health professionals can understand the health problem.

There is no one right way to portray the health problem or to make a health problem statement, as is evident in *The Guide to Community Preventive Services: What Works to Promote Health?* (Zaza, Briss, & Harris, 2005). The *Guide* has chapters on nine health problems. Each of those chapters has a conceptual framework or model of the health problem, but each model looks different. The one consistency across the diagrams is the attention to the explanation of what causes the problem in a way that facilitates choosing an effective intervention.

Diagramming the Health Problem

In health program planning, the understanding of what causes a health problem and how those causes lead to the problem is portrayed in a diagram or conceptual model that organizes key factors along a general sequential time line. Each health problem will have its own unique set of precursors given the specific context. The model of the health problem is distinct from a logic model, which is discussed in full detail in Chapter 8. The key distinction is that a logic model focuses on organizing the delivery of the program, whereas the model of the health problem focuses on understanding what causes the health problem. Attention to the causes and consequences of the health problem is critical if program planners are to select the best point of intervention and the appropriate intervention for that point. In this way, the model of the health problem contributes not only to the development of a logic model, but also to tailoring the programmatic intervention and to designing the evaluation of the program's effect.

Elements of a Causal Theory

The model of the health problem brings together, in a visual display, the key factors that were identified from the community health assessment as being important to the health problem. The combination of these factors is intended to explain or hypothesize about what causes the health problem. For this reason, it is called a causal theory. For some health problems, an existing causal theory may be applicable to the current circumstances. If not, a new causal theory will need to be created. The decision of what to include in the causal theory and what to intentionally exclude from the model has ramifications through the program planning and evaluation cycle: It guides the intervention choice, establishes the parameters for the evaluation of the program effect, and influences the statistical analyses of the evaluation data.

Throughout this textbook, the same approach to displaying a causal theory (shown in Figure 5.1) is used for the sake of illustration. Each program, reflecting the unique perspective of its set of stakeholders, is likely to develop its own approach to visually displaying a causative theory. The template presented in this chapter has been carefully crafted to include four key elements to be considered in developing any causal theory: existing factors, causes, mediating factors, and moderating factors. Factors, conditions, variables, and elements that may exist but are not immediately relevant to the health problem or that are so complex that they are not contenders for programmatic intervention are not included in the causal theory. In other words, the process of developing the causal theory also is a process of narrowing in on the

Figure 5.1   Generic Model of a Causal Theory

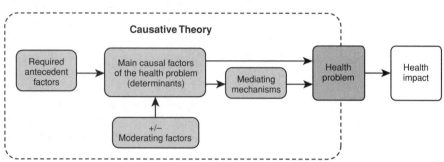

problem and of prioritizing. As with all processes, the creation of the causal theory is an iterative, evolving, and ongoing process that cannot be completed in a single short session.

Precursors can be thought of as existing physical or contextual factors, as well as the causes of the health condition. *Required antecedent factors* are those elements that must be present for the health problem to come into existence or are direct precursors of it. For example, required factors may include genetic predisposition, being in the right place at the right time, prior exposure and vulnerability, or legal or policy conditions. From an asset perspective, required factors might also include variables such as the political clout of the local representatives or the existence of economic empowerment zones. The predisposing factors of health services utilization models (Anderson, 1995; Anderson & Aday, 1978; Green & Kreuter, 1991) generally fall into the required antecedent factors category.

Causal factors are those elements that influence whether the health problem will manifest itself, given the presence of the required antecedents. Depending on the health problem, causal factors might be exposure to the health hazard, susceptibility, or the virulence of the hazard. From an asset perspective, causal factors might include health knowledge, the existence of healthy food choices in local grocery stores, the existence of environmental pollutants, the existence of road safety features (intersection lights), or the accessibility and availability of local health and social service agencies. These causal factors could also be called the determinants of the problem, given that they are directly responsible for outcomes. In recent years, however, the term "determinants" has been more widely applied to encompass a host of social and ecological factors that lead to health problems. To avoid confusion and to be more specific, the term "causal factors" is used throughout this textbook to refer specifically to the factors identified from the community assessment as leading directly to the health problem.

Causal factors include, for example, the water that determines whether a seed will sprout; the hole in a boat that determines whether the boat will sink; and the presence of potassium in the blood that determines whether the heart muscles will contract. Nevertheless, as these concrete examples suggest, the situation involves both required antecedent factors and factors that lead one to say "yes, but. . . ." Those "yes, but" factors can be sorted into two types: moderating factors and mediating factors.

Moderating factors are those elements that have the potential to either exaggerate or lessen the presence of the health problem. Again, depending on the health problem, these factors might consist of laws and policies or social support. Such factors generally act to affect the causal factors. Complex and interacting relationships exist among required antecedents, causal factors, and moderating factors. In a model of the causal theory, moderating factors are shown as possibly influencing the identified causal factors. By their nature, moderating factors can either increase, potentiate, exaggerate, and stimulate or, alternatively, lessen, diminish, and suppress the presence or strength of the causal factors. Factors that would be classified as enabling and reinforcing factors (Anderson, 1995; Anderson & Aday, 1978; Green & Kreuter, 1991) must be reevaluated for their role in the causal theory, as many are likely to function as moderating factors.

Mediating factors come between causes and outcomes. In fact, without the mediating factor, the causes will not result in the health outcome. In other words, without this process or mechanism, the causal factors cannot cause the health outcome. Depending on the health problem, there may not be any mediating factors. For example, if an individual has the genetic mutation that causes cystic fibrosis, the disease will appear—there is no mediating variable. However, if the health outcome is defined as longevity for persons with cystic fibrosis, mediating factors would include quality of health care and individual response to treatments. In contrast, if someone has a stroke, both morbidity and mortality depend on the response time and quality of the emergency medical care, which are mediating factors.

Examples

Table 5.4 shows how data collected during the community assessment can be presented in a tabular format. It contains examples of information for the five health problems identified in the community assessment of the imaginary Layetteville. Possible required antecedent factors, causal factors, moderating factors, and mediating factors that lead to five different health problems are given. The information that is included in a table such as Table 5.4 and in a causal theory diagram is based on the data collected during the community health assessment, including the scientific literature related to the health

Table 5.4   Existing Factors, Moderating Factors, Key Causal Factors, Mediating Factors, and Health Outcome and Impact for Five Health Problems in Layetteville and Bowe County

Required Antecedent Factors or Conditions	Moderating Factors or Conditions	Key Causal Factors	Mediating Factors	Health Outcome	Health Impact
Age, existing health conditions, pathogens in environment	Knowledge about adult immunizations, media attention, quality of medical care	Motivation to be vaccinated, fear of the communicable disease, perceived susceptibility	Vaccine supply and distribution, vaccine cost	Vaccination	Preventable hospitalizations
Age, food availability, type of employment genetics	Knowledge about folic acid, taking prenatal vitamins, genetic counseling	Inadequate intake of folic acid, quality of prenatal care, genetic counseling	Preconception nutritional status, biological processes	Presence of neural tube defect	Rate of congenital anomalies
Psychological development, physical developmental stage	Media messages, knowledge, family support, availability of birth control	Sexual activity, sexual self-efficacy, partner and peer pressure	Use of birth control methods	Diagnosis of pregnancy	Child abuse rate
Developmental stage, local history of violence, local lack of jobs, state gun laws	Parental supervision, school antiviolence program, community action	Lack of conflict resolution skills, school dropout rate, local gang activity, gun availability	Individual resilience, inadequate policing, quality of emergency care	Death from gunshot wounds	Adolescent death rate due to gunshot wounds
Genetic predisposition, age, race, safe place to exercise	Knowledge about diabetes prevention, family support for self-care	Specific health behaviors (e.g., exercise), quality of medical supervision	Physiological processes	Diagnosis of type 2 diabetes	Morbidity due to chronic illness

problem. These hypothetical details of the five health problems are used to demonstrate how a causal theory diagram might look using the data from the table. These five health problems are carried throughout the textbook at the subsequent stages of the planning and evaluation cycle.

One example is the health problem of adult immunizations. Not surprisingly, we want the rate of adult immunizations to increase. The rate of immunizations is based on individuals actually receiving the vaccine. What causes an adult older than age 55 to seek immunization is motivation. However, even a motivated individual cannot be vaccinated if no vaccine is available or if the cost is too high. The level of motivation varies depending on the person's knowledge about adult immunizations, the amount of media attention given to the importance of adult immunizations, and the quality of medical care in terms of having a provider who recommends getting immunized. Fortunately, Allsup, Gosney, Haycox, and Regan (2003) found that quality of life for those aged 65–74 is not affected by immunization. Ultimately, the need for adult immunization and the degree of motivation is based on the person's age, current health condition, and the presence of the pathogens in the environment.

The factors listed in Table 5.4 related to deaths from adult immunization rates, adolescent death rates, and rates of congenital anomalies are shown as causal theory diagrams in Figures 5.2, 5.3, and 5.4, respectively. These examples use hypothetical data, but findings from the literature were used to substantiate those data: Hwang and Jaakkola (2003) found an association between exposure to chlorination and birth defects; and Calhoun, Dodge, Journel, and Zahnd (2005) used police records and gun sales records as part of their assessment. The important consideration here is to gain confidence in pulling the diverse community assessment data together in a coherent, systematic, and scientifically defensible manner.

Writing a Causal Theory of the Health Problem

Community diagnosis, a diagnosis-type formula, was suggested by Muecke (1984) as one technique for synthesizing needs assessment data into a statement that can be understood by various health disciplines. Since then, the term *community diagnosis* has been used to encompass the data collection as well as the planning and is the basis for graduate courses (Quinn, 1999) and for preparedness (Matsuda & Okada, 2006; Okada et al., 2006). Given that these definitions might more aptly describe the community health assessment process, the focus here is on developing a coherent statement that is the equivalent of the diagram of the causal theory of the health problem. The value in writing the causal theory statement is that it complements and extends the value of the diagram as a reference point for planning the intervention, writing objectives, and planning the evaluation. It also serves as a reference point if the

Figure 5.2   Diagram of Causal Theory of Receiving Immunizations, as Contributing to Adult Immunization Rates, Using the Layetteville Example

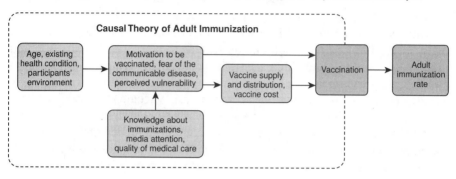

Figure 5.3   Diagram of Causal Theory for Deaths from Gunshot Wounds, as Contributing to Adolescent Death Rates, Using the Layetteville Example

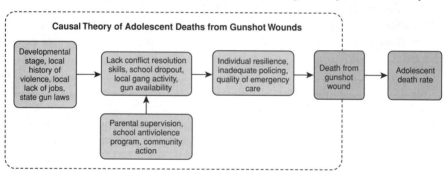

Figure 5.4   Diagram of Causal Theory of Neural Tube Defects, as Contributing to Rates of Congenital Anomalies, Using the Bowe County Example

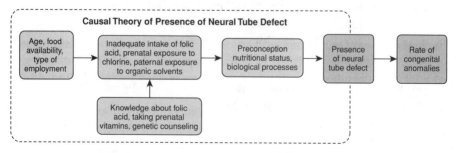

planning and evaluation process begins to drift away from the original health problem and factors identified in the community health assessment.

The causal theory statement adds two elements to the causal theory diagram. The full statement includes both the "who" in reference to the health problem and the relevant health indicators. The elements of the causative theory are used to develop the causal theory statement. The basic format is as follows:

Basic Template

Risk of [*health problem*] among [*population/community*] is indicated by [*health outcome indicators*] and results from [*causative factors*].

Note that the population or community is the "who" of the community health assessment.

Using the example gun violence as described in the Layetteville community health assessment, the basic causal theory would read as follows:

Example

Risk of [*death from gunshot wounds*] among [*adolescents of Layetteville*] is indicated in the [*high rate of admissions for gunshot injuries at the local hospitals and police reports*] and results from [*lack of conflict resolution skills, being a school dropout, local gang activity, and gun availability*].

The basic template can be modified to incorporate findings about existing factors and mediating factors. The resulting template has more of a public health tone. However, the template does not yet include a way to incorporate assets or strengths of individuals, families, or the community. If we consider that assets and resources have the potential to modify the causative factors' ability to result in the health problem, then including assets identified through the community needs assessment statement is key. Thus the final full causal theory statement template is as follows:

Causal Theory Statement Template

[*Health problem*] among [*population/community*], indicated in [*health outcome indicators*], is caused by [*causative factors*], but is mediated by [*mediating factors*] given that [*moderating factors*] moderate the causes and that [*required antecedent factors*] exist prior to the causes.

Continuing with the Layetteville community example, the community diagnosis template statement would read:

Causal Theory Statement A

Risk of [*death from gunshot wounds*] among [*adolescents of Layetteville*], indicated in the [*high rate of admissions for gunshot injuries at the local hospitals and police reports*], is caused by [*lack of conflict resolution skills, being a school dropout, local gang activity, and gun availability*] but is mediated by [*individual resilience, adequacy of policing, and quality of emergency medical care*], given that [*community action, parental supervision, and school antiviolence programs*] moderate the causes and that [*adolescent developmental stage, local history of violence, lack of job opportunities, and state laws*] exist prior to the causes.

The community health assessment is likely to identify or uncover numerous health problems or conditions that potentially need to be addressed. For each health problem, a community health statement can be developed. The factor identified through the community assessment can be used to develop the community needs statement. For example, a community health statement can be written for the birth defects health problem:

Causal Theory Statement B

Risk of [*birth defects*] among [*residents of Bowe County*], indicated by the [*rate of neural tube defects and congenital anomalies*], is caused by [*low folic acid intake, parental exposure to organic solvents, and prenatal exposure to chlorine*], but is mediated by [*preconception nutritional status and biological processes*], given that [*genetic counseling, use of prenatal vitamins, knowledge about folic acid, and cultural practices*] moderate the causes and that [*the mother's age, type of employment, and availability of food high in folic acid*] exist prior to the causes.

A causal theory statement ought to convey information about the health problem in such a way that it stands as a well-articulated base from which to engage in the prioritization and subsequent program designing processes. The statements can be used in priority setting, as will be seen in the next section of this chapter. Statements about health problems can be compared with regard to the extent to which the required antecedents, causal factors, and moderating and mediating factors are amenable to change, as well as the level of seriousness or importance of the health problem. Although a health problem initially might be considered a high priority, data from the community health assessment might, in fact, potentially lead to a reprioritization of the problem. In short, prioritization and assessment are often iterative processes, rather than a straightforward linear process. The nature of these processes hints at the extent to which community assessors and health planners need to be flexible and act as guides throughout the planning–assessment process.

In summary, the elements contained in the causal theory statement are related to both program design and program evaluation as shown in Table 5.5. The causal theory diagram and the corresponding causal theory statement become the basis for developing the program theory with the corresponding logic model, as discussed in Chapter 6. One point is critical to understand at this juncture: The program interventions that will be developed can be targeted at either reducing *or* enhancing key factors.

Table 5.5   Relationship of Problem Definition to Program Design and Evaluation

Diagnosis	Problem →	Program →	Evaluation
Risk of:	Health problem or condition	Program goal	Outcome variables
Among:	At-risk population or group, target audience	Recipients	Intervention group
As demonstrated in:	Health indicators	Program objectives	Outcome and impact variables
Resulting from causal factors:	Specific processes, conditions, and factors	Interventions or treatments for the target population	Outcome evaluation
But is mediated by:	Factors that must be present for the health problem to occur	Possible intervention	Possible control variables
Given moderation of the causes by:	Factors that increase or decrease the potency of the causative factors	Possible intervention	Possible control variables
And required existing factors of:	Socio-demographic characteristics and social ecological factors	Program eligibility criteria	Control variables or comparison groups

PRIORITIZING HEALTH PROBLEMS

The final problems to be addressed by a program are those selected from among the many health concerns identified through the needs assessment. A highly rational approach to prioritization is presented here, because the decision process generally begins as a rational approach. As discussed in Chapter 3, individuals with inclinations toward other planning approaches may alter this process accordingly. Nonetheless, health professionals involved in a community health assessment need to have the skills to guide the decision process in a way that does not ignore the data and that results in a plan with the highest overall potential to improve the health status of the community and target community.

Nominal Group Technique

The nominal group technique is not strictly a health planning or prioritizing method, but rather is more typically used in small-group processes and in research. Because it is widely used and can easily be applied to stakeholders who have little experience, it is included in this section as a prioritization approach. The nominal group technique has been used for a wide variety of prioritization needs, ranging from workforce competencies (Davis, Turner, Hicks, & Tipson, 2008), to environmental changes for physical activity (Lee, Altschuld, & White, 2007; Lees et al., 2007), to relative ranking of health interventions under resource constraints (Makundi, Kapiriri, & Norheim, 2007).

This technique involves a round-robin series of voting and narrowing lists based on the results of the voting. In essence, the process begins with the complete, usually long list of health problems identified from the community health assessment. Each member of the planning group is given three votes to be used to select which problems to address. The problems with the most votes are kept, and the problems with the fewest votes are eliminated. Next, the voting is repeated with each member of the planning group having only one vote. The health problem with the most votes becomes the problem to be addressed. The results may or may not be logical, but they often stimulate dialogue and discussion about why the highest priority problem emerged.

For the nominal group process to be successful in selecting and prioritizing health problems, participants must agree before voting that the results will be honored and used as the basis for moving forward in the program planning. It is also important to give the group adequate background information so that they can make informed decisions when they cast their votes.

Basic Priority Rating System

A more systematic approach was developed by Hanlon (1973), whose model now has a history of being used or adapted in efforts to formulate a community health plan (New York Department of Health, 2006; Sogoric et al., 2005). An overview of this process provides some initial insight into the depth and breadth of the data that are needed for making decisions about program directions.

Hanlon's approach to planning public health programs has been codified into a deceptively simple formula known as the basic priority rating system (BPRS). This method entails prioritizing health problems based on the magnitude of the problem, the severity or importance of the health problem, and the potential effectiveness of interventions. A key part of the process involves assigning values to each of these three factors. The formula is

$$\text{Basic priority rating} = (A + 2B) \times C$$

where A is the score for the magnitude of the problem, B is the score for the seriousness of the health problem, and C is the score for the potential effectiveness of the intervention.

Unfortunately, the scores assigned to the problem magnitude, seriousness, and intervention effectiveness (Table 5.6) can be biased by the personal preferences of those involved in the planning process. By going through a group process to arrive at a score for each factor, however, members of the planning group are forced to make explicit the assumptions underlying their assignment of values. This understanding, in turn, helps establish consensus and consistency within the group.

The first factor to determine is the magnitude of the health problem (A). Magnitude is reflected in expressed need, such as the demand for and utilization of services. It is also demonstrated through normative needs—namely, what health professionals view as being a deviation from a baseline or normally acceptable level. Normative need is reflected in epidemiological measures, such as mortality and morbidity rates, incidence, prevalence, and relative risk. One difficulty with using mortality rates as the sole criterion for determining the size of a health problem is that mortality data are medical, making them less helpful in planning that focuses on behavioral or social health problems. In addition, disability, pain, and quality of life are just as important considerations as death, as we have seen with regard to QALYs and DALYs. Thus the size of a health problem and the factors leading to its manifestation ought to be viewed from various angles and incorporate a diversity of measures or indicators.

Table 5.6 Criteria for Rating Problems According to the Basic Priority Rating System

BPRS Factor	A			B		C
	Size	Urgency	Severity	Economic Consequences	Willingness or Involvement of Others	Intervention Effectiveness
Rating scale	1 (small) to 10 (endemic)	1 (not at all) to 10 (extremely urgent)	1 (low) to 10 (high)	1 (low) to 10 (high)	1 (low) to 10 (high)	1 (low) to 10 (high)
Factors to consider in the rating	Stability of incidence or prevalence over time	Rate of spread	Extent to which QALYs and DALYs are affected; virulence of health problem	Healthcare costs; extent to which YLL and YPLL are affected	Political support for addressing the problems; popular awareness of the health problem	Recalcitrance to change; entrenchment of contributing factors

Not all health problems are equally serious (*B*), where seriousness encompasses the degree of urgency for addressing the problem, the degree of severity of the health problem, the degree of economic losses possible from the health problem, and the degree to which others can be motivated to become involved. Each of these four elements of seriousness can be rated on a scale of 1 (at the lowest end) to 10 (at the highest end). Again, the specific data derived from the community assessment are used to score each element. The severity of a health problem or condition is also related to its virulence.

Seriousness is best determined by examining information from experts, the scientific literature, and input from key stakeholders on the long-term consequences of the health problem. The degree of economic loss focuses on individual loss due to disability and death, but it also might include the societal costs of providing care and the loss of revenue from disabled individuals. Utility measures that capture individuals' preferences for different states of health also play a role, implicitly or explicitly, in determining seriousness.

Intervention effectiveness (*C*) is the third element in the BPRS. Scoring the effectiveness of the interventions that might be used to address a health problem also utilizes a scale of 1 to 10. Interventions for which considerable favorable evidence exists would be rated highest, where "favorable" means having a clinically and practically significant effect on the health problem. The choice of an intervention deserves considerable attention, in terms of whether and how it has the potential to affect causal or other factors (Figure 5.5). The effective and efficient (lower-cost) interventions can be viewed as contributing to the extent to which it is possible to change the health problem. Naturally, at the point that the prioritizing process occurs, the planning group may not have complete data on intervention effectiveness. In this situation, some data gathering may be necessary, with subsequent rescoring.

Propriety, Economics, Acceptability, Resources, and Legality (PEARL) System

A more complex approach to deciding which health problems are appropriately addressed is the PEARL system. PEARL is an acronym for propriety, economics, acceptability, resources, and legality (CDC Sustainable Management Development Programs, 2005). *Propriety* refers to whether addressing the health problem is the responsibility of those represented by the planning group. The *economic* aspect relates to the economic feasibility of addressing the problem. *Acceptability* is assessed in terms of the culture's and population's preference for the potential intervention. *Resources* refers to the availability of all types of resources. Naturally, resources available for addressing a health problem is a concern that affects prioritization. The *legality* element reflects whether there are legal constraints or mandates in addressing the

Figure 5.5   Causative Theory Model with Elements of the BPRS Score: Size, Seriousness, and Interventions

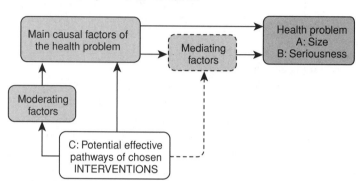

health problem. Each health problem being considered for program planning is evaluated on the five dimensions and scored as either yes (1) or no (0).

Applying the PEARL approach to prioritizing among health problems may not be possible until sufficient data about the health problem and characteristics of the community are known. In other words, it may not be possible to apply the PEARL scoring until a substantial amount of information has been collected about the sociopolitical context of the health problem. The need to revisit priorities when new information is uncovered is likely to be frustrating for everyone involved in the priority setting, but it is a reality of program planning.

Prioritizing Based on Importance and Changeability

A simpler approach to understanding the priority of a health problem is to consider only whether an intervention can actually make a change in the health problem and whether the health problem is important or worth addressing. The importance of a health problem can be assessed through the use of utility measures or through reliance on the *Healthy People 2010* objectives, which indicate whether the health condition is sufficiently important to warrant national attention. The changeability of a health problem or condition is the degree to which any intervention has the potential to alter its course.

When multiple health problems or conditions are being considered as targets for an intervention or health program, each of the health problems can be rated with regard to its degree of importance and changeability. Using these two dimensions, program planners can use the high and low changeability and high and low importance parameters to form four quadrants of a 2 × 2 matrix into which health problems can be sorted (Table 5.7). Health problems

Table 5.7   Program Prioritization Based on the Importance and Changeability of the Health Problem

	Highly Important Health Problem	**Less Important Health Problem**
Highly Changeable Health Problem, More Effective Intervention	High priority for developing a program	Low priority, unless resources are available for developing a program
Less Changeable Health Problem, Less Effective Intervention	High priority, if an innovative program can be developed	No program development is warranted

classified as having both high changeability and high importance ought to be addressed first. In contrast, health problems in the low changeable, low importance quadrant are either at the bottom of the list or off it entirely.

ACROSS THE PYRAMID

In this chapter, the community health assessment process, problem statement development, and prioritization process have been described as though they constituted a linear set of activities. This is not the reality. These activities are iterative processes that must be adapted to the local situation. Reflecting on whether the data gathered during the assessment process are representative of the levels of the public health pyramid can be helpful in identifying gaps in the assessment and prioritization.

Table 5.8 provides a few examples of how prioritization data can be sorted by level of the pyramid. Note that, across all levels of the pyramid, the determination of the effectiveness of proposed interventions ought to come from the scientific literature or existing, rigorously conducted program evaluations. Table 5.9 shows the elements of the causal theory and illustrates how health problem statements incorporate data from across the pyramid.

At the direct services level of the public health pyramid, the data for prioritization come mostly from individual patients through surveys or from provider, clinic, and hospital archival data. Accordingly, the information that is incorporated into the health problem statement tends to be personal, episodic, and specific to a small, highly homogenous target audience. At the individual level, the health problem statement resembles a very comprehensive medical diagnosis that incorporates sociocultural determinants.

Table 5.8   Examples of Sources of Data for Prioritizing Health Problems at Each Level of the Public Health Pyramid

These examples correspond to the five example health problems in Layetteville.

| | Level | | | |
	Individual and Direct Services	Community and Enabling Services	Population-Based Services	Infrastructure
Health problem	Non-immunized adult, infant with neural tube defect, diagnosis of pregnancy, diagnosis of diabetes, death from gunshot wound	Insufficient parenting support services, lack of diabetes management classes	Cultural acceptance of obesity as normal, lack of media messages about safe sex for adolescents and diabetes prevention	Availability of guns, inequities in vaccine distribution, lack of school-based clinics, insufficient inspection of workplaces for teratogens
Data sources for size (A)	Vital records data, clinic or service provider data, hospital discharge data, police records, survey	Census data, waitlists, human services sources of data	Epidemiological data, acute care and outpatient discharge data	Personnel records
Data sources for seriousness (B)	Medical literature on course of the health problem, literature on associated DALYs, YLL, and YHL	Advocacy group pressure, local media on health problem	Statistical trends, Medicaid and Medicare cost data	Regulatory requirements, lawsuits, effects on capacity requirements
Data sources for intervention effectiveness (C)	Scientific literature; professional associations' practice guidelines	Scientific literature, existing health program evaluations	Scientific literature, existing health program evaluations	Scientific literature, existing health program evaluations

Table 5.9   Examples of Required Existing, Causal Factors, and Moderating Factors Across the Pyramid

These examples correspond to the five example health problems in Layetteville.

Factors	Level			
	Individual and Direct Services	Community and Enabling Services	Population-Based Services	Infrastructure
Required existing factors	Genetic predisposition, health beliefs, attitudes, values	Local economic empowerment zones, safe places to exercise and play	Deep cultural practices and beliefs	Legal or policy conditions, organizational mission, workforce capacity
Causal factors	Lifestyle and health practices, individual physiology, quality of medical supervision, exposure to toxins	Road safety features, local gang activity	Exposure to environmental toxins	Resources allocated, capacity
Moderating factors	Lifestyle practices, family, norms, patterns of health services utilization	Culture, accessibility and availability of local health and social service agencies	Income level, educational level	Health workforce competence, needs assessment and planning, information systems
Mediating factors	Quality of emergency medical care	Police presence in community	Vaccine supply and distribution	

At the enabling services level of the pyramid, the data used for prioritization need to be applicable to the aggregate of concern. Accordingly, the assessment data are from community sources, such as local news media and groups advocating for the aggregate. Other sources of data may be gathered by unobtrusive means, such as walking through a park to determine its level of safety. A key archival source of data at the enabling level is the list of existing services, which would be informative with regard to the urgency for creating a program that does not exist. The various data collected can be sorted into the elements of the health problems, perhaps as first step toward determining which data ought to be woven into the final health problem statement.

At the population-based services level of the public health pyramid, data for the prioritization process are more typically drawn from epidemiological data sources, and trend analysis may be necessary to determine the urgency of the health problem. As for the elements of the health problem statement, the factors at the population level would apply to the entire population and, therefore, are not specific to individuals or aggregates. Additionally, the factors affecting the health problem are likely to environmental (either social or physical).

Lastly, at the infrastructure level of the pyramid, sources of data for prioritization come from the organization, relevant legal jurisdiction, and workforce records. As at the other pyramid levels, relevant characteristics of the infrastructure can be sorted into the elements of the health problem statement. Doing so serves as a nice double check on barriers and facilitators to the proposed program.

DISCUSSION QUESTIONS AND ACTIVITIES

1. Which statistical tests would be used to determine statistical significance, and which statistical tests would be used to determine the variance from a population mean? Give a brief description of their key differences.

2. Imagine that you are part of a community health assessment and planning group. Your group believes it is important to know the rate of type 2 diabetes in the three census tracts being assessed. However, the only data available are the county statistics. Describe the process by which you would create a synthetic estimate of the rate of type 2 diabetes for whites, blacks, and Hispanics in the three census tracts.

3. Using the hypothetical data in Table 5.4, create a causal theory diagram for either morbidity due to chronic illness or for child abuse rates. Which decisions did you make in developing the diagram?

4. Create priority scores for the health problems in Table 5.4, using the BPRS. If you had scored these problems as though you were the state health officer, how might the scores be different?

INTERNET RESOURCES

University of North Carolina

At UNC, students' community assessment papers are made public at this website: http://www .hsl.unc.edu/phpapers/phpapers.cfm. A perusal of the papers may help generate some ideas of what is involved and what a needs assessment can yield.

San Diego County

San Diego County has posted community need assessments that were done there over the past 10 years. These informative assessments provide insights into not only how a community's needs change, but also how the approach to the assessment changes over time. Find these documents at http://www.sdchip.org/work_teams/wt_na/chipNeedsAssessment07.html.

Statistical Tests

These two websites list freeware that is available to perform the most commonly used statistical tests. Both websites give brief descriptions and links to the downloads: http://www .healthcarefreeware.com/calc.htm and http://statpages.org/.

Community Tool Box

The Community Tool Box (http://ctb.ku.edu/tools/assesscommunity/index.jsp) provides resources and guidance on conducting community assessment with a focus on building health communities. The "Tools" section includes an entire area dedicated to community assessment.

REFERENCES

Allsup, S., Gosney, M., Haycox, A., & Regan, M. (2003). Cost–benefit evaluation of routine influenza immunization in people 65–74 years of age. *Health Technology Assessment, 7*, 1–65.

Anderson, R. (1995). Revisiting the behavioral model and access to medical care: Does it matter? *Journal of Health and Social Behavior, 36*(1), 1–10.

Anderson, R., & Aday, L. A. (1978). Access to medical care in the U.S.: Realized and potential. *Medical Care, 16*, 533–546

Baker, S. P., & Haddon, W., Jr. (1974). Reducing injuries and their results: A scientific approach. *Milbank Memorial Fund Quarterly, 52*, 377–389.

Baker, T. D., & Reinke, W. A. (1988). Epidemiologic base for health planning. In W. A Reinke (Ed.), *Health planning for effective management* (pp. 117–130). New York: Oxford University Press.

Calhoun, D., Dodge, A. C., Journel, C. S. & Zahnd, E. (2005). The supply and demand for guns to juveniles: Oakland's gun tracing project. *Journal of Urban Health, 82*, 552–559.

Cawley, J., Schroeder, M., & Simon, K. I. (2006). How did welfare reform affect the health insurance coverage of women and children? *Health Services Research, 41*, 486–506.

CDC Sustainable Management Development Programs. (2005). Healthy plan-*it* is. . . . Retrieved March 18, 2008, from http://www.cdc.gov/smdp/healthyplanit.htm

Davis, R., Turner, E., Hicks, D., & Tipson, M. (2008). Developing an integrated career and competency framework for diabetes nursing. *Journal of Clinical Nursing, 17*, 168–174.

Dever, G. E. (1980). *Community health assessment.* Germantown, MD: Aspen Systems.

Dever, G. E. (1997). *Improving outcomes in public health practice: Strategy and methods.* Gaithersburg, MD: Aspen Systems.

Dietz, P. M., Adams, M. M., Spitz, A. M., Morris, L., & Johnson, C. H. (1998). Live births resulting from unintended pregnancies: An evaluation of synthetic state-based estimates. *Maternal and Child Health Journal, 2*, 189–194.

Dijkers, M. (1999). Measuring quality of life: Methodological issues. *American Journal of Physical Medicine and Rehabilitation, 78*, 286–300.

Fos, P. J., & Fine, D. J. (2000). *Designing health care for populations: Applied epidemiology in health care administration.* San Francisco: Jossey-Bass.

Green, L., & Kreuter, M. (1991). *Health promotion planning* (2nd ed.). Mountain View, CA: Mayfield.

Haddon, W., Jr. (1972). A logical framework for categorizing highway safety phenomena and activity. *Journal of Trauma, 12*, 193–207. Cited in Grossman, D. C. (2000). The history of injury control and the epidemiology of child and adolescent injuries. *Future of Children, 10*(1), 23–52.

Handler, A., Rosenberg, D., Kennelly, J., & Monahan, C. (1998). *Analytic methods in maternal and child health.* Vienna, VA: National Maternal and Child Health Clearinghouse.

Hanlon, J. J. (1973). Is there a future for local health departments? *Health Services Report, 88*, 898–901.

Hwang, B. F., & Jaakkola, J. J. (2003). Water chlorination and birth defects: A systematic review and meta-analysis. *Archives of Environmental Health, 58*, 83–91.

Jia, H., Link, M., Holt, J., Mokdad, A. H., Li, L., & Levy, P. S. (2006). Monitoring county-level vaccination coverage during the 2004–2005 influenza season. *American Journal of Preventive Medicine, 31*, 275–280.

Kaplan, R. M. (1996). Utility assessment for estimating quality-adjusted life years. In F. A. Sloan (Ed.), *Valuing health care: Costs, benefits, and effectiveness of pharmaceuticals and other medical technologies* (pp. 32–60). Cambridge, UK: Cambridge University Press.

Lee, Y. F., Altschuld, J. W., & White, J. L. (2007). Problems in needs assessment data: Discrepancy analysis. *Evaluation and Program Planning, 30*, 258–266.

Lees, E., Taylor, W. C., Hepworth, J. T., Feliz, K., Cassells, A., & Tobin, J. N. (2007). Environmental changes to increase physical activity: Perceptions of older urban ethnic minority women. *Journal of Aging and Physical Activity, 15*, 425–438.

Lopez, A. D., Mathers, C. D., Ezzati, M., Jamison, D. T., & Murray, C. J. L. (2006). Global and regional burden of disease and risk factors, 2001: Systematic analysis of population health data. *Lancet, 367*, 1747–1757.

Makundi, E., Kapiriri, L., & Norheim, O. F. (2007). Combining evidence and values in priority setting: Testing the balance sheet method in a low-income country. *BMC Health Services Research, 7*, 152.

Matsuda, Y., & Okada, N. (2006). Community diagnosis for sustainable disaster preparedness. *Journal of Natural Disaster Science, 28*, 25–33.

Mausner, J. S., & Baum, A. K. (1974). *Epidemiology: An introductory text.* Philadelphia: W. B. Saunders.

McKenna, M. T., Michaud, C. M., Murray, C. J. L., & Marks, J. S. (2005). Assessing the burden of disease in the United States using disability-adjusted life years. *American Journal of Preventive Medicine, 28,* 414–423.

Muecke, M. (1984). Community health diagnosis in nursing. *Public Health Nursing, 1,* 23–35.

New York Department of Health. (2006). Building on community health assessment: Workshop agenda. Retrieved December 7, 2007, from http://www.health.state.ny.us/statistics/chac/agenda2_bcha.htm

Okada, N., Yokomatsu, M., Suzuki, Y., Hagihara, Y., Tatano, H., & Michinori, H. (2006). Urban diagnosis as methodology of integrated disaster risk management. *Annals of Disease Prevention Research, 49,* 1–7. Retrieved August 28, 2008, from http://www.dpri.kyoto-u.ac.jp/dat/nenpo/no49/49c0/a49c0p01.pdf

Paronen, O., & Oje, P. (1998). How to understand a community: Community assessment for the promotion of health-related physical activity. *Patient Education and Counseling, 33*(suppl), S25–S28.

Quinn, S. T. (1999). Teaching community diagnosis: Integrating community experience with meeting graduate standards for health education. *Health Education Research, 14,* 685–696.

Radloff, L. S. (1977). The CES-D scale: A self-report depression scale for research in the general population. *Applied Psychological Measurement, 1,* 385–400.

Sogoric, S., Rukavina, T. V., Brborovic, O., Vlahugic, A., Zganec, N., & Oreskovic, S. (2005). Counties selecting public health priorities: A "bottom up" approach (Croatian experience). *Collegium Antropologicum, 29,* 111–119.

Ware, J. E. (2000). SF-36 health survey update. *Spine, 25,* 3130–3139.

Ware, J. E., Kosninski, M., Bayliss, M. S., McHorney, C. A., Rogers, W. H., & Raczek, A. (1995). Comparison of methods for scoring and statistical analysis of the SF-36 health profile and summary measures: Summary of results from the Medical Outcomes Study. *Medical Care, 33s,* AS264–AS279.

Webb, E. J., Campbell, D. T., Schwartz, R. D., & Sechrest, L. (2000). *Unobtrusive methods* (rev. ed.). Thousand Oaks, CA: Sage Publications.

Webb, E. J., Campbell, D. T., Schwartz, R. D., Sechrest, L., & Grove, J. B. (1981). *Non-reactive measures in the social sciences* (2nd ed.). Boston: Houghton Mifflin.

Yu, H., Meng, Y., Mendez-Luck, C. A., Jhawr, M., & Wallace, S. P. (2007). Small-area estimation of health insurance coverage for California legislative districts. *American Journal of Public Health, 97,* 731–737.

Zaza, S., Briss, P. A., & Harris, K. W. (Eds.). (2005). *The guide to community preventive services: What works to promote health?* Oxford, UK: Oxford University Press.

Section 3

Health Program Development

CHAPTER 6

Program Theory and Interventions Revealed

After developing statements about health problems that have been ranked as a high priority, the next steps in health program planning involve a more intellectual and creative effort to articulate an explanation of what caused the problem. This is a critical step toward identifying which intervention or group of interventions will be most effective in addressing the health problem. Wild guesses, past experience, and personal preferences might be used as the basis for decision making, but a more rational approach is to identify existing scientific knowledge and theories that can be used to develop a program theory.

A *theory* is a description of how something works. It is a set of statements or hypotheses about what will happen and, therefore, contains statements about the relationships among the variables. We use working theories in everyday life, usually in the form of working hypotheses, such as "If I ask the children to clean their rooms, they are not likely to do it." We also use theories based in science. For example, based on theories of thermodynamics and heat conduction, we can predict how long the turkey needs to roast.

With regard to planning a health program, a primary consideration is to specify what is to be explained or predicted with a theory. The health problem is what needs to be explained, from a programmatic perspective. To explain how to change or affect the health problem, a theory must contain relevant variables, or factors, and must indicate the direction of the interactions among those variables related to the health problem. Identifying the relevant antecedent, contributing, and determinant factors of the health problem gives planners the foundation for developing a working theory of how the programmatic interventions will lead to the desired health outcome. A difficult part of this task is to identify where a health programmatic intervention can have an effect on those factors. As more details and more factors are included in the explanation of the health problem and beliefs about how the programmatic interventions will work, the theory becomes increasingly more complex.

The theory development phase of program planning requires thinking rather than doing, so it often receives less attention than is needed to fully develop an effective health program. However, using a systematic approach to develop a program theory and to engage stakeholders in the development of the theory has big and long-term payoffs that outweigh any delay or costs associated with developing the theory.

PROGRAM THEORY

A sound basis for developing the health program and for guiding the program evaluation is the use of a program theory. Rossi, Freeman, and Lipsey (1999) acknowledged that the need for a program theory has long been recognized by evaluators in the social sciences. Only recently, however, has a program theory been advocated for as useful in public health program development (Potvin, Gendron, Bilodeau, & Chabot, 2005). *Program theory* is a conceptual plan, with some details about what the program is and how it is expected to work. The comprehensive overview of how the program is to work has various names; other names include logic model, causal model, outcome line, program model, and action theory. These names all refer to a conceptional plan of how the program will work. Whether one is developing a new health program or designing an evaluation for an existing health program, understanding and articulating the program theory is essential.

There are two main components of program theory, as shown in the top half of Figure 6.1. The theory about resources and actions is called the *process theory*, and the theory about interventions and outcomes is called the *effect theory*. The concept of program theory is used throughout this textbook rather than the more widely used term "logic model," as discussed in Chapter 8. The key difference is that a full program theory, as compared to a logic model, contains a far more explicit explanation of the relationship of the factors related to the health problem with the interventions. These relationships are the effect theory. Similarly, the process theory offers a more explicit and detailed description of the resources used than is normally found in a logic model. The major similarity is that both a logic model and the program theory provide road maps to creating a successful program. The development of a program theory and its components leads to a stronger program and a more convincing argument for the program's existence.

Process Theory

The process theory includes three components: the organizational plan, the service utilization plan, and specifications of their outputs (Rossi et al., 1999).

Figure 6.1   Model of Program Theory

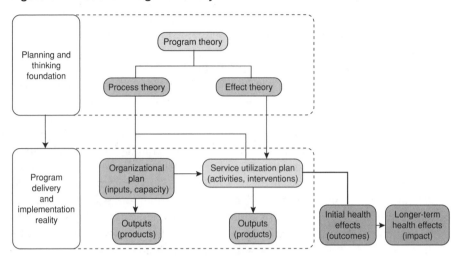

Source: Adapted from Rossi, Freeman, and Lipsey, 1999.

Process theory can be integrated with the current public health language of inputs, which are part of the organizational plan; activities, which are part of the service utilization plan; and outputs, which are by-products of the organizational and service utilization plans.

The *organizational plan*, according to Rossi et al. (1999), encompasses the nature of the resources needed to implement and sustain the program. As such, it includes specifications about personnel, the organization of resources to be used in the program, and elements of capacity, such as infrastructure, information technology, fiscal resources, and personnel. It covers all the "behind the scenes" work needed to provide a program. The organizational plan implicitly contains "if–then" statements. For example, if program staff are adequately supported with regard to supplies and managerial support, then program staff will deliver the interventions as planned. These "if–then" statements are useful not only for checking the logic behind requesting specific resources, but also for guiding the portion of the evaluation plan that focuses on the processes behind the delivery of the health program.

The *service utilization plan*, according to Rossi et al. (1999), specifies how to reach the target audience and deliver the programmatic interventions and services to that audience. It constitutes the nuts and bolts of providing the program and of implementing the program plan. The service utilization plan includes specifics about social marketing of the program, accessibility and availability of the program, screening procedures, and other logistics of providing the program. Development of the service plan ought to reflect cultural sensitivity and appropriateness of the services and intervention given the target audience.

Within the context of planning a program, the organizational plan needs to be in place before the program can begin. Both the organizational plan and the service utilization plan need to be developed using the results of the organizational and community health assessments, particularly with regard to incorporating existing resources into the plans and addressing structural issues that can affect the delivery of the program. The organizational plan is influenced by the service utilization plan to the extent that the planned intervention must be adequately supported by the resources outlined in the organizational plan. As a consequence, the development of the organizational and service utilization plans is an iterative process, with considerable back-and-forth adjustments as each element is more fully explicated. Likewise, the service utilization plan evolves as the effect theory is revised, which then leads to adjustments in the organizational plan. Thus the process theory elements are continually adjusted throughout this phase of planning for the program. Although the time it takes to make adjustments and revisions may be frustrating, it is much easier to make the adjustments at this stage of planning than it is to do so after the program has begun.

Effect Theory

The *effect theory* consists of the explanations of how the programmatic interventions will affect the causal factors and moderating or mediating factors of the health problem and describes the relationship between the programmatic interventions and the desired immediate and long-term outcomes for program participants. Three sets of relationships, or theories, are part of the effect theory (Figure 6.2): the causal theory (introduced in Chapter 5) and the intervention and impact theories (discussed in this chapter). Depending on the health problem, it can be useful to develop each of these theories. Often these theories are implicitly stated and understood by health professionals and program staff. By explicitly expressing and discussing these theories, however, program planners can refine programmatic interventions, thereby increasing the likelihood of program success.

This set of three theories and the associated informally stated hypotheses constitute the effect theory portion of the program theory. The term "effect theory" makes it clear that this part of the program theory deals with both outcomes and impacts. Generating each of the theories that constitute the effect

Figure 6.2   The Effect Theory Showing the Causal Theory Using Community Diagnosis Elements

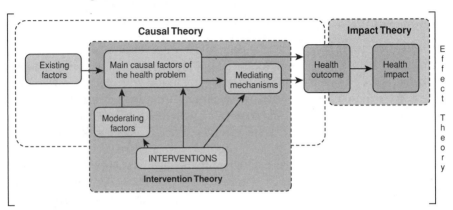

theory may seem complicated. Program experts agree on the complexity of constructing an effect theory as well as its central role in program evaluation (Patton, 1997; Rossi et al., 1999; Rossi & Freeman, 1993).

INTERVENTIONS

Interventions are those actions that are done intentionally to have a direct effect on persons with the health problem. In other words, interventions are the verbs that tell what is being done to make a change in program recipients. Using this definition allows for the inclusion of a broad range of actions, such as medical treatments, pharmacological treatments, and education, as well as psychological strategies and policy formulation. Such a broad definition also allows for the inclusion of strategies not typically considered treatments, such as providing transportation (an enabling service) or community development (an infrastructure-level intervention). Clearly identifying and labeling the interventions as such not only makes developing the intervention and outcome theories easier, but also facilitates developing outcome objectives and helps distinguish outcome and impact objectives from process objectives.

In some presentations about program planning, such as the United Way of America book (1996), interventions are couched in terms of "activities," so that they become indistinguishable from the myriad of activities done as part of the organizational or service utilization plans; the latter activities are supportive of the interventions but are not actions that will make a difference on the health problem. Interventions are the heart of all health programs. A clear understanding and statement of the role of interventions is made in the intervention theory.

Finding and Identifying Interventions

Selecting and then articulating the chosen interventions are cornerstone activities of health program planning. It is important when planning a health program to draw upon existing knowledge in multiple disciplines. A literature review, for example, can generate ideas and information with regard to existing theories that have been used to explain what leads to the health problem, as well as explanations of why some interventions have been effective and others have not.

The use of existing theories can expedite the development of the effect theory and lend it credibility. Heaney and van Ryn (1996) provided a nice example of this phenomenon. In their case, the health problem was worksite stress. These authors wanted to develop a health program to reduce worksite stress but were concerned that existing programs had been designed for a target audience of middle-class employees within the cultural majority. Recognizing this fact, Heaney and van Ryn sought to improve the effectiveness of worksite stress-reduction programs for employees of low status or of a cultural minority. Their premise was that the potential exists for different subgroups to vary in both their participation in and benefit derived from a program.

Heaney and van Ryn (1996) began by reviewing the literature on stress and coping. From this literature, they constructed a theoretical model of stress and coping and identified the major variables, along with the direction of the interaction among those variables. They also reviewed the literature on the content of worksite stress-reduction programs and the sociological literature on status, class, culture, and stress. From their literature reviews, they were able to identify program interventions that might potentially alter specific variables in the stress and coping model. This information became part of their effect theory for the worksite stress-reduction program for low-status minority workers.

Unfortunately, for many health problems, widely accepted theories are not available to guide the development of an effect theory or the selection of interventions. However, health program planners and the planning team have options for how to proceed.

Types of Interventions

A simple starting point for thinking about types of interventions is to consider the levels of prevention. In the most common typology in public health, prevention activities are classified into three levels: primary, secondary, and tertiary. *Primary prevention* includes those activities that are done to prevent a disease or illness from beginning. Getting adequate exercise, having good nutrition, being immunized, and wearing seat belts are examples of primary prevention. *Secondary prevention* involves screening for undiagnosed problems so that a disease can be treated before it manifests itself. Blood pressure screening at health fairs, fecal occult blood tests, and cholesterol tests are all secondary prevention activities. *Tertiary prevention* involves activities to limit the extent of an existing disease. For example, it includes taking blood pressure medications, receiving physical rehabilitation after an injury, and taking stress management classes for individuals with cardiac problems. The three levels of prevention provide a starting point, but are not sufficiently detailed to provide guidance in the development of programmatic interventions.

Another approach to thinking about types of interventions is to consult one of the various classification schemes of interventions that have been developed across the health disciplines. In medicine, the Current Procedural Terminology (CPT) Codes (American Medical Association, 2008) enumerate the various procedures that physicians perform. Excluding diagnostic procedures, all other procedures can be thought of interventions, in the sense that they are intended to affect the health of an individual. In nursing, the equally detailed Nursing Intervention Classification (Johnson et al., 2006) may be used to categorize interventions. Given the highly clinical nature of these intervention classifications, they would be helpful only in the development of health programs at the individual level. Nevertheless, their use with electronic medical or health records is a big advantage in subsequent program monitoring.

A more global intervention typology is needed to identify interventions across the public health pyramid levels. One such typology, as developed by Grobe and Hughes (1993), had seven categories of interventions; an eighth category was added by Issel (1997) when studying case management of pregnant women. This typology, by providing an encompassing perspective, can aid in identifying which activities are programmatic interventions.

Each of the eight types of interventions exists at the direct services, enabling services, and population levels of the public health pyramid (Table 6.1). The typology also accommodates both secondary and tertiary prevention, as these are activities of health professionals undertaken with the intent of having an effect on the health of the program participant. Primary prevention is not included in the typology, because providers cannot "do primary prevention" for or to the participant. Rather, primary prevention is a rubric for a variety of interventions: Individuals receive education about primary prevention, are encouraged to engage in primary prevention behaviors, and might be monitored for the extent to which they practice primary prevention behaviors. This is one example of how such a typology of interventions forces program planners to be

Table 6.1   Examples of Interventions by Type and Level of the Public Health Pyramid

Intervention Type	Direct Services Level	Enabling Services Level	Population Level
Treating	Medical or dental procedures, medications, physical manipulations, tertiary prevention, aromatherapy	Respite care, exercise classes or groups	Water treatment and fluoridation, mass immunizations
Assessing	Determination of needs and preferences by asking individuals, secondary prevention	Determination of needs and preferences by needs assessment	Use of epidemiological data to identify trends and rates of illnesses and conditions
Coordinating	Care coordination, client advocacy, referral, linking to services	Case coordination, local provider networks and collaborations	Systems integration, records and data sharing, disaster response planning
Monitoring	Reassessment, follow-up	Local trends and news reports	Trends analysis
Educating	Skills building, information giving	GED programs, job training programs	Media campaigns
Counseling	Psychotherapy, emotional support, marital counseling, cognitive behavioral therapy	Group counseling, family counseling, grief counseling for groups	News alerts and advice
Coaching	Role modeling, motivational interviewing, empowerment, encouragement, stress management	Community development	Policy formation
Giving tangibles	Giving vouchers for food or clothing	Medical supplies loan programs	Income supplements, insurance supplements

specific about the actions (as reflected in verbs in the written plan) that are undertaken to affect the health condition or situation of the target audience.

Specifying Intervention Administration and Dosage

Many health program interventions differ from medical interventions in that they are thought of in more general terms, such as "hand out informational flyers" or "provide emotional support." Nonetheless, health program interventions also need to be thought of in terms of dosage, route of administration, and site of administration.

Dosage refers to the amount and strength of the intervention required to have an effect, whether measured in terms of hours of education, days of respite, micrograms of fluoride, or weeks of counseling. We normally think of dosage in terms of a medication regimen or an exercise program. However, each intervention strategy that is included in a health program needs to be developed and tailored with regard to the dosage of the intervention exposure for the program participants. For example, Morone, Greco, and Weiner (2008), when providing a stress-reduction mindfulness program, described the dosage in terms of practicing the meditation three times per week, for a minimum of 50 minutes each time, over an eight-week period. Specifying the dosage is important for achieving the optimal program for the target audience; it also provides the information needed to adequately and appropriately develop the process theory. Once the dosage is specified, that information is incorporated into the service utilization plan and is used to modify the organizational plan to ensure that adequate resources have been allocated.

Dosage consists of five elements: frequency, duration, strength, route of administration, and administration credibility. The first four of these are fairly straightforward. *Frequency* is how often the intervention is received, such as hourly, daily, weekly, monthly. *Duration* specifies over what time period the intervention is delivered, such as one session, eight weeks of classes, or six months of exposure. *Strength of the intervention* refers to its powerfulness or potential for effectiveness. For example, a smoking-cessation mass-media campaign has less strength to stop a person's smoking behavior than smoking cessation counseling by that individual's primary care physician. The strength of an intervention can be determined from the literature and is reflected in a variety of statistics, such as beta weight, correlation coefficient, and difference score. *Route of administration* is the mechanism by which the intervention is delivered or the medium used to deliver the intervention, whether interpersonal communication, public mass media, educational brochures, or injection.

Administration credibility refers to the perceived degree to which the person or agency providing the health program is knowledgeable and believable.

In other words, it involves whether the intervention is provided by a health professional of a particular discipline, a lay health worker, or a paraprofessional. For some health problems, the cultural values attached to a physician may be a key factor in the effectiveness of the intervention, whereas for other health problems and programs, a community member will have more credibility. Thus, among facets of dosage, administration credibility is particularly relevant for health programs.

For many health problems, research reported in the literature or official documents can provide information on which doses are needed to be effective. For example, studies are now showing that a minimum of 30 minutes of moderately intense physical activity on most, but preferably all, days of the week is optimal for physical well-being (Myers, 2003). Stice, Shaw, and Marti (2007), in a meta-analytic review of programs to prevent eating disorders, found that larger effects existed in programs that were selective in their focus, had interactive elements rather than didactic elements, included multiple sessions, were offered only to women, and used professionals for delivering the intervention. Such findings highlight the need to be very specific in the development of not only the intervention, but also the target audience and the format elements of the service utilization plan.

Interventions and Program Components

One key challenge in selecting an intervention strategy is deciding whether a single intervention is warranted or whether a package of interventions would be more effective in addressing the health problem. A program component comprises an intervention or set of interventions, with the corresponding organizational plan. Thus, if a health program includes multiple interventions, each addressing one of several causes of the health problem or one of several moderating or mediating factors for the health problem, and these interventions are grouped in some way that makes sense for either effectiveness or efficiency reasons, then the program has multiple program components.

Using program components is appropriate if, to address the health problem, changes must occur across levels, such as at both the family and the community levels. Levels are nested within other levels, and each can be the focus of the program. It is extremely difficult to develop a single intervention that can affect all or most of the causes and moderating or mediating factors for a health problem at multiple levels. Instead, program components are typically needed. For example, if individuals as well as the community as a whole in which those individuals live are targets for the intervention, then interventions tailored to both individuals and communities will be needed. If, to address the problem of gunshot deaths, both individual behavior and actions of the gun industry are targeted, then different interventions (program components) are needed.

Another reason to include multiple program components is to address micro and macro health problems. Blum (1982) suggested that some health problems or risks require individual behavioral changes, whereas others require group behavioral change. From a public health perspective, an individual behavioral change needed to protect against a health risk is called *active protection;* in contrast, protection that does not require individuals to make a behavioral change but is instituted through policy, laws, or some other means that does not involve the individual is called *passive protection*. Passive protection often occurs at a macro level, in that it encompasses more than a small group of individuals. However, macro-level changes can also involve active protection, such as the immunization of all infants and vulnerable adults. Immunization involves individual healthcare-seeking behavior but is intended to have a population effect. In contrast, fluoridation of the water supply and reduction of factory pollutant emissions as health programs are both intended to provide passive protection of a population. The distinctions between micro and macro programs, as well as between active and passive protection, may be important in developing the interventions and the effect theory. If the health program is intended to be community based or community focused, then it will likely include components at the micro level as well as at the macro level.

Of course, it is important to consider the package of interventions that the recipients actually receive. For example, Harris (2007) used dance and movement therapy as an intervention with African adolescents who were former child soldiers and survivors of torture. The group cohesion that developed during this program was important to the success (i.e., the effectiveness) of the intervention. Similarly, Lipman et al. (2007) identified group cohesion as being critical for program outcome. These examples highlight the synergistic effects of interventions that can occur when they are provided in a group context, as well as the delivery of a psychological intervention that may or may not have been planned. Understanding such interactions and identifying the presence of implicit interventions is critical to later evaluations of what made the difference in health outcomes.

Some interventions are packaged with mnemonics to assist practitioners with remembering the set of interventions. For example, the "five A's" consist of assess, advise, agree, assist, and arrange. Fisher et al. (2005) suggested that these interventions may be helpful in programs for diabetes self-management, in addition to drawing attention to the resources and support needed for successful self-management. Alternatively, for programs targeting diabetes and other chronic illnesses, standards have been developed by national associations that specify recommended interventions. Use of national standards is encouraged, given that national standards tend to be evidence based, updated regularly, and used as the community standard of practice.

Because each program component will have a slightly different effect, acknowledging the individual components is important in subsequent evaluation plans. The intervention and outcome theories will vary slightly for each program component and for each of the different units of intervention of the program.

Criteria for Good Interventions

The final choice of an intervention or a package of interventions can be evaluated against a set of criteria for useful interventions. Having a list of criteria for good interventions is not new (Blum, 1982), but is helpful.

Evidence Based

As studies of health problems and their solutions accumulate, it becomes increasingly important to use interventions that have been shown to be effective. The increased awareness of the need to have an evidence-based practice has resulted in an increase in the number of meta-analyses and literature syntheses that provide a summary of the effectiveness of interventions for a specific health condition or problem. Some reviews provide information on which interventions are effective for a specific health problem (Waddell, Hua, Garland, Peters, & McEwan, 2007); other reviews provide information on the dosage characteristics of effective programs (Stice et al., 2007).

In choosing an intervention based on scientific evidence for its effectiveness, program planners sometimes face the question of what constitutes "evidence." The array of possibilities ranges from meta-analyses of existing studies, a single randomized clinical trial, qualitative reports, or practice guidelines. The other challenge when selecting an evidence-based intervention is dealing with equivocal findings. For example, Van der Molen, Lehtola, Lappalainem, Hoonakker, and Hsiao (2007), in a meta-analysis of interventions to prevent injuries at construction worksites, identified several intervention strategies that have been used, but found that none had been adequately studied. For this reason, they were reluctant to recommend one intervention over others. This ambiguity over the relative effectiveness of interventions is likely to be the case across many health areas.

Tailored to the Target Population

A good intervention is tailored to the characteristics of the target population. Tailoring the intervention encompasses adapting the program for cultural sensitivity, linguistic appropriateness, group similarity, cultural beliefs, and ethnic values. It can occur either through a modification of the intervention to fit the target audience or through screening the target audience for eligibility based on an important characteristic. Either approach achieves the goal of having an intervention that can be readily accepted by the program recipients.

Even widely accepted interventions may need tailoring. For example, Kelly, Baker, Brownson, and Schootman (2007) found that the standard interventions in *CDC's Guide to Community Preventive Services* (Zaza, Briss, & Harris, 2005) needed to be tailored to local conditions and preferences of specific communities. At the individual level, Kreuter and colleagues (2005) found that tailoring breast cancer prevention messages to both behavioral and cultural characteristics of African American women older than age 40 led to their being 2.6 times more likely to adhere to follow-up screening than the comparison control group. However, the difficulty in tailoring interventions—and especially public health prevention messages—can be very difficult, as Perchmann and Reibing (2006) discovered when comparing seven different antismoking messages.

Conducive to Health Gains

A third criterion is that health gains must result from the intervention. That is, the problem must be able to be changed with the available knowledge of how to change it. This criterion acknowledges that some interventions may have unintended consequences or side effects. For example, at the population level, welfare reform had the unintended effect of decreasing access to health services for vulnerable women (Cawley, Schroeder, & Simon, 2006). Other programs are simply ineffective, such as the Drug Abuse Resistance Education (DARE) program, which has been widely adopted but is ineffective (Brown, 2001; Des Jarlais et al., 2006).

This criterion also speaks to an advantage of fully articulating the effect theory. A common tendency among health professionals and program planners is to jump to a favorite solution, albeit one that may not necessarily be a good match for addressing the health problem. One technique that helps avoid this tendency is to specify the mechanisms and processes that would result in the health gains. In some scenarios, interventions could be useful and effective with regard to one type of outcome, but may not lead to the outcome or impact of interest. For example, health education about family planning methods may be effective in reducing the birth rate in a target audience but may not be effective in reducing rates of sexually transmitted diseases. Again, having done the work of developing the effect theory helps program planners be certain that the intervention will lead specifically to the desired health gains.

In addition, the program planners need to have the requisite expertise for designing the intervention and activities so that those activities will actually affect the health problem. As was discussed earlier in terms of prioritizing the health problems, the changeability of a health problem is considered to be one aspect of its importance. In terms of interventions, a more technologically feasible intervention ought to result in a more changeable health problem.

Manipulable

The fourth criterion is that the intervention must be manipulable (Rossi & Freeman, 1993). *Manipulability* refers to the ability of the program planners and program staff to adjust the intervention to the specific needs of the participants. A major element of manipulability is dosage, as discussed earlier in this chapter. If the dosage of the intervention can be tailored to the target audience, then the intervention meets the manipulability criterion. Effective and efficient interventions are customized to some extent to account for the variations among potential participants.

Related to manipulability is the ability to achieve synergy by taking into account other programmatic interventions that are already in place. For example, Guidotti, Ford, and Wheeler (2000) described a project that was specifically designed to be delivered along with existing community initiatives. By building on existing programs and interventions, the new program could mutually reinforce the effects of the other programs. Thus the intervention was manipulated to be compatible with existing interventions. The approach of intentionally developing a program intervention to maximize the effects of all programs being delivered to a community is increasingly important as communities become saturated with health promotion programs.

Another aspect of manipulability is the notion that the intervention must be designed to overcome influences on the health problem that are not directly addressed by the health program. The intervention needs to have sufficient strength to overcome those factors. In some instances, existing theories can be helpful in manipulating the intervention so that it is sufficiently strong.

An example of a theory-based nutritional intervention is the Gimme 5 intervention (Baranowski et al., 2000). Guided by social cognitive theory, the researchers designed this intervention to address interrelated environmental, personal, and behavioral factors. The use of social cognitive theory facilitated manipulating the interventions in ways that increased the likelihood that the interventions would be effective with the school-age children in the program.

Another example is provided by Brenton (1999), who argued for the use of chaos theory in planning prevention and mental health interventions. In chaos theory, critical moments are followed by transitions and then stable states that are better adapted to the existing environment. Based on this theory, Brenton argued that prevention programs could focus on the critical moments, thereby better targeting the groups at risk. Based on the concept of sensitivity to initial conditions, he suggested that programs would have the greatest impact at the beginning of life. Brenton's work is just one example of how a theory that is not typically used by health professionals can nevertheless guide thinking and foster creativity in the selection of interventions and the planning of health programs.

Technologically and Logistically Feasible

Feasibility of an intervention needs to be considered from the point of view of whether it is technologically realistic and logistically doable within the context in which the intervention will be provided. These aspects of an intervention could be determined through a pilot study in which the intervention is provided on a small scale and on a trial basis. For example, Filiatrault and colleagues (2007), before attempting to bring a falls prevention program into the community, conducted a feasibility study. Also, ensuring involvement of the stakeholders—and particularly those likely to be providing the intervention—in the planning can provide insights into the feasibility of providing the intervention within an everyday context.

Another aspect of feasibility considers the technology to be used as part of the intervention. In some settings or situations the availability or acceptability of technology is minimal, limiting the nature of interventions. For example, use of mammography for early detection of breast cancer would not be possible in undeveloped nations, but it also might not be possible in some remote and impoverished regions in the United States.

Reasonable Cost

The sixth criterion is that the cost of the intervention must be reasonable rather than prohibitive. The cost of the intervention will depend on many factors, such as the extent to which the health behavior or problem is resistant to change, the duration of the program, and the number of program components. Estimating the cost of the intervention, generally considered under the organizational plan, is discussed more fully in subsequent chapters.

Politically Feasible

The seventh criterion of a good intervention is that it be politically feasible. Not all interventions are equally acceptable to the target audience, to funding agencies, or to other stakeholders. During the assessment phase, program planners ought to have determined the preferences and willingness of various stakeholders to endorse different types of interventions. Interventions need to be culturally appropriate and sensitive as a first step toward being politically feasible. Various strategies, such as conducting focus groups and pretesting an intervention, can be used to design culturally sensitive and competent health program interventions for use with ethnically or racially distinct target populations.

A corollary to the political feasibility criterion is that meeting this criterion helps the program planner, as well as the program, to survive. Proposing interventions that are not politically feasible can result in the planner being used as a scapegoat and blamed for a "bad" intervention. Worse yet, politically sensitive programs run the risk of not being funded, which will reflect poorly on the qualifications of the program planner.

Addresses Societal Priorities

The last criterion is that the intervention must address societal priorities; in other words, the problem must be important in the larger picture. Sufficient agreement first needs to exist with regard to the importance of the health problem. This consensus should have been established during the priority-setting and assessment phases. A lack of the desired health or a high prevalence of the problem may contribute to its high priority. By contrast, many effective interventions can be used to address trivial problems of low priority.

Health program planners and evaluators might potentially play a role in raising the priority of the issue so that the health problem takes a more prominent place. To some extent, societal priority is set by celebrity spokespersons for specific health problems or by the nightly news covering the current health research. These societal pressures may conflict with the local assessment data. Nevertheless, the intervention must be aligned with the societal priorities assigned to health problems if it is to receive public credibility and backing. Also, the new behavior or health state must be important to the target audience, or else they will not make attempts to change. Although the importance of the health problem to the target audience may have been included as an element in the community needs assessment, this issue can resurface during program theory development in terms of societal versus public health priorities.

OUTCOMES AND IMPACTS IN PUBLIC HEALTH

Just as it is important to carefully consider which interventions will be used in the health program, so too must program planners carefully consider which effects are anticipated from the program. In evaluation science, authors do not seem to follow any convention regarding the use of the words "impact" and "outcome." These terms are not used consistently in the literature, in practice, or in government. Therefore, it is prudent to look beyond the words themselves and ask for definitions.

In this book, *outcome* refers to the immediate effects resulting from an intervention, whereas *impact* refers to the long-term or cumulative effects attributable in part to the programmatic interventions. The term *effect* generically refers to changes or consequences of an intervention, regardless of whether the changes are immediate, proximal outcomes or longer-term, distal impacts.

Several factors can distract program planners from having a clear vision of the relevant effect. For example, a plethora of possible outcomes from programmatic interventions may exist. There may also be many ways to think about changes resulting from programs (Patton, 1997, p. 160). Yet another distraction is that with extensive stakeholder involvement, it is quite possible to become sidetracked and end up with an extensive list of what "our program could do." For these reasons, having the community diagnosis, as written at the conclusion of the community needs assessment, is important because it helps those involved in the planning process stay focused on both the health problem and those health outcomes and impacts that are directly related to the health program.

Further complicating the choice of key health outcomes and impacts is the reality that change is not always the purpose of health programs: some programs are, in fact, intended to stabilize, prevent, or maintain a health state. Because health is multidimensional, Patton (1997) has suggested that changes can occur in multiple arenas: in life circumstances, health or economic status, behavior, functioning, attitudes, knowledge, or skills. This is true if the health problem being addressed has causal factors that are not physiologically based but relate to one of these other arenas.

Behaviors, such as primary prevention behaviors, are often the focus of health and public health programs. If the desired health outcome is a new or modified behavior, criteria must exist for selecting which behavior ought to be changed. Ideally, the behavior ought to be free from outside influences, such as peer groups or economic factors beyond the control of the program. The behavior also ought to be critical to achieving the desired health outcome. In addition, knowledge of how to develop the preferred behavior needs to exist; in other words, the behavioral intervention needs to have a scientific basis. Naturally, the new behavior must be important to the learner, in the same way that a health state ought to be important to the target audience. Experts need to agree that the new behavior is an important link to the health outcome. The pervasive lack of the behavior would be equivalent to a health problem of large magnitude and would influence the choice of the behavior as the focus of a health program.

Another challenge in developing the effect theory is to match the level of intervention with the level of the public health pyramid at which the outcomes and impacts are expected. Target audiences may consist of individuals, families, aggregates, or populations, with effects occurring at each of the levels. Program interventions need to be tailored to reach that specific target audience, essentially matching the level at which the intervention is aimed to the level at which the target audience exists and the level at which the outcome is desired. For example, if the intervention is designed to affect family eating patterns, then the health outcome sought ought to be family nutritional health, rather than reducing anemia in children or increasing the daily consumption of milk in a neighborhood. The latter two effects would be impacts. Being clear about the level or unit for the intervention is pivotal because that unit of intervention becomes the unit of analysis in the evaluation phase (Jackson, Altman, Howard-Pitney, & Farquhar, 1989).

Generate the Effect Theory

After having considered the type of intervention and the criteria for choosing an intervention, the next step is to more fully articulate the effect theory by enumerating the causal, intervention, and impact theories that constitute the effect theory. This iterative process requires going back and forth between the needs assessment, priorities, and intervention choice. Developing or generating the effect theory is guided by several strategies suggested by Patton (1997).

Both inductive and deductive approaches can be used to generate an effect theory. In other words, theory development can proceed through a deductive process that uses reason and existing knowledge, or it can occur through an inductive process that uses experience and intuition. Either approach will lead to an effect theory. In practice, a combination of both inductive and deductive approaches is typically used and yields the optimal results.

Generating an effect theory need not be a daunting task. This process includes several steps, which can be done either in sequence or iteratively. Elements of the effect theory draw upon the community diagnosis developed for each of the high-priority health problems as well as the literature. Recall the template for the community diagnosis: Risk of [*health problem*] among [*population/ community*], indicated in [*health indicators or measures*], is caused by [*causative factors*], but is mediated by [*mediating factors*] given that [*moderating factors*] moderate the causes and that [*exiting factors*] exist prior to the causes. The literature can be particularly helpful in identifying and incorporating mediating and moderating factors. For example, Marcus, Pahl, Ning, and Brook (2007), in studying smoking cessation, identified positive family relationships as an antecedent or existing factor and maladaptive personality attributes as causal factors leading to substance use. This type of research, in combination with the community assessment information, enhances the clarity and specificity of the effect theory.

Causal Theory

The first theory to be developed or understood is the *causal theory*, which is an explanation of the process that currently underlies the health problem. It includes statements or hypotheses that describe which causal factors are directly responsible for the health problem. The causal theory ought to include the factors found present through the community needs assessment and draw upon the scientific literature to justify the causal theory.

For example, we can use the community diagnosis related to deaths from gunshot wounds from Chapter 5 to develop a causal theory. The causal theory states that deaths from gunshot wounds stem from causal factors of local gang activity, lack of conflict resolution skills, being a school dropout, and gun availability. Individual resilience, adequacy of policing, and quality of emergency medical care are mediating factors that determine whether the causal factors actually result in a death. In addition, the adolescent's developmental stage, local history of violence, lack of job opportunities, and state laws, as preexisting forces, influence whether the causal factors exist. Lastly, community action, parental supervision, and school antiviolence programs all have the potential to moderate—either decreasing or increasing—the potency of the causal factors.

Similarly, the community diagnosis for birth defects is the basis for a causal theory of birth defects in Bowe County. The causal theory states that birth defects among residents of Bowe County are caused by low folic acid intake, parental exposure to organic solvents, and prenatal exposure to chlorine. However, preconception nutritional status and biological processes (mediating factors) influence whether the causal factors actually result in a birth defect. In addition, the mother's age, type of employment, and availability of food high in folic acid, as contextual preexisting factors, determine whether the causal factors exist. Lastly, genetic counseling, use of prenatal vitamins, knowledge about folic acid, and cultural practices all have the potential to moderate the influence of the causal factors, by either increasing or decreasing their potency.

Intervention Theory

The *intervention theory* explains how interventions affect the causal factors, or possibly the moderating or mediating factors. It contains hypotheses about the relationships of the programmatic interventions to the factors in the causal theory that the interventions are intended to affect. More importantly, it must address how the intervention alters the causal factors or breaks the chain between causal factors and health outcome. The intervention theory includes statements describing the relationships connecting interventions and outcomes. The intervention might also affect some of the moderating or mediating factors. Thus the intervention theory articulates the connection between the programmatic intervention and the intended effects on the health problem. Having the intervention theory explicitly stated and understood by the program staff contributes to the success of the program. Because clarity about interventions is so important, what the interventions are and how to identify them are discussed in a separate section later in this chapter.

The intervention theory describes how the program "works its magic." Developing an intervention theory is useful to refine the number, types, and quality of interventions that are carried out as part of the health program. Interventions that are not likely to alter or change the key factors in the causal theory can, in turn, be eliminated, which results in a more effective and efficient program.

In the birth defects health problem, planners might identify several possible points at which to intervene to ensure that the causal factors do not lead to neural tube defects. For example, the program might target the moderating factor regarding knowledge about the importance of folic acid. Accordingly, one part of the intervention theory would state that nutritional education [intervention] changes the behavior of the woman with regard to eating dark green vegetables. Another point at which to intervene on the causal factors might be by encouraging the use of prenatal vitamins [intervention] to remove the causal factor of inadequate folic acid intake. Also, screening for occupational exposures followed by an early ultrasound [intervention] could identify fetuses with abnormalities. Together, receiving nutritional education, taking supplements, and making changes in prenatal care can alter the biological processes that result in a neural tube defect.

As this example shows, not all moderating, causal, or mediating factors need to be, or can be, addressed by a single health program. An equally plausible intervention theory might state that education about occupational exposures [intervention] leads to decreased exposures and subsequently fewer infants with neural tube defects. The decision regarding which intervention theory to use as the basis of a program is influenced by the preferences of stakeholders, the mission of the organization, and the science regarding which factors are more readily changeable.

Impact Theory

The final element of effect theory is the *impact theory*, which is akin to the conceptual theory described by Rossi et al. (1999), in which statements about how the outcomes lead to impacts are explicated. Usually, a health program has a very limited number of health outcomes that it seeks to affect. Impact theory helps substantiate the sometimes seemingly wild and wishful claims of program planners about the effects of their program, by specifying the relationship between the immediate outcome of the program and the long-term, ultimate changes to the health problem. It is possible to have multiple impact theories for one long-range impact, especially if multiple intervention theories are used within a single program. Given the complex nature of many health problems and conditions, this is a likely scenario. Continuing with the birth defects example, the impact theory states that fewer infants born with neural tube defects leads to a decrease in the rate of birth defects of all types.

Funding agencies commonly specify program impacts—for example, a decrease in infant mortality or an increase in early detection of preventable disease. These impacts might be stated as program goals that the funded programs are to achieve. In such cases, program planners must essentially work backward to generate the impact theory and the intervention theory. In addition, impact theories show the links and explain the relationships between objectives and goals—an important factor that is discussed in detail in Chapter 7.

In summary, the effect theory encompasses the causal, intervention, and impact theories. These theories are all needed to explain the complexity of a health problem. Figure 6.3 brings together all of the components of the effect theory in the birth defects example.

Involve Key Stakeholders

Generating a program theory is not a solitary task; it is a task that requires brain power, diverse ideas, and sustained energy. Involving key stakeholders not only makes good ideas evident, but also encourages stakeholders to become invested in the health program and to address the health problem. This type of involvement is a critical step toward having a politically feasible intervention.

Potential program participants and providers typically have their own working explanation, or theory, of how a program will affect participants. One type of theory they may advocate is an espoused theory. Agryis and Schon (1974) were among the first to understand the importance of espoused theories. They found that employees had explanations for why things happen in their organizations; these stated explanations are the espoused theories. People know what they are supposed to do or say, regardless of whether they actually do or say it. The espoused theory consists of this stated and repeated explanation. For example, staff providing a diabetes management program may say that the program works because they are teaching the patients what to eat and how to exercise. This contention is the espoused theory of how the program improves participants' control of blood sugar levels.

Agryis and Schon (1974) also found that espoused theories were not always congruent with the behaviors they observed. What people do to achieve their ends is termed their theory-in-use, sometimes called a theory-in-action. The theory-in-use is crucial in program evaluation, because it consists of t he interventions that actually make up the health program and affect participants. Returning to the diabetes management example, if the staff in the diabetes management program become friends with the patients and provide

Figure 6.3   Effect Theory Example: Effect Theory for Reducing the Rate of Congenital Anomalies

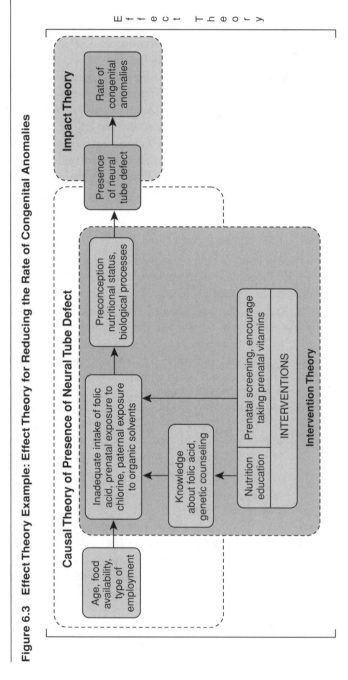

encouragement in a supportive manner but rarely focus on teaching patients, then their theory-in-use is coaching or social support rather than education.

As seen in the diabetes management example, espoused theories and theories-in-use may not be congruent. It is the theories-in-use that denote how the program is implemented and are the source of the effects on participants. One way to avoid incongruity between the espoused theory and the theory-in-use is to explicitly include the theory-in-use in the effect theory. Being aware of the differences among espoused theories, theories-in-use, and effect theories (Table 6.2) can help planners to generate an effect theory that incorporates useful elements of both the espoused theories and the theories-in-use. If the program has been in existence for some time, an alternative is to decide either to incorporate the theory-in-use into the program theory or to explicitly exclude the theory-in-use as an element of the program. Modifying the program theory based on the practical experience gained through the theory-in-use may be efficient and prudent if the theory-in-use has had the desired effect on program participants.

Table 6.2   Comparison of Effect Theory, Espoused Theory, and Theory-in-Use

	Effect Theory	**Espoused Theory**	**Theory-in-Use**
What it is	Explanation of how program interventions affect participants	What staff say about how the program affects participants	What staff do to affect participants
Where it resides	Manuals and procedures; program descriptions	Minds of program staff; program manuals and descriptions	Actions of program staff; on-the-job training
How it is identified	Review of scientific literature, program materials	Listen to staff describe the program, read program materials	Watch what staff do in providing the program
Importance	Guides program and evaluation; basis for claiming outcomes	Becomes what staff, clients, and stakeholders believe and expect of the program	Is the actual cause of program outcomes

Draw upon the Scientific Literature

Program planners should review articles published across the health disciplines for information that can help them generate the theories by providing information on the relationships among the antecedents, causal, moderating, and mediating factors. Abstracts available through online databases are another good source of ideas that can be incorporated into the effect theory. The published literature is also helpful in developing the process theory, particularly with regard to the service utilization elements.

Existing theories from multiple disciplines can be used to develop the effect theory. If the health program is intended to have a physiological effect or address a certain pathology, then theories from genomics, biochemistry, pharmacology, or physiology might be useful. If the health program addresses mental health or family problems, then theories from psychology or social work about psychopathology, stress, coping, or family functioning might be used to explain the health problem. If the health problem is related to the knowledge and abilities of individuals, then theories from psychology, education, decision sciences, or public health about learning, cognition, memory, and attention could be used to explain how knowledge, skills, and abilities are gained and retained. If a health program is intended to foster or maintain lifestyle behaviors and self-care, then theories from nursing, public health, and psychology about motivation, decision making, change, and self-efficacy might be suitable candidates.

Many existing theories can help health program planners develop causal theories for health problems and situations. The examples listed in Table 6.3 are grouped by the domain of health outcomes anticipated by the program, as a reminder that ultimately the program intervention theory must be matched with both the health problem and the desired outcomes of the program. In addition, existing theories can be used in developing the process theory; examples of such theories are shown in Table 6.4.

The theories used by program planners are generally specific to the level of the public health pyramid. In this section, the examples are largely at the individual level. For problems at the other levels of the pyramid, theories can be found in the literature. For example, Gay (2004) relied on the theory of disease transmission as a framework for understanding what is required to develop a program to eliminate measles, an infectious disease. Although measles is an individual illness, the elimination of any infectious disease—whether measles, tuberculosis, or HIV/AIDS—requires thinking in terms of populations as well as individual susceptibility. To change population behaviors related to alcohol use problems, Wallin (2007) reported that the successful program was based on the diffusion of innovation theory.

Table 6.3 Examples of Types of Theories Relevant to Developing Causative Theories Within the Effect Theory, by Four Health Domain Outcomes

Physical Health	Psychosocial Health	Knowledge and Abilities	Self-Care and Lifestyle Behaviors
Pathophysiology	Psychopathology	Learning	Peer pressure
Immunology	Social cognition	Communication	Decision making
Endocrinology	Stress and coping	Cognition	Self-efficacy
Pharmacology	Family functioning	Attention	Self-worth
Wound healing		Memory	Risk taking
Biochemistry	Addiction	Diffusion of innovation	Social stratification
Metabolism	Violence		
	Resilience	Acculturation	Motivational

Diagram the Causal Chain of Events

Drawing or creating a visual representation of the various theories is important, given the complex nature of the causes of health problems and the equally complex systems of services required to address health problems (Joffe & Mindell, 2006). Diagrams that depict the effect theory, the process theory, and the program theory can be created with pencil and paper or by using graphics software. Most software packages include some kind of drawing feature that can be used to create such a diagram.

Table 6.4 Examples of Types of Theories Relevant to Developing the Organizational Plan and Services Utilization Plan Components of the Process Theory

Organizational Plan	Service Utilization Plan
Social network	Social marketing
Communication	Marketing
Leadership	Cueing
Accounting	
Quality improvement	

A picture showing how each intervention changes a characteristic of the participants provides an expedient means of engaging program staff and getting feedback from other professionals in the field. As the scientific literature is reviewed and assimilated, additional relevant variables and their interrelationships can be incorporated into the map of the causal chain of events. Including every possible variable is neither realistic nor desirable, of course; instead, program planners should include only those variables that relate to the essence of the program and that, according to the community health assessment and available scientific literature, are mostly likely to influence the success of the proposed interventions.

In some instances, a health program is started in response to a mandate or a health policy initiative and, therefore, may not have an explicit program theory. If a program has been in existence or is ongoing, the development of a program theory is still possible, and, its creation instead can contribute to program improvements. In such cases, the espoused theory of program staff is a good starting point for the development of a program theory. Observation of program staff would then help identify the theory-in-use. Together with findings from the literature, these elements could be formalized into a program theory. It is quite possible that new areas for program monitoring and evaluation would emerge from such an exercise with program staff. In addition, program staff may come to see the value of their work and become more committed to the program and the participants. Involving program staff in reconciling their espoused theories and theories-in-use can lead to new program approaches and the identification of areas of inefficiencies.

For some health programs, timing is critical, such that some intervention components must be accomplished before other intervention components are implemented. If either the intervention or the outcomes must proceed in stages, these increments need to be reflected in the effect theory of the causal chain of events leading to the health outcome.

Check Against Assumptions

The program theory—and the effect theory in particular—needs to be checked against alternative assumptions about theories. Patton (1997) referred to these points as validity assumptions. One assumption is that the theory is really about the phenomenon of interest. In other words, program planners assume that the program theory truly deals with the health problem or condition that is the focus of the health program. Through the multiple interactions and discussions with stakeholders, this assumption can inadvertently be violated.

Another assumption relates to parsimony. Improving the health of individuals, families, and communities is a complex task, so most health programs address only one aspect of a complex puzzle of factors affecting health. Including too much in a program theory can lead to confusion, diffuse interventions, and frustration, not to mention exorbitant expenditures. Parsimony is a crucial characteristic of a good theory, including a program theory or an effect theory. Relying on the priorities set earlier in the planning process by focusing on the most important factors about the target audience helps achieve parsimony.

FUNCTIONS OF PROGRAM THEORY

Having an articulated theory of how the health program will lead to improved health, and specifically how the interventions will affect participants, serves several purposes (Bickman, 1987) that range from providing guidance and enabling explanation to forming a basis for communication.

Provide Guidance

A program theory that can be stated in one or two sentences provides a description of what is being implemented. To say that a program is helping asthmatic children is less compelling or descriptive than saying that a program teaches children how to be aware of their bodies and thereby avoid situations that may trigger an asthma attack. The latter is a description of how the program works to reduce asthma attacks and provides direct guidance on what to include in the program.

In a world of complex and interactive health problems, identifying the specific health problem and the appropriate target audience for a program can be difficult. Blum's (1982) caution against failure to analyze problems adequately is avoided by developing the program theory, which specifies the problem and the target audience. If the program theory is inordinately difficult to develop, it may indicate that the health problem has not been sufficiently narrowed, the target audience is not specific enough, or too many program components have been included. Having a target audience that is too broad can lead to a program theory that is too complex to be of value in designing and implementing the program.

The program theory guides what to measure in both the process and the effect evaluations of the program. In terms of the process evaluation, it specifies what needs to be measured with regard to the delivery of the intervention. In terms of the effect evaluation, the effect theory specifies the desired effects and, therefore, what needs to be measured. When a health program has several possible outcomes, the effect theory clarifies which outcome is most directly a result of the intervention. This information makes the evaluation of outcomes more efficient and enables program planners and evaluators to design an evaluation that will find those program effects that are arguably the result of the program.

Just as theory is used to guide the development of the health program, so theory can be used to guide the development of the evaluation. For example, Newes-Adeyi, Helitzer, Caulfield, and Bronner (2000) used ecological theory to guide their formative evaluation of the New York State's Women, Infants, and Children (WIC) nutritional program. Their use of ecological theory strengthened the evaluation in terms of its design and ability to explain how the program worked. Their report also serves as a reminder that the same underlying social or psychological theory that guides the effect theory can be applied to the effect evaluation as well.

When a new health program is first provided, its evaluation helps refine the subsequent delivery of the program. A program theory helps identify needed inputs and determine what needs to be evaluated and where improvements or changes in the delivery of the interventions are appropriate.

Enable Explanations

The program theory helps identify which interventions are likely to have the greatest effect on program participants and clarify how the interventions cause the desired effect in program participants. In this way, the theory enables planners and evaluators to more easily explain how the program should and does work.

One task of program planners is to anticipate the unintended. Careful attention to the development of the program theory can help uncover unintended consequences that may result from the program. The development of an effect theory, in turn, helps generate plausible explanations for those unintended consequences. Engaging in this kind of exercise in speculation helps program planners avoid another source of unsuccessful programs: failure to examine and compare relevant possible interventions (Blum, 1982).

A program theory also enables the evaluators to distinguish between process theory failure and effect theory failure (Figure 6.4). If the evaluation results show no effect on program participants, then the evaluator must explain what failed. A successful program sets into motion the interventions (causal processes) that lead to the desired outcome. However, if a program is not effective, the evaluator needs to identify the roots of that failure. A lack of program success can result from the program not being provided—a process theory failure. A lack of program success also can result from an ineffective intervention—an effect theory failure. This distinction between process and effect theory failures, based on the notions of program and theory failure put forth by Weiss (1972), helps evaluators sort out what went wrong or right with the program and explain the evaluation findings to stakeholders.

Figure 6.4   Two Roots of Program Failure

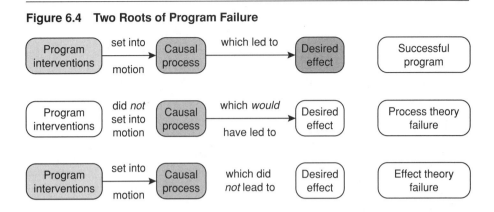

Form a Basis for Communication

Health programs compete for resources. A program theory helps convince organizational or legislative policy makers that the program is worthy and deserving of support. The causal chain of events outlined in the effect theory serves to frame discussions on a more rational basis, leading to a more rational decision-making process about the health program. The effect theory also helps policy makers understand the extent to which the program interventions are ideologically compatible with their stance and are based on science rather than biases and opinions. In other words, the effect theory provides a basis for clear communication of the program intent and content.

Starting and maintaining a program requires that key stakeholders agree on supporting the program. Gaining consensus from stakeholders—whether program staff, administrators, or legislators—is an important step in ensuring the success and acceptance of the health program. If stakeholders understand the program theory, it becomes easier to gain consensus on the usefulness of the program. Having gone through the exercise of developing the causal, intervention, and impact theories, the program planners are in the position of being better able to anticipate questions and provide alternative rationales for the health program. As mentioned earlier, stakeholders can be included in the development of the program theory as a way to gain consensus on the program interventions. For controversial programs, such as those dealing with sexuality education or family planning for adolescents, consensus on the program theory could be critical to the program's survival.

Make a Scientific Contribution

In a sense, every health program is an experiment that tests the program theory. In other words, every evaluation has the potential to contribute to our understanding of human nature and health. Evaluations based on the program theory can be used to modify existing theories relevant to the target population and types of interventions used.

ACROSS THE PYRAMID

At the direct services level of the public health pyramid, because the health problems are related to specific individuals, the relevant theories will focus on individual behavior and intra-individual responses to treatment or pathology. In other words, the focus is on the micro level. As a result, the interventions delivered are one-on-one, with providers directly delivering the interventions to their clients. (Examples of direct services interventions appear in Table 6.1.) If the program will have subcomponents, those components would involve different types of interventions that are delivered directly to individuals.

At the enabling services level, because the health problems are related to aggregates of individuals, the relevant theories will focus on the interactions of individuals with family or community characteristics. Because enabling services are still provided to individuals, the focus continues to be at the micro level. Hence, interventions are delivered on a one-on-one basis, as well as to groups with similar characteristics. Different intervention types can be applied at the enabling services level (Table 6.1).

At the population level, because the health problems are related to entire populations, the relevant theories will focus on group responses that lead to the health problem, cultural theories that explain behaviors and beliefs related to the health problem, and social theories about interactions among groups. Liddle and Hogue (2000), for example, described an intervention for high-risk adolescents. One key feature of their intervention model was that the theoretical foundation included risk and protection theory, developmental psychopathology theory, and ecological theory. This blend of theories is consistent with the intent of the program. In terms of the public health pyramid, however, the use of ecological theory reflects the theoretical awareness of the program planners that the population level influences both the enabling level (i.e., the family) and the individual level. At the population level, the interventions are designed and intended to have a universal focus. Such interventions are more likely to be delivered though the mass media or to involve policy formation. Although having program components at the population level may create synergies that enhance the intervention, such components may be prohibitive in terms of feasibility, manipulability, and cost.

At the infrastructure level, because the problems are related not to individuals but rather to processes and structures that enable the delivery of health programs, relevant theories might focus on organizational behavior, management and leadership style, personnel motivation, political action, and communication. The interventions can be delivered one-on-one with personnel, as well as with groups of workers or entire organizations. Because workforce capacity building is a key focus at the infrastructure level, it may be appropriate to use individual-level theories. For example, Kirk, Tonkin, and Burke (2008) used the theory of planned behavior as the basis for enhancing genetics literacy among health professionals.

DISCUSSION QUESTIONS AND ACTIVITIES

1. Select a health program with which you are familiar.
   a. Briefly state the hypotheses that constitute the effect theory of the program.
   b. What are the intervention components and the specific interventions?
   c. Develop an effect theory of the program theory used by the program.
   d. Do a brief literature search to determine whether the scientific evidence supports the interventions used.

2. What are the relationships among the possible functions of effect theory and the selection of optimal interventions?

3. Which of the theories that make up the effect theory are likely to be affected by the cultural, ethnic, or racial differences of target populations? In what ways might you make those theories culturally appropriate or sensitive?

4. Identify possible primary, secondary, and tertiary prevention interventions for each level of the public health pyramid.

5. Figure 6.4 shows a possible effect theory, with the interventions, to address the health problem of congenital anomalies. It builds on the causal theory shown in Figure 5.4. Try developing an effect theory diagram for one of the other health problems presented in Chapter 5: (a) vaccine-preventable hospitalization, (b) child abuse rate, (c) adolescent death rate due to gunshot wound, or (d) morbidity due to chronic illness.

INTERNET RESOURCES

University of Iowa, College of Nursing

This website (http://www.nursing.uiowa.edu/excellence/nursing_knowledge/clinical_effective ness/index.htm) provides an overview of standard nursing interventions (NIC) and outcomes (NOC). The detailed list can be helpful to show the level of specificity for interventions, which may be needed for some programs.

International Development Research Centre

A notable amount of health program planning and evaluation occurs in an international context. This website (http://network.idrc.ca/ev.php?ID=28377_201&ID2=DO_TOPIC) has a focus on international programs, and the content is applicable globally.

Understanding Change and Theories Critical in Developing Program Theory

The following websites focus on understanding and generating change. For example, the Change Project (http://www.changeproject.org/) has some interesting and practical applications in health. The chapter found at http://cancer.gov/cancerinformation/theory-at-a-glance/page8 is part of a short, online text and nicely summarizes the theories often used in public health. If you want to broaden your repertoire of change theories, then the information at the Communication Initiative Network (http://www.comminit.com) would be helpful.

Social Marketing Institute

This article (in pdf format) is provocative and addresses the ethical issues in developing change programs: http://www.social-marketing.org/papers/carrotarticle.pdf.

Community Guide to Preventive Services

This website lists interventions for various health topics and the degree of scientific evidence for the use of the intervention: http://www.thecommunityguide.org.

REFERENCES

Agryis, C., & Schon, D. A. (1974). *Theory in practice: Increasing professional effectiveness.* San Francisco: Jossey-Bass.

American Medical Association. (2008). *CPT 2009: Professional edition.* Chicago, IL: Author.

Baranowski, T., Davis, M., Resnicow, K., Baranowski, J., Doyle, C., Lin, L., et al. (2000). Gimme five fruit, juice, and vegetables for fun and health: Outcome evaluation. *Health Education and Behavior, 27*(1), 96–111.

Bickman, L. (1987). The functions of program theory. *New Directions for Program Evaluation, 43,* 5–18.

Blum, H. L. (1982). Social perspective on risk reduction. In M. M. Farber & A. M. Reinhart (Eds.), *Promoting health through risk reduction* (pp. 19–36). New York: Macmillan.

Brenton, J. J. (1999). Complementing development of prevention and mental health promotion programs for Canadian children based on contemporary scientific paradigms. *Canadian Journal of Psychiatry, 44*(3), 227–234.

Brown, J. H. (2001). Youth, drugs and resilience education. *Journal of Drug Education, 31,* 83–122.

Cawley, J., Schroeder, M., & Simon, K. L. (2006). How did welfare reform affect the health insurance coverage of women and children? *Health Services Research, 41,* 486–506.

Des Jarlais, D., Sloboda, Z., Friedman, S. R., Tempalski, B., McKnight, C., & Braine, N. (2006). Diffusion of the D.A.R.E. and syringe exchange programs. *American Journal of Public Health, 96,* 1354–1358.

Filiatrault, J., Parisien, M., Laforest, S., Genest, C., Gauvin, L., Fournier, M., et al. (2007). Implementing a community-based falls-prevention program: From drawing board to reality. *Canadian Journal of Aging, 26,* 213–225.

Fisher, E. B., Browston, C. A., O'Toole, M. L., Shetty, G., Anwuri, V. V., & Glasgow, R. E. (2005). Ecological approaches to self-management: The case of diabetes. *American Journal of Public Health, 95,* 1523–1535.

Gay, N. J. (2004). The theory of measles elimination: Implications for the design of elimination strategies. *Journal of Infectious Diseases, 189*(1S), S27–S35.

Grobe, S. J., & Hughes, L. C. (1993). The conceptual validity of a taxonomy of nursing interventions. *Journal of Advanced Nursing, 18,* 1942–1961.

Guidotti, T. L., Ford, L., & Wheeler, M. (2000). The Fort McMurray Demonstration Project in social marketing: Theory, design, and evaluation. *American Journal of Preventive Medicine, 18,* 163–169.

Harris, D. A. (2007). Dance/movement therapy approaches to fostering resilience and recovery among African adolescent torture survivors. *Torture, 17,* 134–155.

Heaney, C. A. & van Ryn, M. (1996). The implications of status, class, and cultural diversity for health education practice: The case of worksite stress reduction programs. *Health Education Research, 11*(1), 57–70.

Issel, L. M. (1997). Measuring comprehensive case management interventions: Development of a tool. *Nursing Case Management, 2,* 3–12.

Jackson, C., Altman, D. G., Howard-Pitney, B., & Farquhar, J. W. (1989). Evaluating community-level health promotion and disease prevention interventions. In M. T. Braverman (Ed.), *Evaluating health promotion programs* (pp. 19–32). San Francisco: Jossey-Bass.

Johnson, M., Bulechek, G., Butcher, H., Maas, M., Moorhead, S., & Swanson, E. (2006). *NANDA, NOC, and NIC linkages: Nursing diagnoses, outcomes, and interventions.* St. Louis, MO: Mosby.

Joffe, M., & Mindell, J. (2006). Context of causal process diagrams for analyzing health impacts of policy interventions. *American Journal of Public Health, 96,* 473–479.

Kelly, C. M., Baker, E. A., Brownson, R. C., & Schootman, M. (2007). Translating research into practice: Using concept mapping to determine locally relevant intervention strategies to increase physical activity. *Evaluation and Program Planning, 30,* 282–293.

Kirk, M., Tonkin, E., & Burke, S. (2008). Engaging nurses in genetics: The strategic approach in the NHS national genetics education and development center. *Journal of Genetic Counseling, 17,* 180–188.

Kreuter, M. W., Sugg-Skinner, C., Holt, C. L., Clark, E. M., Haire-Joshu, D., Fu, Q., et al. (2005). Cultural tailoring for mammography and fruit and vegetable intake among low-income African-American women in urban public health centers. *Preventive Medicine, 41,* 53–62.

Liddle, H. A., & Hogue, A. (2000). A family-based, developmental–ecological preventive intervention for high-risk adolescents. *Journal of Marital and Family Therapy, 26,* 265–279.

Lipman, E. L., Waymouth, M., Gammon, T., Carter, P., Secord, M., Leung, O., et al. (2007). Influence of group cohesion on maternal well-being among participants in a support/education group for single mothers. *American Journal of Orthopsychiatry, 77,* 543–549.

Marcus, S. E., Pahl, K., Ning, Y., & Brook, J. S. (2007). Pathways to smoking cessation among African American and Puerto Rican young adults. *American Journal of Public Health, 97,* 1444–1448.

Morone, N. E., Greco, C. M., & Weiner, D. K. (2008). Mindfulness meditation for the treatment of chronic low back pain in older adults: A randomized controlled pilot study. *Pain, 134,* 310–319.

Myers, J. (2003). Exercise and cardiovascular health. *Circulation, 107*(1), e2–e5.

Newes-Adeyi, G., Helitzer, D. L., Caulfield, L. E., & Bronner, Y. (2000). Theory and practice: Applying the ecological model of formative research for a WIC training program in New York State. *Health Education Research, 15*(3), 283–291.

Patton, M. Q. (1997). *Utilization-focused evaluation* (3rd ed.). Thousand Oaks, CA: Sage Publications.

Perchmann, C., & Reibing, E. T. (2006). Antismoking advertisements for youths: An independent evaluation of health, counter-industry, and industry approaches. *American Journal of Public Health, 96,* 906–913.

Potvin, L., Gendron, S., Bilodeau, A., & Chabot, P. (2005). Integrating social theory into public health practice. *American Journal of Public Health, 95,* 591–595.

Rossi, P., & Freeman, H. (1993). *Evaluation: A systematic approach* (5th ed.). Newbury Park, CA: Sage Publications.

Rossi, P., Freeman, H., & Lipsey, M. (1999). *Evaluation: A systematic approach* (6th ed.). Thousand Oaks, CA: Sage Publications.

Stice, E., Shaw, H., & Marti, C. N. (2007). A meta-analytic review of eating disorder prevention programs: Encouraging findings. *Annual Review of Clinical Psychology, 3,* 206–231.

United Way of America. (1996). *Measuring program outcomes: A practical approach.* Alexandria, VA: Author.

Van der Molen, H. F., Lehtola, M. M., Lappalainem, J., Hoonakker, P. L., & Hsiao, H. (2007). Interventions for preventing injuries in the construction industry. *Cochrane Database of Systematic Reviews* (Online), 4: CD006251.

Waddell, C., Hua, J. M., Garland, O. M., Peters, R. D., & McEwan, K. (2007). Preventing mental disorders in children: A systematic review to inform policy-making. *Canadian Journal of Public Health, 98,* 166–173.

Wallin, E. (2007). Dissemination of prevention: Community action targeting alcohol use-related problems at licensed premises. *Substance Use and Misuse, 42,* 2085–2097.

Weiss, C. (1972). *Evaluation.* San Francisco: Jossey-Bass.

Zaza, S., Briss, P. A., & Harris, K. W. (Eds.). (2005). *The guide to community preventive services: What works to promote health?* Oxford, UK: Oxford University Press.

CHAPTER 7

Program Objectives and Setting Targets

L. Michele Issel, PhD, RN, and Deborah Rosenberg, PhD

In this chapter, the focus is on setting the parameters by which the program is judged as successful—in other words, developing goals and objectives for the program. Setting goals and objectives is informative in terms of forcing further clarity and specificity about implementing the program and later evaluating its effects. After a logic model has been developed, it is the next step in program planning.

PROGRAM GOALS AND OBJECTIVES

"Goals" and "objectives" are terms that are widely used in program planning and evaluation. *Goals*, in a strict sense, are broad, encompassing statements about the impact to be achieved, whereas *objectives* are specific statements about outcomes to be achieved and are stated in measurable terms. Funding bodies do not use the terms "objectives" and "goals" in a consistent manner, so program planners and evaluators must understand the difference. Making the distinction between objectives and goals is key to subsequently making conceptual distinctions between short-term outcomes and long-term impacts of the program.

Goals and their corresponding objectives flow from the logic model and the program theory. Involving the stakeholders and program staff in the development of the program objectives and goals can be useful in gaining their support, stimulating good ideas, and reaching a consensus on what will constitute the program. However, the process of reaching a consensus, particularly on objectives, can be a bit of a struggle if stakeholders have vested interests in achieving particular health outcomes for their constituents. In addition, program planners often must cope with tight schedules for preparing a program

211

proposal, making timely involvement of stakeholders a considerable challenge. The efforts devoted to arriving at a set of clearly articulated goals and objectives do pay dividends, however; they lay the foundation from which to develop the evaluation and establish standards against which to assess the success of the program.

Goals

Goals are always statements about the health impact or status of the target audience, but generally apply to a longer time horizon, such as five years. Typically, goals do not incorporate a quantifiable measure but instead refer in broad terms to the most important anticipated effect of the program. A program will have at least one goal, and a well-focused program with several components may have more than one. In general, however, the number of goals is quite low. The use of creative activities, stories, and clear communication can make writing goals a positive experience.

Good goals are congruent with and contribute to the strategic plan, whether it consists of a national (e.g., *Healthy People 2010*), state, or local health plan or the healthcare organization's strategic plan. The extent to which the program goals and objectives are compatible with the strategic or long-term plan of the organization can affect the priority given to the program and hence the fiscal support provided for, and organizational approval of, the program. For health programs being developed by local health agencies or local community-based organizations, this larger context of health programs can be crucial in achieving synergies within the program as well as between programs with complementary foci.

On a cautionary note, Friedman, Rothman, and Withers (2006) provocatively remind evaluators that using goals for evaluation creates a paradox. Goals implicitly or explicitly embody values. The paradox arises when goals are used to guide an evaluation, because the evaluation then also embodies those values. This is not necessarily a bad thing, but it serves as a reminder that who is involved in developing and approving the goals is important.

Foci of Objectives

Development of objectives begins with having conceptual clarity regarding whether the objective is related to the program's process theory or effect theory. This section explores the distinction between process and effect objectives. The next step is to identify and select appropriate indicators for the objectives. This section concludes with a review of the characteristics that distinguish well-constructed goals and objectives.

An easy format that helps in remembering the parts of a good objective is this: "by when, who will achieve what, by how much." For example, one objective may be "By 2012, the Layetteville Innovation—Adolescent Preventing Pregnancy (i-APP) Program will reduce the pregnancy rate among program participants by 20% compared to girls not participating." The "by how much" portion of the objective, or the target value, is the quantifiable measure that distinguishes an objective from a goal. The target value is the essence of the objective; without it, no objective exists.

The statement "The percentage of pregnant adolescent girls among girls enrolled in the Layetteville i-APP Program during 2010 will be reduced" is a goal, not an objective. A goal may have several objectives that delineate more precisely what achieving the goal entails. Thus adding a target value would yield the following for reaching that goal: "The percentage of adolescent girls who become pregnant among girls enrolled in the Layetteville i-APP Program during 2010 will be 8%." The "8%" quantifies the reduction and is measurable.

The time frame used in the objectives needs to be short term and well within the life span of the program. For direct services and enabling services, objectives generally are set with a one- or two-year time horizon. This time line contrasts to that for objectives for population services, which are more likely to have five- or ten-year horizons that are aligned with the national *Healthy People* targets set for a particular decade.

Process Objectives

The process theory component of the program theory—and specifically the organizational plan and the service utilization plan—provides a framework for stating process objectives (Figure 7.1). Because the process theory describes how the program is designed and delivered, the process objectives serve to focus the activities of the program staff on implementing and sustaining the health program. Following the format for writing objectives, process objectives would then state, "by when, which staff will do what, to what extent" (Table 7.1).

Process objectives focus on the activities of the program staff, rather than on the benefits of the program for the participants. The organizational plan and service utilization plan provide insights into what ought to be included in each process objective, particularly for the "do what" portion. The "to what extent" portion will be determined based on past experience with the capabilities of the staff and on the amount of work to be done within the time frame. Objectives can be identified for the capacity of the infrastructure, as is commonly done in terms of personnel qualifications. Capacity objectives are best considered as objectives about the organizational plan. Thus a process objective might be, "By month 6, 100% of program staff will have participated in training on health education modules being used in Layetteville's i-APP Program."

Figure 7.1   Using Elements of Program Theory as the Basis for Writing Program Objectives

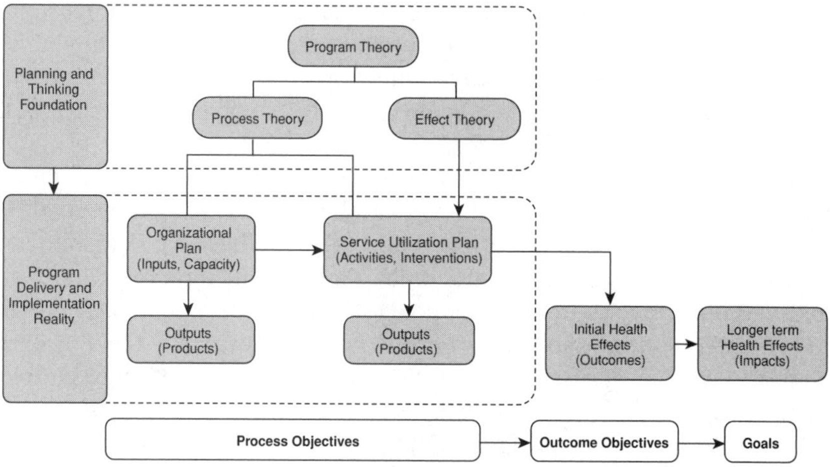

Table 7.1   Aspects of Process Objectives as Related to Components of the Process Theory

	Organizational Plan	Service Utilization Plan	Process Theory Outputs
Objective	By when, who will obtain or organize how much of which types of resource in what ways	By when, who will do what, how many interactions with participants of what type	By when, how many of what types of outputs or products will be created or finalized by whom
Objective Examples	By [date], the program manager will secure funding for three new computers with electronic clinical record software. By [date], the medical director will provide 20 staff with 4 hours of training about community gang violence.	By [date], the health educator will identify three evidence-based interventions for improving self-management of diabetes.	By [date], staff will distribute 100 brochures to women receiving genetic counseling at the clinic.

Effect Objectives

Effect objectives focus on the program participants and the benefits they will experience as a result of receiving the program interventions. Following the formula for writing objectives, effect objectives would state, "by when, how many of which program participants will experience what type of health benefit or state and to what extent."

The effect theory—most notably, the intervention, causal, and impact theories—provides the basis for stating intervention, outcome, and impact objectives, remembering that impacts are more appropriately called goals (Figure 7.2). In most program literature, all three types of objectives are referred to as outcome objectives. The purpose of distinguishing among the three types is to ensure that, during the planning process, connections between the planned interventions and health changes are made explicit. Being explicit at this phase of the planning will facilitate subsequent development of the evaluation, particularly with regard to which changes, benefits, or health outcomes should be measured. Because funding agencies generally require objectives dealing with effects, intervention objectives can be included with outcome and impact objectives.

The format for writing good objectives can be used to write objectives in terms of increasing or reducing the level of a certain outcome compared to some benchmark level. The earlier example, "By 2010, the Layetteville i-APP Program will reduce the rate of pregnancy among program participants by 20%

Figure 7.2   Diagram Showing Relationship of Effect Theory Elements to Process and Outcome Objectives

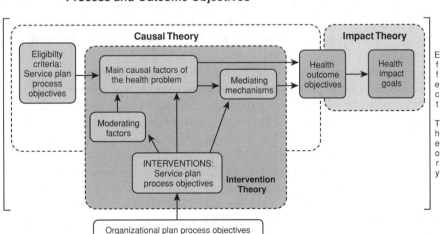

compared to girls not participating," uses nonparticipants as the comparison—that is, the benchmark. Another approach to writing an outcome objective is to have the "by how much" parameter reflect a preferred level of achievement or a target value that the program seeks to achieve. An objective written in this way might state, "During 2010, participants enrolled in the Layetteville i-APP Program will have a pregnancy rate of 8%." Regardless of how the "by how much" parameter is stated, the objectives need to reference a time frame, the program participants to be affected, a health outcome related to the program interventions, and a quantifiable target value for that health outcome. Clearly stated objectives that include these components serve as clear guideposts in designing the evaluation of program effect.

Objectives and Indicators

One aspect of developing objectives is to consider indicators. Like so many other terms in program planning and evaluation, *indicator* has many uses and interpretations. It can refer to the "what" portion of the objective, to the variables used to measure that "what," or to performance benchmarks used to determine the failure or success of a program. There is no easy way to distinguish among these uses or to prescriptively state that one is better than the others. It is, however, important to be aware that the results of the evaluation regarding "by how much" can be influenced not only by the program's true effect, but also by the sensitivity of the measure (indicator) selected. For example, if an outcome objective concerns improvement in cognitive functioning of children with special healthcare needs, indicators of cognitive functioning might consist of a score on a standardized scale such as the Bayley Scales of Infant Development or the Denver Developmental Screening Test, or a parental report of cognitive functioning. Because the standardized scales are more sensitive and specific than the parental report, they can detect a smaller true change.

By choosing—or at least considering—indicators when developing objectives, planners and evaluators can set reasonable target numbers for how much change is projected, given the indicator chosen. For full-coverage programs at the population level, it may be more appropriate to think of indicators in terms of benchmarks. For example, the national standard for a healthy birth weight could be used as an indicator, as in the objectives for infants born to women in the Women, Infants, and Children (WIC) nutrition program.

Most health programs address one or more domains of health or well-being. Typically, these domains encompass physical, mental, cognitive, behavioral, knowledge, social, and financial issues. For each of these domains of health, specific variables (indicators) are used to measure the program effect on that domain. Table 7.2 lists some commonly used variables for each health or well-being domain. The developers of a health program would need to select those indicators that reflect the specific health domain targeted by that program. Reliance on the effect theory and identification of the antecedent,

Table 7.2   Domains of Individual or Family Health Outcomes with Examples of Corresponding Indicators and Standardized Measures

Outcome Domain	Examples of Indicators (Variables) to Measure Objectives
Physical health	General measures: cardiovascular fitness, weight, dental diagnosis, medical diagnosis of acute illness, medical diagnosis of chronic illness Standardized measures: normal range on laboratory tests, ICD-10, *DSM-IV*
Mental health	General measures: motivation, values, attitudes, emotional bonding, medical diagnosis of mental illness, medical diagnosis of addiction, stress Standardized measures: CES-D, Edinburgh Postnatal Depression Scale, Daily Hassles Scale
Cognitive processes	General measures: decision making, judgments, problem-solving ability, cognitive development, cognitive impairment Standardized measures: Bayley Scales of Infant Development, IQ tests
Behavior	General measures: smoking, exercise, acts of aggression, wears seat belt, food purchasing behavior, specific parenting behavior, risk-taking or risk-seeking behaviors
Knowledge	General measures: skill, ability, performance, education of others, recall of facts, synthesis of facts
Social health	General measures: marital status, social network, recreation activities, volunteerism Standardized measures: Norbeck Social Support Questionnaire
Resources	General measures: income, insurance source, housing situation, employment status, education level Standardized measures: Hollingshead Index, dissimilarity index

causal, moderating, or mediating factors of the health problem being targeted may also suggest the optimal indicators of program effect.

A variety of criteria can be applied when selecting indicators. The first and foremost criterion to consider is any indicators that are required or mandated by the funding agency. For example, the Maternal and Child Health Bureau (MCHB) of the Health Resources and Services Administration (HRSA) requires that all grantees of Title V funds use its set of 18 performance measures, 6 outcome measures, and 8 capacity-related objectives. MCHB Title V indicators include measures such as the rate at which children are hospitalized for asthma, the percentage of women with a live birth who have had an adequate number of prenatal visits according to the Adequacy of Prenatal Care Utilization index (Kotelchuck, 1997), and the percentage of live births where the newborns weigh less than 2500 grams (Maternal and Child Health Bureau, n.d.). Although some of the MCHB indicators could be considered related to process, grantees must use these indicators as outcomes.

Another criterion for selecting indicators includes the requirement that the data for the indicator, if it is a variable, must be feasible to collect and easy to analyze. Indicators such as variables also ought to be scientifically defendable—hence the use of standardized or existing questionnaires and tools. Indicators of any type also ought to be relevant to users, such as the program managers and program stakeholders. Finally, indicators (measures) need to be relatively easy to analyze. It is pointless to rely upon an indicator (measure) that is so difficult to analyze that it is not used in program management or improvement.

Indicators may also be selected by returning to the community health diagnosis statements developed about health problems. In those statements (see Chapter 5), the health status indicator can be directly applied to the outcome objectives. For example, for each the five health problems identified as being a high priority in Bowe County, indicators or variables are used in the objectives (Table 7.3). Table 7.4 provides examples of intervention, outcome, and impact objectives for the goal of reducing birth defects, and Table 7.5 provides examples of intervention, outcome, and impact objectives for adolescent pregnancy. In each example, the objectives are derived from, and thus correspond to, the intervention, causal, and impact theories.

Good Goals and Objectives

Obviously, good goals and objectives are both meaningful and useful (Patton, 1997). Of course, the objectives need to be distinctly related to either process or effect. Likewise, both process and effect objectives need to be tailored to the specific health program being planned. Thus program planners are

Table 7.3   Bowe County Health Problems with Indicators, Health Outcomes, and Health Goals

Health Problem	Indicator of Health Problem	Health Outcome	Health Goal or Impact
Vaccination	Rates of under-immunization, by age group	Vaccine-preventable illness	Decrease vaccine-preventable hospitalizations
Presence of neural tube defect	Rates of neural tube defects and congenital anomalies	Absence of neural tube defect	Reduce current rate of congenital anomalies
Diagnosis of pregnancy	Pregnancy rate, by age group	Diagnosis of pregnancy	Reduce child abuse related to unwanted pregnancy
Hospital admissions for gunshot wounds	Rate of admissions for gunshot injuries at local hospitals, number of police reports	Adolescent death rate due to gun-shot wounds	Reduce adolescent death rate due to gunshot wounds
Diagnosis of type 2 diabetes	Incidence rate of diabetes, prevalence rate of diabetes	Rates of amputa-tion and vision loss due to diabetes	Reduce morbidity due to chronic illness

encouraged to adapt—rather than plagiarize—objectives from similar programs. Each objective ought to convey only one idea, so that each statement can be related to only one measure. Ideally, the objectives will be understandable to any stakeholder who might read them.

Goals and objectives are often written using language that indicates a direction, such as *improve* or *reduce*. Using a direction in the objective can be confusing and misleading. For example, "improving birth outcomes" as a goal includes both reducing congenital anomalies and increasing birth weight. Especially for objectives, the target value gives a more precise direction because it is based on baseline data. To the extent possible, objectives and

Table 7.4   Effect Objectives for the Intervention, Impact, and Outcome Theory, Using Congenital Anomalies as an Example

	Intervention Objective from Intervention Theory	Outcome Objective from Causal Theory	Impact Objective from Impact Theory
Format of objective	By when, what proportion of recipients will have how much effect from program interventions on which causal factors that lead to the health problem	By when, what proportion of recipients will have how much effect from program interventions on the immediate health problem	By when, long-term or global health change or status among target population
Example	By [date], [target #] women in the program will have a decrease by [target %] in exposure to environmental hazards that are teratogenic. By [date], [target #] women in the program will increase dietary folic acid intake so that ADA standards for pregnant women are met.	By [date], [target #] women in the program will have normal newborns (no neural tube defects).	By [date], [target] rate of congenital anomalies among residents of Bowe County.

goals ought to be written to reflect the final rate or state of health, not the change needed to get there.

Another important consideration is the ability to imagine that without the program, whatever is stated in the objective would not occur. This projection offers a way to double-check that the program is directly responsible for the elements addressed in the objective. Similarly, the program goals and objectives need to be reviewed for alignment with the needs, problems, and assets identified through the community health assessment.

Table 7.5   Effect Objectives for the Intervention, Impact, and Outcome Theory, Using Adolescent Pregnancy as an Example

	Intervention Objective from Intervention Theory	Outcome Objective from Causal Theory	Impact Objective from Impact Theory
Format of objective	By when, what proportion of recipients will have how much effect from program interventions on which causal factors that lead to the health problem	By when, what proportion of recipients will have how much effect from program interventions on the immediate health problem	By when, long-term or global health change or status among target population
Example	By 2009, 100% of adolescents in the i-APP program will be able to describe what constitutes safe sex (use of condoms).	By 2010, 95% of sexually active adolescents in Bowe County will practice safe sex (use of condoms).	By 2012, the incidence of infant abuse will be 8.0 per 1000 among residents of Bowe County.

Although this chapter presents the development of the goals and objectives as being derived from the logic model and the program theory, in actuality, discussions that develop about objectives may prompt the program planners and the program stakeholders to revise the logic model or the program theory. Similarly, the process of selecting indicators for objectives may cause the objectives to be revised. These iterations ought to be viewed as a positive sign that ways to strengthen and streamline the health program are being identified and attempts to do so are occurring during the planning phase, rather than after the program has been implemented.

Sooner or later someone will mention the acronym SMART in reference to objectives. SMART stands for five qualities of a good objective: specific, measurable, achievable, realistic, and time. Specific refers to the "what" that is to be achieved. Measurable refers to the metric or measure being used to determine whether the objective was met. Achievable is a reality check ensuring that the target being set can actually be achieved or attained. Realistic asks whether, given the resources and conditions, it is plausible that the objective will be achieved. Time refers to the time frame for achieving the objective. In developing objectives, it can be helpful to reflect on the SMART qualities to ensure that the objective is good.

USING DATA TO SET TARGET VALUES

All types of objectives, whether related to process theory or effect theory, have the "by how much" portion for each "what." A critical step in developing a meaningful objective is choosing a numeric value as the target for the "by how much" portion of the objective.

For process objectives, the procedure for establishing target values for the "by how much" portion generally means using data from the organizational and marketing assessments. National standards or objectives are not always available for use as a guide. Nevertheless, professional standards can often be used, particularly for organizational plan objectives. For example, legal and professional standards have been established for minimum qualifications for personnel. These standards can be used as a starting point for setting targets— say, for the percentage of program staff with a given certification.

For effect objectives, the target-setting process relies on the effect theory. The assumption is that as long as the objectives are consistent with the program theory and the level of programmatic effort, targets can be achieved. What is achievable, of course, depends on a host of factors both internal and external to the program. Having reasonable target values will directly influence the extent to which a program is perceived as successful, particularly with regard to outcomes and impacts. Consequently, the measurement of success must be scientifically credible. During the development of the objectives and their corresponding targets, planners and evaluators will want to agree on a strategy that accounts for both the program theory and any extraneous factors, and they will also want stakeholders to become involved during this crucial initial stage.

Developing a rational target-setting strategy, instead of using mere guesstimation, is more likely to lead to targets that are meaningful from a programmatic perspective and that are achievable to the extent that they represent an outgrowth of the program theory and are based on empirical data. It is certainly possible to choose reachable target values without having a clear analytic strategy, but doing so emphasizes looking successful over measuring the effect due to the program theory. To use an extreme example, a target value of 0.0% change among program recipients could be chosen, and achieving this target would for all intents and purposes be guaranteed. Nevertheless, choosing this target value would undermine the integrity of the target-setting process, not to mention that of the program evaluation.

The target-setting approaches outlined here begin with the process of establishing guidelines based on a decision framework and then move to choosing one or more relatively simple statistical procedures to yield target values consistent with the decisions. These approaches are best suited for setting target values for effect objectives. The framework described in the next section was developed by Rosenberg (1999) as an outgrowth of an effort by the MCHB to provide states with enhanced skills for program planning and evaluation.

Decisional Framework for Setting Target Values

The first and most basic element in developing a target-setting strategy is deciding how program success will be defined. This decision is best made prior to selecting target values. Success can be defined as meeting or exceeding a target, or as making meaningful progress toward the target but not necessarily meeting it. If success is defined as meeting a target, then targets will probably be chosen more cautiously than if success is defined less strictly. If program planners and staff wish to claim success even when a target value is not achieved, then "making meaningful progress" must be quantified, in addition to setting the target value itself. Either definition of program success is acceptable, but the definition to be used in the later program evaluation needs to be agreed upon and, more importantly, made explicit to all relevant parties during the planning stage.

The way in which program success is defined will influence whether targets are chosen primarily according to past or baseline indicator values or whether more emphasis is placed on the values of longer-term objectives for the program. This difference in perspective can have a dramatic effect on a final target value. Referencing targets to past or baseline values is typically a more cautious approach, because the target values will tend to be set to a level that represents a very modest improvement in the health outcome being measured—in other words, a minimum expectation for program effectiveness. In contrast, referencing targets to longer-term objectives is a bolder approach, often resulting in target values that will be somewhat more difficult to reach but that will challenge program managers to continually examine the program implementation and to advocate for changes if necessary. Both approaches are appropriate, and a decision needs to be made as to which focus is more important to the particular program under consideration.

Once program success is defined and a consensus has been reached regarding the relative importance of past, present, or future indicator values, program planners can begin developing a specific methodology for incorporating indicator values into the target. Sometimes only current data values are used in setting a target; sometimes a combination of current values and trend data is considered; and sometimes current values, trend data, and a local or national standard are all incorporated into the target-setting process. For example, if data have already been collected over time and a well-established objective or national standard specifying a long-term outcome exists, it may be important to set a target based both on the trend in the data and on the distance between the existing standard and the desired outcome.

Table 7.6 shows a matrix depicting combinations of patterns over time and relationships to a long-term objective. A different target value might be selected depending on which cell is relevant to the outcome of interest. For example, if

Table 7.6   Matrix of Decision Options Based on Current Indicator Value, Population Trend of the Health Indicator, and Value of Long-Term Objective or Standard

Population Trend of Indicator	Current Value of the Health Indicator in the Target Audience		
	Better Than Long-Term Objective or Standard	Meets Long-Term Objective or Standard	Worse Than Objective or or Standard
Improving	Set target to *maintain* current level; better than the long-term objective and limits to further improvement	Set target to *surpass* the long-term objective; continuing the improving trend	Set target to a *better* level; accelerate improving trend to approach the long-term objective
No change	Set target to slightly *better level;* better than the long-term objective, but want to see improving trend	Set target to *surpass* the long-term objective; begin improvement in trend	Set target to a *moderately better* level; begin improvement in trend
Deteriorating	Set target to *maintain* current level; stop the worsening trend	Set target to *maintain* current value; stop the worsening trend	Set target to *maintain* current level or adjust it slightly downward; stop or slow the worsening trend

a program is being implemented for a target population that has been experiencing worsening conditions over time and that has a current indicator value far from a long-term objective, the target value might be set more cautiously than if the program is being implemented for a target population that has been experiencing gradual improvement and that has a current indicator already fairly close to the long-term target value.

Another component of making decisions about target setting is choosing which types and sources of data will be used. A wide variety of data sources are often available and appropriate for assessing health programs and measuring objectives. Ideally, multiple data sources will be used in setting target values, because each source contributes slightly different information to the target-setting process. For example, one source of data might consist of police reports on the use of guns, and another source might be medical diagnoses of gunshot wounds in emergency departments. The statistics reported by each of these sources might be similar, but they might also be different. Having access to both data sets would be useful in setting a reasonable target for the rate of intentional gun violence in Layetteville.

Both the number of data sources available and the consistency of the data across these sources influence the target-setting process. Table 7.7 shows the

Table 7.7   Framework for Target Setting: Interaction of Data Source Availability and Consistency of Information

	One or Only a Few Sources	**Many Sources**
Consistent Information Across Sources	Need to consider whether the available data are of high quality. Need to consider whether it is relevant to the program and objective target being considered.	Can use any of the data sources.
Inconsistent Information Across Sources	If the one data source is markedly different from the literature, need to either change the objective or verify the data.	Need to decide which data source to use, given the strengths and weaknesses of each data source. Need to consider which data source is most relevant to the program and the objective being considered.

intersection of these two dimensions. For example, if many data sources are available and their data are in reasonable agreement, then arriving at a target value is relatively straightforward because it will reflect the consistent values. In such a case, similar target values would be reached no matter which data sources are used. If, however, many data sources are available but the information is inconsistent or conflicting, then decisions must be made regarding which data source should be given precedence or which combination of data sources will be used. These decisions should be based on the strengths and weaknesses of each data source, including its sample size, data completeness, and other aspects of data quality. The goal is to integrate the data and the information in a way that permits arriving at one target value.

The choice of data source also needs to be congruent with or to correspond to the target population or audience. For example, if a target value is being developed for effect objectives for a full-coverage, population-level program with a goal of improving birth outcomes, an appropriate data source would be vital records data. In contrast, for the Layetteville i-APP program, which is a partial-coverage program geared toward a smaller target audience with the goal of reducing adolescent pregnancy, appropriate data sources might include medical records and surveys of the women who are program recipients, as well as the county vital records data.

The data sources for setting the target may or may not be the same as the sources of the evaluation data or the data for the community needs assessment. The choice of data source for each of these program planning and evaluation activities always must correspond to the purpose for which the data will be used. Also, if different sources of data are used, then the program planners and evaluators need to agree that the different sources yield the same information.

Another factor to consider in the decision-making process is the extent to which disparities exist across or within the target populations. During the community health assessment, some sense of the disparities ought to be evident. If the disparities exist by income or race/ethnicity or geographic location, the data may need to be stratified by those factors. When available data are not stratified, indicator values are simply averages that may mask very different outcomes for different population groups. Left unstratified, for example, the rate of adolescent pregnancy in a community might appear relatively close to the *Healthy People 2010* objective of 43 per 1000. When pregnancy is stratified by neighborhood, however, it may become clear that the rate of adolescent pregnancy in one area is far from the national target value and much different from the rate in another area. Target values may or may not be chosen based on stratified data, but program evaluators should certainly incorporate stratified values into their interpretation of why targets are or are not met. With respect to the program theory, the preexisting factors or moderating factors may include factors that can be stratified. Continuing with the adolescent pregnancy example, an antecedent factor, such as cognitive development or family income, or a moderating factor, such as school-based sex education, may be a variable that can be stratified.

It is not always possible to stratify data in the way that evaluators may want. Data sources related to the indicator of interest may not include data for the variables to be stratified. For example, data from emergency department records are not likely to include information on the educational level of the patient, and data from police reports are not likely to include information on the severity of the injury.

Stratification may also result in only a few individuals being grouped within some strata, which poses statistical and interpretation problems. One approach to addressing this problem of small numbers is to minimize the number of strata by combining data across multiple years, across multiple geographic areas, or even across sociodemographic characteristics, if appropriate. For example, while it might be desirable to stratify a population or target audience based on age, broad (rather than narrow) age strata might be defined to ensure adequate numbers in each group. This problem of small numbers is particularly challenging for programs in rural areas or for target audiences with rare health needs or problems.

One technique for explicitly organizing and documenting the process of setting targets is to use logic statements. These statements can be written as the decision-making process is unfolding as a way to keep the decisions explicit and the discussions focused. Logic statements are written in "if, then;" or "otherwise, if, then" format. For example, thinking about how to integrate different data sources, a logic statement for gun violence might be as follows:

If the emergency department data and the police department data do not agree, **then** the [one or other of the data sources] will be given precedence in setting the target value.

To integrate different types of data about gun violence, a logic statement might be something like the following:

If trend data for gun violence show steady improvement, but the current value is still far from a long-term objective,
then the target value will be set to reflect an increase in the rate of improvement;
otherwise, if the trend in gun violence shows steady improvement and the current rate is already close to a long-term objective,
then the target value will be set to reflect a continuation of the existing rate of improvement;

otherwise, if no trend data are available,
then the target value will be set to reflect an improvement in the current
    value of X percent.

Sets of such statements can be drafted for each indicator about which decisions are being made, such as data sources, data consistency, data types, existing or perceived disparities, and resource availability. These statements should
incorporate information obtained during the community health assessment,
along with input from stakeholders.

Although some target-setting decisions can be applied to all of the program
objectives, other decisions may vary depending on the objective. Objectives for
different health outcomes will rely on differing pools of data sources and may
exhibit differing trends over time, differing patterns of disparities, and differing
importance within a larger context. In addition, objectives for population-based
and full-coverage programs will require a target setting strategy that differs
from that developed for a direct services level program that addresses a specific health domain within individuals. Program planners must also recognize
that target setting is an iterative process, taking place over the life of a program.
Rarely are target values set beyond one year, making it necessary to revisit the
targets on an annual basis for health programs that are institutionalized or that
are planned to last for a longer period of time.

Options for Calculating Target Values

Many options for calculating target values are available, each of which may
be appropriate in some circumstances but not in others. The fact that target
values for any one health problem can be calculated in so many ways underscores the importance of having established a consensus on the underlying
logic reflected in the "if, then" statements that lead to a particular value. Ten
options for calculating target values are described here. The calculations can
easily be done using a calculator or a spreadsheet.

Figures 7.3, 7.4, and 7.5 show the calculations for a program whose goal is to
reduce adolescent pregnancy in Bowe County. For this program, outcome objectives are needed regarding the extent to which that goal is being met.

In planning some health programs, very limited information may be available on which to base the calculations for some target values. This is often the
case, for example, for innovative programs, programs addressing rare health
problems, and programs that are highly tailored to the location in which they
are delivered. In such cases, only one piece of information from the community health assessment may be relevant—namely, a numeric value for the current level of the health problem. Four options for calculating a target value can

Figure 7.3   Calculations of Options 1 through 4 Using a Spreadsheet

	A.	B	C	D	E	F	G	H	I	J	K	L
1			Long Term									
2	Current Value	% Change	Target Value	Number of Years	Population at Risk		Option	Description	Formula	Target Value	Absolute Change	Percent Change
3	37.6				16,556		1	Default	(none)	37.6	0	0.0%
4												
5	37.6				16,556		2	Use statistically significant change (approx.)	A5−(SQRT(2*(A5*(1000−A3))/E5)*2)	33.5	4.1	−10.9%
6												
7	37.6	−0.02			16,566		3	Use current trend as change desired	(B7 * A7) + A7	36.8	0.8	−2.0%
8							4	Use meeting long-term objective				
9	37.6	−0.04	30	5	16,556							
10												
11								then, Yr 1	(B9 * A9) + A9	36.1	1.5	−4.0%
12								then, Yr 2	(B9 * J11) + J11	34.6	1.5	−4.0%
13								then, Yr 3	(B9 * J12) + J12	33.2	1.4	−4.0%
14								then, Yr 4	(B9 * J13) + J13	31.9	1.3	−4.0%
15								then, Yr 5	(B9 * J14) + J14	30.6	1.3	−4.0%
16								Total improvement			7.0	18.6%

Figure 7.4 Calculations of Options 5 Through 8 Using a Spreadsheet

	A	B	C	D	E	F	G	H	I	J	K	L
1	County	Size of Population at Risk	Number of Teen Births	Teen Birth Rate per 1000		Option	Description	Formula	Current Value	Target Value	Absolute Change	Percent Change
2	O	793	9	11.3					37.6			
3	P	2785	66	23.7			*Not considering sample size:*					
4	Q	859	22	25.6		5	Mean rate	Average (D2:D11)	37.6	**33.8**	3.8	–10.2%
5	R	2205	64	29.0		6	Median of the rates	Midpoint between County S and T:D6+((D7-D6)/2)	37.6	**31.0**	6.6	–17.4%
6	S	1338	40	29.9								
7	T	994	32	32.2								
8	*Subtotal/Rate for Approx. 50% of Population*	**8974**	**233**	**26.0**			*Considering sample size:*					
9	U	708	24	33.9		7	Rate for "best" 50% of population	50% = B14 x 0.50 = 8,278. Sum sizes until reach 8278, O,P,Q,R,S,T				
10	V	2664	106	39.8				(C8/B8)*1000	37.6	**26.0**	11.6	–30.9%
11	W	302	15	49.7								
12	*Subtotal/Rate for Approx. 75% of Population*	**12,648**	**378**	**29.9**		8	Rate for 75% of population (Counties P to	75% = B14 x 0.75 = 12,417. Sum sizes until reach 12,417, P,Q,R,S,T,U,V,W				
13	X	3908	244	62.4				(C12/B12)*1000	37.6	**29.9**	7.7	–20.5%
14	*Total/Overall Rate*	**16,556**	**622**	**37.6**								

Figure 7.5   Calculations of Options 9 and 10 Using a Spreadsheet

	A	B	C	D	E	F	G	H	I	J	K	L
1	Strata	Size of Population at Risk	Number of Teen Births	Teen Birth Rate per 1000		Option	Description	Formula	Current Value	**Target Value**	Absolute Change	Percent Change
2	Poverty											
3	Yes	2533	148	58.4		9	Rate for best strata	(none)	37.6	**33.8**	3.8	−10.1%
4	No	14,023	474	33.8		10	Overall rate based on strata specific rates	**Step 1. Use Option 2 formula per strata**				
5	Total	16,556	622									
6								10% decrease for Poverty = (−0.1 * 16) + 16	58.4	**52.6**	5.8	−10.0%
7								2% decrease for No Poverty = (−0.02 * 17) + 17	33.8	**33.1**	0.7	−2.0%
8								**Step 2. Calculate final target, weighting by % of population in each group**				
9												
10								(J6*(B3/B5))+(J7*(B4/B5))	37.6	**36.1**	1.5	−4.0%

be used in developing the outcome objective under these conditions. Table 7.8 summarizes the conditions under which each of the ten options would be best and outlines the advantages and disadvantages of each option.

Option 1 assumes that no change will occur because of the program. This is equivalent to accepting the current level or value. As a default position, it provides a starting point, particularly if the health program is in its first year and minimal empirical information is available regarding how much change is realistic or possible. This approach may also be appropriate for health programs that are mature and are seeking to maintain the current value because it is already at an acceptable, healthy level. The formula is as follows:

Target value = current value

In other words, the target value for the birth rate per 1000 female adolescents ages 15 through 17 is stated in the objective as 37.6 per 1000. This target value is used in the program objective as the "how much" value.

Option 2 identifies a value that, when compared to the current value, results in a statistically significant improvement. This option would be appropriate if the data source is credible, the program has a rigorous intervention, or policy makers need to be convinced that the program is a worthwhile investment. Because change may happen by chance, not just because of the health program, planners must be able to argue that the amount of change is greater than would occur by chance alone, and hence is attributable to the program. An approximate Z-test can be used to derive the amount of change needed to be statistically significant. Typically, the significance level is set at $p = .05$, meaning that the probability of reaching that target by chance alone is less than 5 in 100, or 5%. The .05 significance level translates into a Z score of 1.96, which is used in the formula to estimate the target value. The formula is quite complex but has been simplified somewhat here so that it can be used with a spreadsheet:

$$\text{Target Value} = \text{Current Value} - \left(\sqrt{\frac{2 \times \text{Current Value} \times (\text{multipler} - \text{Current Value})}{\text{Population at Risk}}} \times 1 \right.$$

This formula assumes that the current value is an integer—that is, it is a percentage or a number per 1000, 10,000, or whatever the usual units are for reporting the indicator. The multiplier, then, is that unit value. In the adolescent birth rate example, the current value is 37.6 and the multiplier is 1000. In addition, the formula is written so that the target value will be less than the current value. If improvement in an indicator translates into a target value that is larger than the current value, then the minus $(-)$ sign in the formula will change to a plus $(+)$ sign.

Table 7.8 Summary of When to Use Each Option

Option	Description of Option	Type of Program for Which Is Ideal	Advantages of Option	Disadvantages of Option
1	Default, no change	Mature, stable program	Does not require historical data	Does not require improvement
2	Change based on results of statistical test	Population based or program with large numbers of recipients	Supports argument that improvement was more than by chance	Sensitive to sample size; may result in unreasonable target; requires some statistical knowledge
3	Percentage change in health problem based on current trend, literature, or hopeful guess	Stable program; stable target population	Very straightforward and easy to understand; can easily take into account trend data if available	Must know the trend
4	Use existing benchmark or standard to project target values for several years	Program must show improvement	Comparable programs can be compared	Requires existence of long-term objective or standard; requires long-term program
5	Mean rate across geographic areas	Population based	Easily understood	Requires having data for each area
6	Median of rates across geographic areas	Population based	Easily understood	Requires having data for each area

Table 7.8   Summary of When to Use Each Option (continued)

Option	Description of Option	Type of Program for Which Is Ideal	Advantages of Option	Disadvantages of Option
7	Overall rate for best 50% across geographic areas	Population based or multisite	Takes into consideration the best and worst values in the target population; moves entire target population to an achievable value	Requires having data for each area; may be more difficult to understand; overlooks sample size
8	Overall rate for best 75% across geographic areas	Population based or multisite	Takes into consideration the best and worst values in the target population; moves entire target population to an achievable value	Requires having data for each area; may be more difficult to understand
9	Rate for best stratum using sociodemographic groupings	Population based or diverse target audience with evidence of disparities	Takes into consideration the best and worst values in the target population; moves entire target population to an achievable value	Requires having data for each group; may be more difficult to understand
10	Overall rate based on differential targets for each stratum	Population based or diverse target audience with evidence of disparities	Program must show improvement; more intense program intervention aimed at group with the most need for improvement	Requires having data for each group; may be more difficult to understand

Any test for statistical significance is very sensitive to sample size. For a full-coverage program using population data, the number of recipients is typically large, so even a modest improvement in the current value can lead to a statistically significant result. If the number of participants or recipients is small, as is likely in a partial-coverage program using data for only the program recipients, it is likely that an unrealistically large target would be needed to achieve statistical significance.

In the adolescent pregnancy example, the statistical test is based on more than 16,000 adolescents, so a reasonable target value of 33.5 would result in a significant result. In contrast, suppose that this method were to be used in a program serving only 500 adolescents. In this case, a target value of 14.0 would be required to result in statistically significant improvement—clearly an impossible target to meet. Statistical testing, then, should really be used as an aid to understanding what a reasonable target value might be, rather than for determining the target value per se.

Option 3 is to select a desired percentage decrease in the health problem or, conversely, a desired percentage increase in the healthy counterpart. This option is the most straightforward approach and can be understood intuitively by stakeholders. It can be used with health programs that are situated at any level in the public health pyramid and in any health domain. The percentage change can be chosen based on information gained from published literature, or it may merely be a hopeful guesstimate. The formula is as follows:

Target value = (% change desired $\times$ current value) $\pm$ current value

If trend data exist for the health outcome, then the percentage decrease (or increase) can be refined based on past and recent experience. The percentage change can be chosen to reflect either a continuation of the observed trend or a change in the trend (i.e., either an acceleration of improvement or a slowing of deterioration, depending on the health outcome of interest).

In the example of the adolescent birth rate, trend data indicate an average 2% annual decrease. Using this percentage in the formula for option 3, the target value for the birth rate per 1000 female adolescents is 36.8 per 1000 (see Figure 7.3). If program planners decide that a 4% decrease is more appropriate—that is, if they assume that the program can accelerate improvement—the target value for the birth rate per 1000 female adolescents would be 36.1. The target value chosen for this calculation is then used in the program objective as the "how much" value.

As this exercise reveals, although a 4% decrease in adolescent births may require considerable programmatic resources to achieve, the reduction in the rate may be barely noticeable. It may be useful to repeat the calculation with slightly different percentage changes and consider which elements in the organizational plan and service utilization plan would need to be modified to achieve those other percentage changes.

Option 4 is used when programs are ongoing, are multiyear projects, or are expected to have long-term effects. For such programs, the "by when" portion of the objective may be several years into the future. In this case, it becomes necessary to have annual target values that cumulatively reach the desired long-term target value. Essentially, the total amount of change is dispersed across the time period for the program. For this reason, the target values for each year will be affected by the anticipated length of the program and the starting or current value. Option 4 can be used for programs at any level of the public health pyramid, but it is appropriate only for objectives related to a long-term goal. To use option 4, health program planners' first decision is to select an existing benchmark or standard, such as a *Healthy People* objective that identifies the desired target value for the health problem that is to be achieved over the long term.

Calculating annual target values requires first estimating the amount of annual change needed to get close to the long-term target. This annual percentage change is then used in calculations like those in option 3 to find the target value for each subsequent year. The following set of formulas is used in sequence to carry out option 4:

Annual % change = [(long-term objective – current value) / current value] / number of years

Next-year target value = (annual % desired change × current value) ± current value

Subsequent-year target value = (annual % desired change × past year value) ± past year value

As seen in Figure 7.3, an annual 4% decrease results in an adolescent birth rate of 30.6 per 1000 at the end of five years, for an overall decrease of 7 births per 1000. This decline represents an 18.6% decrease in the birth rate among adolescents. In this example, a rate of 30 births per 1000 was the long-term objective; thus, using the method described here, the final target value was not exactly met because the rate of improvement was maintained at 4% each year. To reach the long-term objective, the rate of improvement would have to increase slightly each year. The question for discussion among the planning team, however, is whether a 4% decrease every year for five years is possible for the program, and whether the 18.6% decrease over five years will be acceptable to funding agencies and other stakeholders. Program planners must also consider whether the change can be identified using the methods currently chosen for use in the effect evaluation.

Options 5 through 10 are relevant for population-based and multisite programs when the data can be stratified, either by geographic area or by some characteristic such as age, race/ethnicity, or income. The adolescent pregnancy example is a population-based program, using data from all high schools in Bowe County as well as data on whether the adolescents' family income is below or above the poverty level. When stratification is used for target setting, the planners often assume that some sites may already have reached a very desirable level and, therefore, would not be expected to improve dramatically when the program is implemented. A corollary is that some sites will likely be drastically far from any target that might be set, which means they must make radical improvements to reach any reasonable target. The extent to which a site may already be at an ideal level warrants attention from the planning team and ought to be reflected in the logic statements and the subsequent decisions about selecting target values.

Option 5 sets the target value as the mean of the rates across the sites, and *option 6* sets the target value as the median of the rates across the sites. Options 5 and 6 are likely to give very similar target values, especially if the rates of the health outcome across the sites are normally distributed. Conversely, if there is not a normal distribution, they may not yield similar values. In the adolescent (females ages 15–17 years) birth rate example (see Figure 7.4), the county birth rates range from 11.3 per 1000 adolescent females to 62.4 per 1000 adolescent females, with the mean of all high school rates being 33.8 and the median being 31.0. A disadvantage of these two options is that they do not take into account the differing sizes of the target population in each group, such as in each county or in each clinic. If the sites have very different adolescent birth rates and target population sizes, and if those data are not normally distributed, then options 5 and 6 may not be the optimal approaches.

Options 7 and 8 take into account the population sizes in the area targeted by the program. The overall rate of 37.6 births per 1000 adolescent females for all schools combined (the value used in options 1 through 4 as the current value) is the mean for the whole population. Nevertheless, because it combines the data for all schools, it obscures the school-by-school information. Options 7 and 8, by contrast, also calculate overall current values; rather than using all schools, however, each option uses only a portion of the population with the "best" outcomes. Options 7 and 8 are based on the idea that the rate achieved by a certain portion of the target audience should be reachable by the whole target audience, so the target value ought to be set based on that existing rate.

Options 7 and 8 use what is called a "pared means method" (Kiefe et al., 1998). This approach reinforces the idea that the target value for a program should aim to move the entire target population to a value already achieved by a portion of the target population. In other words, for options 7 and 8, the target value for the objective would be for the adolescent birth rate in the schools to improve to match the birth rate already achieved by the schools encompassing 50% or 75% of adolescents.

The difference between options 7 and 8 lies in the proportion of the target population that is used to calculate the target value: option 7 is based on 50% of the target population, whereas option 8 is based on 75% of the target population. The pared means method can actually be used with any proportion of the target population. The higher the proportion, the easier it will be to reach the target; the lower the proportion, the more difficult achieving that the target will be. Choosing 50% means that half of the target population has already achieved the target but the other half will have to improve; choosing 75% is more conservative approach, because improvement will have to occur only in 25% of the population.

Continuing with the example, to calculate the target value according to option 7, program planners would take as many schools as necessary to incorporate 50% of all of the adolescents in the ten schools that have the lowest (best) birth rates. They would then calculate the overall birth rate for this subset of schools. In this example, the calculation must include six of the ten schools so as to include 50% of female adolescents. The calculation is as follows:

Target value = number with the health outcome in the top 50% / number in target population in the top 50%

Using these data gives a target value of 26.0 births per 1000, which is a 30.9% decrease from the overall, current rate of 37.6. In comparison, if the counties that have 75% of the adolescents are used in the calculation (option 8), then the target value is 29.9, or a 20.5% change.

Options 9 and 10 are examples of approaches to using stratified data (see Figure 7.5). If data are available on the health status or rates of groups within the target population, then it is possible to use those rates to calculate target values for those groups. Option 9 is simply an extension of the pared means method used in options 7 and 8; it uses the "best" rate of the two groups as the overall target. In contrast, option 10 starts with two separate targets, based on the two strata, by choosing different percentage decreases or increases for each. The different percentages chosen may reflect a more intense programmatic effort aimed at the group with the most urgent need for improvement. Thus distinct, stratum-specific targets are calculated, but these can then be combined into a single target value for the whole population by calculating an average weighted by the size of the population in each group. The formula for this calculation follows:

Target value$_{\text{Group 1}}$ = (% change desired $\times$ current value) $\pm$ current value

Target value$_{\text{Group 2}}$ = (% change desired × current value) ± current value

Overall target = (% of population in group 1 × Target value$_{\text{Group 1}}$)
  + (% of population in group 2 × Target value$_{\text{Group 2}}$)

In summary, a variety of techniques can be used to calculate the target value to be used in the effect objectives. Each calculation technique results in a different value (Table 7.9). In the example cited here, the potential target value for the rate of births to adolescents ranges from a low of 26.0 births per 1000 using option 7 to a high of 37.6, which is the current value, using option 1. This range of possible and reasonable target values underscores the importance of having a decisional framework for target setting, including developing

Table 7.9   Range of Target Values Derived from Options 1 Through 10, Based on the Data from Figures 7.3 Through 7.5

Option	Description	Resulting Target Value
1	Default, no change, overall rate	37.6
2	Result of statistical testing	33.5
3	Percentage change in health problem: based on trend data	36.8
4	Use existing benchmark or standard to project target values for several years: first-year target	36.1
5	Mean of rates across geography/sites	33.8
6	Median of rates across geography/sites	31.0
7	Overall rate for best 50%	26.0
8	Overall rate for best 75%	29.9
9	Rate for "best" stratum (i.e., adolescents not living in poverty)	33.8
10	Overall rate based on stratum-specific rates	36.0

explicit logic statements, to realistically define what constitutes the success or effectiveness of a health program.

Which target value is ultimately chosen depends on the program theory, the availability of resources, and the strength of the intervention. Although options 2 and 5 through 10 are best suited to population-based programs, they can be adapted to very large programs at the direct services and enabling services levels of the public health pyramid. To use these options, sufficient data must be available for each site and enough sites must have reasonable numbers in the groups. Options 3 and 4 are straightforward and can be used for any program.

CAVEATS TO THE GOAL-ORIENTED APPROACH

All aspects of planning, implementing, and evaluating a program are open for critique and reflection. Although goals and objectives may seem noncontroversial, at least three caveats highlight the need to be self-critical during these processes: the tenuous effectiveness of using objectives to guide work, the need for spontaneity, and the messy interface of objectives and performance measures.

First, the high degree of emphasis placed on having objectives—both process and effect—warrants some reflection on its history and a cursory review of the evidence of the usefulness of objectives. The concept of management by objectives (MBO) was developed and popularized in the 1950s by Peter Drucker, a management scholar, based on a theory of goal setting as being motivational for workers. MBO was subsequently adopted by the Nixon administration (Dahlsten, Styhre, & Willander, 2005), and it has since become an entrenched expectation, particularly in federal and state governmental agencies. The purpose of MBO is to motivate individuals to work toward a common organizational goal, thereby keeping the organization focused and internally well coordinated.

Since its introduction, relatively little research has focused on the effectiveness of MBO. Poister and Streib (1995), in a survey of governmental agencies, found that MBO is widely used but inconsistently implemented. Dinesh and Palmer (1998) commented that MBO is effective, but only when it has been implemented as intended. Specifically, they contended that MBO is unsuccessful in practice because it is partially implemented, and the human relations aspect of MBO has been forgotten over the years. As a consequence, MBO is seen as a older fad (Gibson & Tesone, 2001), albeit with some potential relevance for the present. The use of objectives as the basis for decision making, whether for a program or an organization, must be complemented and supplemented with attention to gaining staff acceptance of and support for the objectives, deploying human resources in a manner that supports the activities necessary to achieve the objectives, and using a reward system that makes achieving the objectives meaningful.

Second, being guided by goals and objectives is a logical, linear, systems approach to planning a health program. By contrast, the growing body of scientific literature on complexity theory suggests that in many workgroup settings, greater flexibility and spontaneity lead to more productive work teams. If a health program is being designed and provided in response to community needs and a controlled evaluation of the program is deemed unnecessary, then allowing for self-organizing teams could lead to a "better" program. This approach certainly will not be feasible for health programs that are, say, federally funded. Nonetheless, health program planners and managers may find situations in which less control—in other words less reliance on objectives—leads to a better program.

Finally, too often the list of objectives, once created, is forgotten and becomes disconnected from the ongoing program oversight. This is more likely to be the case for programs that emerge in response to community demands or are provided on an inconsistent basis. For the most part, in health care, health outcome objectives are linked to performance measures, which are used for quality improvement. The relationships among objectives, performance measures, and program monitoring are discussed in detail in Chapter 10.

ACROSS THE PYRAMID

At the direct services level of the public health pyramid, process objectives are likely to focus on how providers interact with program participants and how the program supports those providers in their involvement with the program. Effect objectives for programs at the direct services level will focus on individual client behavior or health status change. Setting targets for direct services programs may involve translating national objectives into local program objectives. Although national targets may or may not be appropriate for local programs, the national targets need to be considered at least as an accepted benchmark or goal.

At the enabling services level, in addition to the foci at the direct services level, process objectives are likely to include a focus on the involvement of community resources in the program, as well as emphasis on interagency collaboration and cooperation. Effect objectives for the enabling services level are likely to address changes in the behavior or health status of families and other aggregates, such as students in a school or residents of a public housing project. Setting targets for enabling services can be more challenging because national or state data regarding the problem being addressed likely will not exist. For enabling services, past experience, experiences of similar programs, and data from the community needs assessment may be the only data available for health program planners to use with a rational approach to setting the target numbers.

At the population services level, process objectives will need to include an emphasis on the coordination of efforts necessary to implement the health program, and on the garnering of adequate and appropriate resources to provide a population-based health program. The effect objectives can have either an outcome or impact focus, and the "who" portion will consist of the community or a specific population. Processes for setting targets for population-based services—particularly those provided to state and metropolitan populations—will draw heavily upon national data.

At the infrastructure level, process objectives will dominate. The infrastructure, by virtue of its nature, emphasizes developing and sustaining an organization and obtaining and managing the resources needed to implement a health program. Nonetheless, effect objectives can be written in relation to the infrastructure, most probably about the effectiveness and efficiency of services. For example, Allison, Kiefe, and Weissman (1999) proposed using a pared means benchmark method to arrive at a target value for the best-performing physicians in terms of patient outcomes. Effect objectives may also more directly apply to the infrastructure itself. For example, effect objectives might address impacts from and educational training for staff, or outcomes from employee screening programs.

DISCUSSION QUESTIONS AND ACTIVITIES

1. The organizational plan and the service utilization plan may include many elements and processes. What would you use as criteria for developing a set of objectives about the process theory? Would you set targets for process objectives?

2. For effect objectives at each level of the public health pyramid, which sources of data might be commonly used for establishing targets?

3. Imagine that you have been asked to explain to your colleagues in 10 minutes how to set targets for program objectives. Develop an outline of the steps involved.

4. Which of the ten options for setting targets would be best suited to developing targets for the other four health problems in Layetteville and Bowe County? Provide some rationale for your choice. Try using

your choice of target setting based on the following data: the adult immunization rate is 30%, with 25 hospitalizations per 1000 adults for influenza-related pneumonia; for children younger than 1 year old, the incidence of maltreatment is 14.0 per 1000 children (University of California at Berkeley Center for Social Services Research, http://cssr.berkeley.edu/CWSCMSreports); 1.2 adolescents are discharged with a diagnosis of gunshot wounds for every 1000 hospital admissions; the neural tube defects rate is 18 per 100,000 (National Center for Health Statistics); and new diagnosis of diabetes is 7.5 per 1000 (Centers for Disease Control and Prevention).

INTERNET RESOURCES

For fun, here are examples of goals and objectives related to natural resources:

The Indiana Department of Education

The Indiana Department of Education's document (pdf) on writing goals and objectives: http://www.prm.nau.edu/prm423/goals_and_objectives_lesson.htm.

A nifty checklist: http://ideanet.doe.state.in.us/sdfsc/pdf/writing-gos.pdf.

Taxonomy of Educational Objectives

Attention to Verbs: Bloom's Taxonomy (Bloom, B., et al. (1956). *Taxonomy of educational objectives: Handbook I: Cognitive domain.* New York: Longman) is a classic and worth knowing if the intervention relates to knowledge: http://www.roundworldmedia.com/cvc/module4/bloomtaxx.html.

Rapid Bi

This business-oriented page on writing SMART objectives has some useful tips: http://www.rapidbi.com/created/WriteSMARTobjectives.html.

REFERENCES

Allison, J., Kiefe, C. I., & Weissman, N. W. (1999). Can data-driven benchmarks be used to set the goals of *Healthy People 2010? American Journal of Public Health, 89*(1), 61–65.

Dahlsten, F., Styhre, A., & Willander, M. (2005). The unintended consequences of management by objectives: The volume growth target at Volvo Cars. *Leadership and Organization Development Journal, 26,* 529–541.

Dinesh, D., & Palmer, E. (1998). Management by objectives and the Balanced Scorecard: Will Rome fall again? *Management Decision, 36,* 363–369.

Friedman, V. J., Rothman, J., & Withers, B. (2006). The power of why: Engaging the goal paradox in program evaluation. *American Journal of Evaluation, 27,* 201–218.

Gibson, J. W., & Tesone, D. V. (2001). Management fads: Emergence, evolution, and implications for managers. *Academy of Management Executive, 15,* 122–133.

Kiefe, C. I., Weissman, N. W., Allison, J., Farmer, R., Weaver, M., & Williams, O. D. (1998). Identifying achievable benchmarks of care: Concepts and methodology. *International Journal for Quality in Health Care, 10*(5), 443–447.

Kotelchuck, M. (1997). Adequacy of prenatal care utilization. *Epidemiology, 8,* 602–604.

Maternal and Child Health Bureau of the Health Resources and Services Administration. (n.d.) *Title V Information System.* Retrieved February 3, 2008, from https://perfdata.hrsa.gov/mchb/mchreports/Search/core/MeasureIndicatorMenu.asp

Patton, M. Q. (1997). *Utilization-focused evaluation* (3rd ed.). Thousand Oaks, CA: Sage Publications.

Poister, T. H., & Streib, G. (1995). MBO in municipal government: Variations on a traditional management tool. *Public Administrative Review, 55,* 48–57.

Rosenberg, D. (1999). *Performance and outcome measurement: Methods for setting annual targets.* Retrieved October 17, 2007, from http://www.uic.edu/sph/cade/citymatch99/targets/slideshow/sld001.htm

Implementing and Monitoring the Health Program

CHAPTER 8

Program Implementation

Implementation of the health program requires acquiring and overseeing adequate resources to provide the program in a manner that is consistent with the program theory and purpose of the program. The amount of effort needed at each stage of the planning and evaluation cycle varies throughout that cycle. Implementation of the health program requires the most and longest sustained effort of all the phases of a health program (Figure 8.1).

This chapter introduces the logistics associated with managing a health program, with special attention being paid to budgeting and general managerial issues. These logistics fall within the organizational plan and the services utilization plan portions of the process theory (Figure 8.2). The operational logistics of implementing a program tend to be straightforward but do require attention to ensure proper implementation of the health program.

Health programs are projects that can be viewed as miniature organizations. In the management literature, the organizational plan and the services utilization plan would be considered elements of the tactical plan. A common frame of reference for thinking about organizations and health programs is to consider inputs, throughputs, outputs, and outcomes (Turnock, 2009). In the process theory, various inputs into both the organizational plan and the services utilization plan are specified. In addition, specific outputs of both the organizational plan and the services utilization plan are expected. Distinguishing between the inputs and outputs of these plans aids in acquiring the appropriate resources and in being able to communicate both programmatic needs and successes. The chapter concludes by relating the various process theory elements to the logic model format.

ORGANIZATIONAL PLAN INPUTS

The organizational plan encompasses the program inputs and resources, as well as the way in which those resources are organized. The type and amount

Figure 8.1   Amount of Effort Across the Life of a Health Program

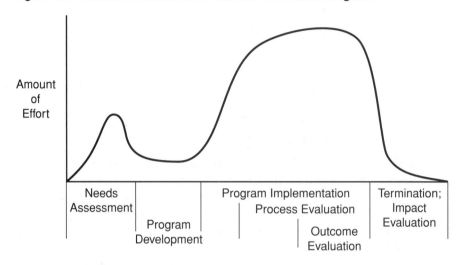

of resources required for a health program vary with the interventions to be used. Nonetheless, the expertise of personnel, the characteristics of the target audience, and the degree of attention to acquiring and managing resources all affect the potential to have a successful program. The organizational plan objectives serve as a guide to which are the most critical organizational plan activities for implementing a health program. Many aspects of the organizational plan will not be in the organizational plan objectives, yet still need to be addressed. This section presents an overview of the key inputs and outlines the rationale for considering them as key.

Human Resources

Human resources encompass the quantity and quality of personnel needed to carry out the program, in terms of their expertise, experience, and capabilities. Human resources come at a cost, of course, and personnel costs are almost always the largest portion of any program budget. The dollar cost of personnel includes not only wages (amount paid hourly) or salaries (amount paid monthly), but also fringe benefits as a percentage of the wage or salary. Estimating the dollar cost of personnel is a rather straightforward arithmetic problem, as explained later in the discussion of budgeting.

Figure 8.2 Diagram of the Process Theory Elements Showing the Components of the Organizational Plan and Services Utilization Plan

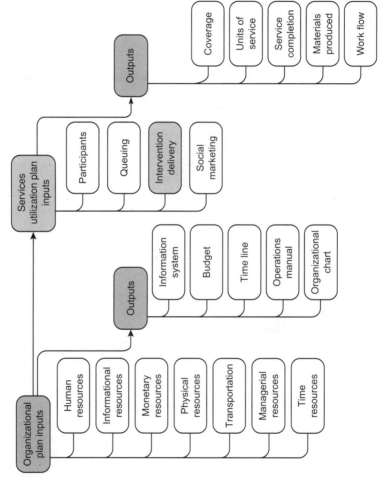

Licensure and Statutory Regulation of Health Professionals

In Chapter 2, Table 2.3 lists the major health professionals who are likely to be managing or delivering health programs. Table 8.1 builds on that information by indicating whether individuals from each of the health disciplines are subject to legal and state statutory regulation with regard to their practice. The legal parameters of practice for each of the licensed health disciplines ought to influence who is hired into which position. Some familiarity with the state regulations of scope of practice is important for matching the program needs

Table 8.1   List of Health Professionals with a Summary of Typical Legal and Regulatory Considerations

Health Discipline	State Licensure Required	State Regulation of Scope of Practice	Professional Certification Exists
Dentistry	Yes	Yes	Yes
Community health worker	No	No	Certificate programs
Dietitian	Yes, as Registered Dietitian	Yes	Yes
Health administration	No (except for long-term care administration)	No	Yes
Health education	No	No	Yes
Industrial hygiene	Yes	Yes	Yes
Medicine	Yes	Yes	Yes
Nursing	Yes, as Registered Nurse	Yes	Yes
Physical therapy	Yes	Yes	Yes
Social work	Varies	Yes, for those with licensure	Yes

with the qualifications of program personnel. In addition, for some health disciplines, professional associations oversee certification of individuals. For some health programs, it may be wise or important to ensure that the program services are provided by individuals with specialty certification, which serves as an indicator of advanced or specialized knowledge and skills.

Training for Program Delivery

Training staff and volunteers for their roles in the program implementation is a key aspect of human resources management. Training costs include both staff time for this activity and the trainer's time. In addition, costs are incurred for the materials used during training, such as handouts, equipment, or audiovisual materials. These costs may quickly mount, but such training is nevertheless necessary for ensuring the standardized delivery of the program interventions. Without this standardization of the intervention through training, the actual intervention delivered can deviate from what was intended program, depending on the personal preferences of the individuals providing the intervention. In other words, training helps align the theory-in-use and the espoused theory with the effect theory. This has serious implications for achieving the desired outcomes and, subsequently, for ensuring the long-term sustainability of the program.

Training is also necessary to maintain the morale and self-efficacy of the staff. Receiving training helps program staff members feel valued, trusted, and capable of providing the interventions. These feelings contribute to the sense of having a higher ability to carry out the intervention as designed—in other words, they promote greater task self-efficacy. This is an especially important ingredient in the delivery of a complex intervention to a target and recipient audience that is resistant or difficult to change.

A separate consideration with regard to human resources is workforce cultural diversity. As health programs are increasingly targeted to audiences with specific cultural and racial characteristics, it becomes important that program staff are not only culturally competent with regard to the target audience, but more ideally are members of the target audience. While having program personnel who are culturally diverse may help in the delivery of the intervention, it can sometimes lead to other problematic issues among staff members. Program managers must be attentive to signs of interracial or cross-cultural tensions among program personnel and address these issues as soon as they surface.

Volunteers as Human Resources

Community involvement in the development and implementation of health programs can occur through the establishment of advisory committees and boards, councils, or consortia. Through such groups, community members have a formal venue through which to participate in the program delivery. To maximize the benefits of having these groups, the best are considered or approached as being volunteers and human resources input.

Volunteers are widely used to deliver health program interventions. For example, volunteers have delivered a physical activity program for women in Iran (Pazoki, Nabipour, Seyednezami, & Imami, 2007), provided free surgery to children with physical abnormalities in Nevada (Landis & Loar, 2007), and collected evaluation data for a school hand washing program in Illinois (Tousman et al., 2007).

The use of volunteers in health programs makes them a key human resource requiring particular attention, especially if they create a synergy between themselves and the program recipients (Hintgen, Radichel, Clark, Sather, & Johnson, 2000). In other words, volunteers gain from the experience even as participants benefit from their service in terms of personal attention. Evidence suggests that use of volunteers who are peers of the program recipients (in other words, volunteers who are themselves members of the target audience) may lead to a greater achievement of desired health outcomes than would the use of professionals (Schafer, Vogel, Viegas, & Hausafus, 1998).

Volunteers are motivated by factors that are different from those that motivate paid employees. Altruism is a major motivation to be a volunteer (Bowen, Kuniyuki, Shattuck, Nixon, & Sponzo, 2000; Roessler, Carter, Campbell, & MacLeod, 1999). Other motivators include personal gains in terms of pre-employment experience and references, being accepted by the program staff, being valued as an important team member (Roessler et al., 1999), and having personal concerns related to the health condition that is the subject of the intervention (Bowen et al., 2000). Older adults are likely to perceive the opportunity to engage in a new endeavor as the strongest reason to volunteer, although a sense of life satisfaction, a need to be productive, and social interaction are also important reasons to volunteer (Morrow-Howell, Kinnevy, & Mann, 1999).

Recruitment of volunteers can be accomplished through a variety of techniques. In a study of volunteers for one cancer prevention program, Bowen and associates (2000) found that half of the volunteers were recruited through media, such as television, radio, or newspapers, and from work-related sources. Although these methods are similar to those used to recruit employees, the messages for recruiting volunteers will be different. Specifically, these messages will focus on motivating factors such as those mentioned previously.

Despite having sincere and honorable motives, volunteers often come without adequate training or experience with the target audience. This makes training volunteers particularly critical to the success of the health program.

Volunteers need not only the skills to effectively implement the intervention, but also emotional support in dealing with challenging clients and knowledge about the clients and the health condition. Volunteers in programs for high-risk clients may be particularly vulnerable themselves, including being subject to police harassment (Bluthenthal, Heinzerling, Anderson, Flynn, & Kral, 2008). Another human resources issue arises from the fact that the source of satisfaction and work-related stress are different for volunteers than for employees (Ferrari, Luhrs, & Lyman, 2007).

One issue germane to community health programs and the use of volunteers was identified in the study by Trettin and Musham (2000), who found a difference between program developers and community volunteers in their perceptions of the role of volunteers. This finding hints at an undercurrent in the relationship between program planners and the community—namely, the perception that individuals are being exploited under the guise of being volunteers. This undercurrent will be more evident and influential in determining the success of a health program in some communities.

Physical Resources

Physical resources include material resources, facilities, supplies, and equipment (Kettner, Moroney, & Martin, 1999).

Material resources are those tangible items that are needed to provide the intervention and to provide program support. Intervention equipment might, for example, include blood pressure cuffs, syringes, or imaging machines. Space—usually called facilities—is another material resource needed for both the intervention and the program support. The costs associated with having or renting a classroom, auditorium, community meeting room, waiting room, examination room, and offices need to be taken into account. *Supplies* constitute another material cost. They encompass miscellaneous office supplies (i.e., paper, stationery, pens, clips, computer supplies), specific resources for program staff (i.e., journal subscriptions, resource or reference manuals), and any items needed related to the intervention (i.e., tote bags, clip boards, stop watches, Band-Aids, flip charts). Physical resources may be needed for the evaluation as well—generally office supplies and storage space for data collected. Maintaining adequate supplies, without hoarding, is the function of inventory control; having too many unused supplies drains monetary resources that may be needed for other expenses.

A large category of physical resources is office equipment: computers, printers, cables, fax machines, and photocopiers. If the costs of these items exceed an amount set by the organization, the purchase of the item will be considered a capital expense and will require special approval and possibly special ordering procedures. Also, some funding agencies look unfavorably on the purchase of standard office equipment if it exceeds a certain amount. For these reasons, many program managers minimize purchases that are considered capital expenditures.

Transportation

Transportation is a separate type of resource and expense. Transportation must be thought of from the perspective of program staff and program participants. For staff, the issue is one of reimbursement for any travel related to providing the program. For example, if the health program includes an outreach component, then staff members need to carefully document their mileage or keep track of expenditures for public transportation. From the perspective of program participants, the issue is accessibility of the program site given the usual mode of transportation used by potential program participants. Thus, in a rural program the transportation issue might be one of travel time required to get to the program site, whereas in an urban program the issue might be proximity to a major mass-transit stop.

Informational Resources

Computer hardware and software costs are always included in the budget, usually as physical resources. By contrast, information is a key intangible resource. The knowledge and expertise of the staff must be viewed as a resource to be managed. Increasingly, information possessed by individuals is being considered an asset for the organization and more managerial attention is being devoted to managing knowledge as resource (Freeze & Kulkami, 2007; Orzano, Tallia, McInerney, McDaniel, & Crabtree, 2007).

Information as a resource can be present in the form of professional networks, street smarts that affect program implementation, and professional knowledge and experience. Staff members bring their professional knowledge to the program, and they gain additional knowledge through the training sessions. In terms of health programs, this means the knowledge held by employees involved in the program is valuable to the implementation of the program.

As staff become more qualified for other positions based on their knowledge and experience, it can become difficult to retain those personnel. Consequently, retention of such employees is a key issue for health programs and represents another reason to make efforts to keep the program personnel satisfied with their jobs and the organization. Loss of staff is not just an issue of replacing personnel, but rather is more appropriately thought of as replacing knowledge and expertise—hence the importance of maximizing staff retention and minimizing unplanned staff turnover.

Time

Time generally translates into personnel costs, but it must also be thought of as a separate resource. Time is relevant to the overall timeline for program design and implementation. The sequencing of events, especially in the start-up phase of a program, is very time dependent. Any delay in accomplishing one step could easily affect the overall timeline. If meeting a start date is essential, then additional personnel resources may be required during the start-up phase, which in turn will affect the budget. Time also affects the budget in less obvious ways through depreciation, inflation, and interest. These points are discussed later in this chapter as part of planning via budgets.

Managerial Resources

The qualities and characteristics of the managerial personnel are also key resources. When selecting the project manager, Posner (1995) suggests considering the skills required of a person in the position—namely, organizational abilities, communication skills, team-building skills, leadership qualities, coping skills related to managing complex and ambiguous tasks and environments, and technical skills related to the health program intervention.

Organizational abilities include not only the logistics of juggling multiple tasks and persons, but also the ability to keep track of important dates and information. The ideal program manager will also be able to manage the project in terms of structuring the relationships among project personnel, as is usually reflected in organizational charts that identify the flow of communication, delegation, and responsibilities. A somewhat different, but equally crucial aspect of organizational abilities is the understanding of how the health program fits within the parent organization, and the knowledge of how to position the program for success within the parent organization.

Communication skills are not just the ability to communicate verbally with peers, but also the ability to guide discussions, to communicate nonverbal messages that are consistent with verbal messages, and, perhaps most importantly, to listen and appreciate various points of view. In addition, written communication skills are essential for a health program manager to function in the larger context of grant writing, report generation, and e-mail communication. Another facet of communication skills is the ability to understand who needs what and when. This communication skill is closely linked to the creation and manipulation of information so as to have an effective and efficient health program.

Negotiation is a major component of communication skills required of program managers. During this process, two or more parties reach a decision despite having different preferences with regard to the options (Bazerman, 2005). Much research about negotiation has revealed what we know about how people think and respond to information. Three pieces of information are needed in any negotiation: each party's best alternative to the negotiated agreement, analysis of all the interests of each party, and the relative importance of each party's interests. Armed with this information, the negotiator enters into a process in which strategies are used to arrive at an agreement by breaking out of the existing definitions of differences. These strategies include many actions commonly encountered in good communication—specifically, building trust, asking questions, strategically disclosing information, and simultaneously making many offers (Bazerman, 2005). Program managers will negotiate not only with funding agencies, but also with program staff and community stakeholders. Thus a rudimentary understanding of negotiation techniques is important.

Team building is another essential managerial skill, especially for health programs that are participatory, community-based, or multidisciplinary in nature. Mobilization of a group, fostering group cohesion, and facilitation of teamwork are all key elements of team building. Information about team building and teamwork can be found in both the lay managerial literature available at most bookstores and professional management journals. Managers must consciously attend to the quality of interactions within teams and the quantity of teamwork. Problems can arise quickly, of course, and they must be addressed expeditiously. Otherwise, the team can become dysfunctional and drain resources, rather than being a resource itself.

One critical aspect of team building is the use of stories. As program staff begin to develop as a team, stories will be told about clients, about managers, and about events. These stories, which are ubiquitous in most organizations, serve the function of building team norms and establishing communication among the team members.

Leadership is the ability to inspire and motivate others into action that is purposeful and organized. Program managers are rarely thought of as leaders, yet they must motivate staff, serve as role models of productivity, and generate enthusiasm for the health program. As a consequence, program managers need to be knowledgeable about the motivational process in regard to both staff members and program participants. Motivation of program staff results in all members doing what they were hired to do in a timely, efficient, and high-quality manner.

The technical skills required of program managers consist of skills related to the health program intervention. In most health programs, the manager must have basic scientific or practice knowledge about the health problem and the type of interventions that are provided. In some situations, program staff, program participants, or funding agencies may not view the health program favorably if the program manager does not have some professional credibility. Technical skills are also necessary to supervise the program staff adequately and ensure the integrity of the program intervention.

Monetary Resources

Monetary resources are generally listed on the income side of a balance sheet or budget, because they comprise funding and income generated through fees and billing. Monetary donations are another resource that needs to tracked and included in accounting records. However, if participants are given any cash for participation, then monetary resources are placed on the expense side of the budget.

ORGANIZATIONAL PLAN OUTPUTS

Not all inputs into the organizational plan will be directly linked to specific organizational plan outputs; some will be linked to services utilization plan outputs. The following outputs are examples of outputs that could be measured or at least documented as effective use of the organizational plan inputs.

Time Line

A *time line* is a way to graphically represent the dates, time span, and sequence of events involved in planning, initiating, sustaining, and evaluating the health program. Time lines vary from simple to highly intricate. At a minimum, the time line ought to reflect the activities necessary, be related to the expenses detailed in the budget, and be easily understood by those who will use it (Exhibit 8.1). A time line can be created by using the table function in a word processing program, a spreadsheet, or specific project management software. This communication tool conveys deadlines, helps keep activities coordinated and sequenced, communicates accountability for assigned tasks, and helps program managers estimate personnel and material costs.

Operations Manual

The *operations manual* contains the policies, procedures, guidelines, and protocols related to the health program. It also includes job descriptions and workplace polices and procedures.

Exhibit 8.1   Example of an Abbreviated Time Line for a Short-Term Health Program, Created with the Table Function in Microsoft Word

Activity	Month											
	1	2	3	4	5	6	7	8	9	10	11	12
Convene program planning group	▓											
Conduct community needs and asset assessment	▓	▓										
Translate assessment information into health problem statement and objectives		▓	▓									
Formulate program theory; articulate process theory		▓	▓									
Initiate institutional process regarding human subjects' protection				▓	▓							
Advertise for program personnel				▓	▓							
Hire and train program personnel				▓	▓							
Advertise the health program (social marketing)						▓						
Deliver the health program							▓	▓	▓	▓		
Conduct process evaluation							▓	▓	▓	▓		
Conduct outcome evaluation								▓	▓	▓		
Analyze evaluation data										▓		
Produce reports				▓								▓
Disseminate findings												▓

One element of many health program operations manuals will be a section on safety. For both staff and participants, safety is an issue—safety not only in their cars as they are coming to or from the program site, but also on the street surrounding the program site. In particular, if program staff are outreach workers, their safety must be considered. In such a case, safety strategies need to be part of workers' job training and procedures related to their work.

Organizational Chart

Most organizations construct some sort of graphic representation to depict the relationships among work units, departments, and individuals. As a result of having personnel designated to the health program and having program accountability, health programs will have their own organizational chart. One aspect of the health program organizational chart that may be different from the organizational charts of other work units is the inclusion of any community-based consortium or council that serves as an advisory committee to the health program. Inclusion of such groups is important because it reflects, in a legitimate and visible fashion, the involvement of the community in the health program.

Also, the health program ought to be identified specifically within the appropriate organizational chart. For health programs that are population based, such as state child health insurance, the program ought to appear somewhere in the organizational chart of the state agency. The program also ought to be included in the organizational charts of the community organizations involved in promoting or providing the program.

Information System

The information system has outputs that are part of the organizational plan. Upgraded hardware and software are outputs, just as are reconfigured and programmed computers that accommodate data generated by the health program. New report capacities are also information system outputs.

Budget

Budgets are mechanisms for planning and tools for communicating and refining priorities. They are projections of dollar amounts that enable the program planner to assess the fiscal feasibility of doing a project. Developing a budget for a program highlights which programmatic changes may be needed for the health program to be fiscally responsible and efficient. For example, changes might be needed in the size of the program so that a more efficient participant-to-staff ratio is achieved.

Each organization will have its own particular format for developing budgets, and it may potentially use special software for this task. The financial officer in the organization will set forth the rules and accounting specifics used across programs and departments within the organization. This chapter discusses only the more general budget principles that apply across formats and organizations. The intent here is to introduce basic program budget concepts so that health program planners and managers can communicate with financial personnel, funding agencies, and administrators in a manner that presents the program in a positive light.

Budgeting Terminology

The broadest categories within budgets are expenditures and revenues. Expenditures are classified in various ways: as fixed or variable and as direct or indirect.

Fixed costs do not vary with the number of clients served. Examples of fixed costs include rent, salaries of administrative personnel, and insurance costs. In contrast, *variable costs* do vary with the number of clients served. Examples of variable costs include copying program handouts, program advertising, and refreshments for participants. Depending on how the health program is designed and implemented and how the organization does its accounting, certain costs may be counted as fixed or variable. For example, if program staff are paid regardless of how many clients show up, then personnel wages and salaries represent a fixed cost. Conversely, if the program uses staff on a part-time, as-needed basis, then personnel costs are variable. Budgets prepared based on the distinction between variable and fixed costs are more likely to be useful for program management via fiscal monitoring and for later conducting economic and accounting analyses of the program.

Another way to think about costs is as direct or indirect. In the purest sense, *direct costs* reflect those resources that are used directly in the delivery of the program. Generally, the wages and salaries of staff providing the intervention are a direct cost, as are materials or supplies used with clients. Similarly, in the purest sense, *indirect costs* are those costs not associated with the delivery of the program, but more generally with supporting the program. Utility bills, telephone charges, and staff travel expenses to present the program at scientific conferences are all examples of indirect costs. Indirect costs associated with overhead expenses (e.g., rent, utility, facilities management, shared clerical support staff, office equipment) are typically estimated based on a standard rate that is set by the program funding agency or the organization's financial officer. Indirect costs, as a percentage of direct costs, can vary from 8% as limited by funding agencies up to 51%. Given this wide range, it is important to obtain the correct rate at which indirect costs should be applied to the expenditure side of the budget.

In developing a budget for planning a program, Foster, Johnson-Shelton, and Taylor (2007) remind us that costs associated with time are very important. In their work, they estimated the costs associated with participant recruitment time, staff training time, intervention time of staff and participants, and time of volunteers. The need for this level of detail can be anticipated and the actual expenditures tracked as the program is delivered.

Identifying revenues is a bit simpler. Funds for health programs come mostly from grants from funding agencies, fees collected from program participants, reimbursements from third-party payers, or charitable fund raising. Revenues might also be matched from state or federal agencies for local dollars allocated to the health program. A critical distinction is made between the cost of a service and the charge for that service. The *cost* of the service is the simple sum of all resources required to provide the service. However, clients are asked to pay more than the cost; *charges* typically include the cost plus a profit margin and administrative costs. When budgeting, the program planners must consider both the cost of the service and the charges, given that ultimately the charges influence participation and acceptance of the program.

One source of revenue is often invisible: in-kind donations. Those services are provided to the program free of charge, but the program would have to pay for them if they were not donated. A common example is printing costs given as an in-kind donation; volunteer time is another in-kind donation for staff time. In some not-for-profit agencies, the in-kind donations can be substantial. It is important to track these revenue sources for two reasons. One, use of in-kind donations is looked upon favorably by funding agencies as an indication of community support for the program. Second, if adequate in-kind donations are not received, a contingency plan for paying for those services must be developed and implemented.

Most grant proposal budgets focus on the major categories of direct costs. However, some federal funding agencies have begun to ask for budgets that are more directly linked to the program objectives, while others ask for budgets broken out by levels in the public health pyramid. Such budgets enable the funding agencies and program managers to determine the merit of the budget in terms of what is planned and which outcomes are anticipated. While creating such a budget can be challenging and require some degree of speculation, assigning costs per program objective can be a powerful motivational and managerial tool.

Break-Even Analysis

After the program budget is complete and nearly final, it is possible to do a break-even analysis. A *break-even analysis* is the mathematical determination of the point at which the expenses related to providing the program are equal to or less than the revenues generated for or from the program. This type of analysis uses the price of the service (the charge), the variable costs of program, and the fixed costs of the program. The rather straightforward formula (Finkler, Ward, & Baker, 2007) for a break-even analysis follows:

$$\text{Quantity of services} = \frac{\text{fixed cost}}{(\text{price per client} - \text{variable cost per client})}$$

When the total fixed costs associated with the program are divided by the difference between the amount charged per participant and the variable cost per participant, the result gives the number of services that need to be provided to break-even. Exhibit 8.2 is a narrative example of a break-even quest, and Exhibit 8.3 is the analysis done using a spreadsheet program, Microsoft Excel.

Even programs provided by not-for-profit agencies would be wise to conduct a break-even analysis. This rudimentary process provides useful insights into the amount of funding needed. Unfortunately, all too often public agencies

---

Exhibit 8.2   Example of a Break-Even Analysis

Layetteville's Lighthouse Agency has decided to implement an updated evidence-based program, Bright Light II, to address self-care for elderly diabetes patients, based on the needs identified during the community health assessment. In the past, Lighthouse billed Medicaid and insurance companies $75 for a similar service (Bright Light I, which focuses on community education on diabetes) and plans to charge the same for Bright Light II. Operational expenses for Bright Light I for the past year totaled $4300, but Bright Light II will share those fixed costs with Bright Light I.

Because Bright Light II is an intensive educational program and Lighthouse tries to have a consistent ratio of teachers to clients, the number of teachers varies with the number of clients. For every ten clients, Lighthouse employs one teacher, at a salary of $500. Lighthouse can provide classes to only 100 clients per year.

Based on this information, how many clients must be served, billed, and pay for Bright Light II services if the program is to break even? What recommendation would you make to Lighthouse?

Exhibit 8.3   Example of a Break-Even Analysis for Bright Light II on an Excel Spreadsheet

	A	B	C	D	E	F
1	**Fixed Costs (annual)**		$4,300			
2	Rent	$2,000				
3	Clerical support	$1,200				
4	Cleaning service	$500				
5	Financial service	$600				
6						
7	**Revenue**					
8	Charge per class	$100				
9						
10	**Variable Costs**		$5,000			
11	Teacher per class	$500				
12	Max students per class	10				
13						
14	Quantity to break even = fixed costs / (price per class – variable cost per class)					
15	Quantity to break even = (C1) / (B8 – (C10/100))					
16	Quantity to break even = 86					
17						
18	Lighthouse needs to decide whether to have 9 or 8 classes.					
19						
20				9 classes	8 classes	
21		**Formula**		*Option A*	*Option B*	
22	Fixed costs	C1		$4,300	$4,300	
23	Variable costs	# classes * B11		$4,500	$4,000	
24	Expense subtotal			$8,800	$8,300	
25						
26	Revenue	# classes * 10		$9,000	$8,000	
27		students * $100				
28	Balance	Revenue – expenses	$200	–$300		
29	Conclusion: Assuming that the classes are full with 10 clients, Lighthouse loses money if it chooses Option B (fewer classes) but makes a little money with Option A (more classes).					

and public programs neglect their fiscal accountability and efficiency accountability by not conducting a break-even analysis. If clients are not paying for services, as is often the case in public health programs or mass-media campaigns,
the price an individual might be willing to pay for the service or other such
information can be used in place of the charge or price. For example, if residents of a community are willing to pay only $0.10 for information on how to
prevent sexually transmitted diseases, then a "safe sex" mass-media campaign
will need to reach a very high number of persons to theoretically break even.

Thinking in terms of break-even analysis may seem unethical or contrary
to the public health ethic. A break-even analysis would not be appropriate for
health services that are required to ensure the health and safety of a population, such as a program to ensure that persons infected with tuberculosis take
their medications or a national infant immunization program. In programs
such as these, program participants are not expected to pay and thus the revenue portion of the break-even equation is zero. However, a break-even analysis
could be conducted to understand the fiscal implications of these programs. In
reality, use of a break-even analysis is a fiscally responsible way to make decisions among programs or programmatic options. It also provides a quantifiable
rationale for proceeding or modifying a health program. Importantly, a break-
even analysis may reveal that additional funding is required to provide the program as intended; it is far better to identify this potential problem before the
program is initiated.

Budget for Evaluation

The budget must also include expenses related to the program evaluation.
Whether the program staff will be involved in the evaluation activities or
whether a consultant is hired, funds must be allocated to support the evaluation before the program begins. Retrospectively acquiring funds to conduct an
evaluation can be difficult. In general, program grant proposals and budgets
that do not include evaluation funds receive lower-priority scores.

Evaluation expenses generally fall into the same categories as program
expenses, although material expenses are typically limited to supplies and
copying costs. Incentives given to individuals to participate in the evaluation
can account for a substantial portion of the evaluation budget. As with program
costs, personnel will usually be the largest expense. At a minimum, a meaningful evaluation cannot be done for less than 10% of the direct program costs.

Budget Justification

Budget justification is a requirement for virtually all grant proposals,
although the degree of detail expected varies by funding agency. A safe rule of
thumb is to provide a very detailed budget justification; more detailed budget

justifications demonstrate a more thorough program implementation and evaluation plan. Most budget justifications involve some narrative explanation of why the dollar amounts are requested, but they must also include fairly detailed arithmetic formulas that show the derivation of specific costs. For example, budget narratives typically show the cents per mile paid to staff for travel, the estimated number of miles staff are expected to travel, and the number of staff members traveling those miles. Even if a health program is being sponsored by the parent organization, a budget justification is typically presented to departmental administrators or advising boards when requesting their support.

SERVICES UTILIZATION PLAN INPUTS

Social Marketing

Kotler and Zaltman (1971) were the first authors to advocate social marketing as a method to reach a wide audience with health or social messages. Subsequently, Walsh, Rudd, Moeykens, and Moloney (1993) defined *social marketing* as the design, implementation, and control of the program calculated to influence the acceptability of social ideas.

Social marketing adapts the four P's of classical marketing: product, price, place, and promotion. *Product* refers to the service, tangibles, or ideas that are delivered with the intent of being beneficial to the target audience. Social marketing focuses on the beneficial aspect and understanding from the perspective of the recipient how those benefits are valued and perceived. *Price* in social marketing is the cost, of any type, that poses a barrier to accessing or using the product. Price considerations focus not only on the charge for the service, but also on the secondary costs, such as transportation or loss of peer group status. *Place* refers to where the product is available, whether it is in a clinic, on a billboard, or in a convenient location within a store. Making the product accessible, convenient, and visible are qualities of place that merit attention. *Promotion* is the more visible publicity type of activities, including paid media, public service media, and word-of-mouth sharing by opinion leaders. Social marketing goes beyond these classic four P's to include other P's, such as partnership and policy.

As applied to health programs, social marketing is also called health marketing (CDC, 2008). These principles from social marketing have been used successfully in a variety of health educational programs to get the health program to the target audience. In this way, the development and implementation of the social marketing strategy serve as an input into the service utilization plan, because that strategy enables the health program to reach the target audience.

Eligibility Screening

One of the first decisions facing program planners is to define for whom the program is designed. Although general agreement may exist about who is the focus of the program based on the needs assessment and the logic model, further specificity is required. The *target population* is the entire population in need of the program, whereas the *target audience* is the segment of the population for whom the program is specifically intended. The term *recipient* is used to refer to those individuals who actually receive or participate in the program.

For programs at the population level of the public health pyramid, the target population is also the target audience and, ideally, the recipients. At the direct services and enabling services levels of the pyramid, however, no program can hope to accommodate all those persons in need; thus the program may be designed for a subpopulation. For such programs, "target audience" is a better term.

The distinction between the target population or audience and the recipients is critical in terms of both budgetary issues and program implementation and evaluation issues. The program can have an impact only on the recipients, so the evaluation will focus primarily on this group. Nevertheless, planners also need to quantify the broader target audience to estimate underinclusion and overinclusion in the program and describe how these variations may influence the evaluation.

Inclusion: Underinclusion and Overinclusion

Ideally, only members of the target audience would receive the program. In reality, this ideal can be difficult to achieve, resulting in overinclusion or underinclusion of individuals in the program.

Overinclusion occurs when some participants in the program are not part of the target audience. It can be minimized by developing procedures to correctly exclude individuals who are not members of the target audience. For example, in a dental sealant program, children who are younger than 2 years of age, as well as children who are between the ages of 5 and 14 and who already had sealant treatment, might be excluded to avoid overinclusion.

Underinclusion occurs when some members of the target audience do not receive the program. It can be minimized by developing procedures to correctly include members of the target audience for whom the program is designed. Underinclusion in the dental sealant program would be seen as having fewer children of the appropriate age receive the dental sealant than the number of children of that age who need the sealant and who are within the catchment area of the dental clinic. Underinclusion can occur if the program is not well publicized, if some characteristic of the program is unappealing to the target audience, or if a barrier prevents members of the target audience from accessing the program.

Neither overinclusion nor underinclusion is desirable, and the program should be tailored to avoid both possibilities. In terms of program expenditures, overinclusion can result in a shortage of funds, whereas underinclusion can result in unspent funds that may need to be returned to the funding agency. Underinclusion and overinclusion are also undesirable from the perspective of the program evaluation.

Providing services to individuals who do not need the program (overinclusion) can decrease the measurable effect of the program on participant outcomes. That is, the extent of change experienced by those individuals who do not need the program is likely to be less than that experienced by those individuals who do need the program. This diffusion of the program's effects will translate into a decrease in the average amount or degree of change found when all participants in the program are considered. In addition, overinclusion may artificially inflate the normative need for the program. If current enrollment or requests for participation in the program are used for future planning of the program, overinclusion will falsely increase the apparent number in the target audience. Overinclusion also can lead to a decreased availability of funds to include true target individuals in the program. This result is particularly likely if members of the true target audience are more likely not to be the first persons to enroll in the program.

Underinclusion can also affect evaluation results, particularly for programs designed for and delivered at the population level. Having too few members of the target audience in the program: (1) could make it difficult to find significant small-numbers effects; (2) could increase the amount of program services received by individual participants and thereby falsely inflate the program effects; and (3) will definitely increase the cost per participant. At any level of the public health pyramid, underinclusion can lead to biased evaluation results if members of the target audience who do and do not participate in the program differ from one another in ways that are related to the program's effectiveness.

Several steps can be taken to help minimize overinclusion or underinclusion. The first step comes in developing the process theory, in terms of specifying how those in need of the program get into the program; this is part of the services utilization plan. Another step is to have a solid, thoughtful marketing plan, which is another element in the services utilization plan.

Once the target population or audience has been clearly specified, screening tests that are both highly sensitive and specific can be used to minimize both overinclusion and underinclusion (Table 8.2). Test *sensitivity* refers to the probability that the screening test will be positive when an illness, need, or

Table 8.2   Relationship of Test Sensitivity and Specificity to Overinclusion and Underinclusion

	Specificity	
Sensitivity	High	Low
High	Ideal inclusion and coverage; minimal overinclusion and underinclusion	Overinclusion
Low	Underinclusion	Overinclusion and underinclusion

Specificity identifies ineligibles, or those not in need; sensitivity identifies true eligibles, or those in need.

existing risk factor is actually present. Using a highly sensitive screening test to identify individuals who are eligible for the program increases the likelihood that more individuals will be in the program who actually need it, thereby reducing underinclusion. Test *specificity* refers to the probability that the test will be negative when there is no illness, need, or risk factor. Using a highly specific screening test to identify individuals who are not eligible for the program results in fewer individuals in the program who do not need it, which reduces overinclusion.

In practice, it is never possible to have a screening test that is both 100% sensitive and 100% specific. Typically, a trade-off must be made between sensitivity and specificity, with the screening test being either more sensitive or more specific. Nonetheless, a screening mechanism is often the best way to minimize overinclusion and underinclusion.

Scope: Full and Partial Coverage

The distinction between target population, target audience, and recipient is also critical in determining whether the program has partial or full coverage (Rossi & Freeman, 1993). This distinction between partial- and full-coverage programs has implications for public health and health policy.

Partial-coverage programs are designed to serve some portion of the target population, and participation in the program is based on a set of criteria that focuses recruitment strategies and takes into account limited resources. During the planning stage, the decision to have a program provide only partial coverage generally stems from having limited capacity to serve all those in the target population. Partial-coverage programs are likely to occur at the direct care or enabling services levels of the public health pyramid. Examples of such programs include early childhood intervention programs for children at developmental risk, or hospice care for those dying who choose that service.

Full-coverage programs are delivered, or are intended to be delivered, to the entire target population. By definition, these programs are more likely to occur at the population services level of the public health pyramid. Examples of full-coverage programs include seat belt laws and water fluoridation.

Some programs are less readily identified as providing full or partial coverage because, although the program is designed with the population level in mind, the target population is restricted to those meeting the criteria for participation, such as income level for state child health insurance programs, federal Women, Infants, and Children (WIC) nutrition programs, or Medicare. Because these programs are intended to serve the entire target population, they could be considered full-coverage programs, although the eligibility criteria are such that they are partial coverage programs. Across the public health pyramid, both partial- and full-coverage programs reflect whether the program is primarily designed to make changes at the individual, aggregate, or population level (Table 8.3).

Making a distinction between full- and partial-coverage programs during the planning phase may not be so easy. Stakeholder issues may potentially arise and advocacy positions potentially may be taken regarding whether a program ought to provide full or partial coverage. Some vocal activist groups may want the health program to serve an entire population at risk or in need, regardless of budgetary or logistical issues. The positions of these groups must be taken into account and reconciled with issues of feasibility if the program is to be successful in gaining their support or endorsement. Also, if the health program is to provide partial coverage, program planners must establish eligibility criteria and procedures for prioritizing and enrolling potential recipients. This issue, of course, can lead to considerable debates over the particulars of the cut-off criteria chosen for program eligibility. The other reason to consider whether the health program will provide full or partial coverage is that the scope of the program affects the design of the evaluation and potentially the cost of conducting an effect evaluation of the program.

In addition, the scope of the program needs to be considered with respect to underinclusion or overinclusion. Overinclusion is much more difficult to detect in a full-coverage program than in a partial-coverage program because the presumption in the former type of program is that the intended program recipients are the members of an entire target population. Given that a full-coverage program by its nature is likely to have a large number of recipients, it

Table 8.3   Examples of Partial and Full Coverage Programs by Level of the Public Health Pyramid

Pyramid Level	Partial Coverage (for Segment of Target Population)	Full Coverage (for Entire Target Population)
Individual— direct services	Dialysis for portion of those with kidney failure, early-childhood intervention programs for children at developmental risk, hospice care for those dying who choose the service	Ambulance and emergency medical care for all individuals, immunization clinics available to all individuals
Aggregate— enabling services level	Needle exchange programs for some substance abusers, Medicare services for the disabled and homebound, Head Start for low-income children	Medicaid coverage for dialysis of those with kidney failure
Population-based level	WIC program for low-income families, state child health insurance plans (SCHIP) for low-income families	Seat belt laws, Medicare coverage for all individuals older than age 65, fluoridation of the water supply for all residents
Infrastructure level	Laptop computers for nurses making home visits	Licensure for all physicians, nurses, and dentists; national cancer registry

will be difficult to identify those few recipients who are not members of the target population. By contrast, in a partial-coverage program, overinclusion is more likely to occur than underinclusion.

The interaction of the scope of a program with the appropriateness of inclusion may have implications that need to be considered, especially when developing the program marketing plan and the program budget. It will also be a consideration in establishing the eligibility criteria and screening procedures. In addition, an awareness of the potential for this interaction may help explain later findings during evaluations of either the process or program effect.

Screening

Having a procedure to actually screen for program eligibility is another services utilization plan input. Such a procedure is necessary to ensure that the program is provided to members of the target audience, thereby minimizing underinclusion or overinclusion. Despite the inclination to want to provide the program to anyone interested, screening enhances the efficiency and the effectiveness of the program. Efficiency is enhanced by providing the program to only those participants to whom the intervention is tailored, thereby making it less likely that the program intervention will need to be individually tailored. Effectiveness is enhanced because only those who need the program, and thus are more likely to experience the benefits of the program, are included in the outcome and impact evaluations.

Queuing

Waiting to be seen for services, being on hold, and having to wait until services become available are all aspects of being put in a queue. Waiting lines and wait times reflect the degree of match between the capacity to provide the service and the demand for the service. The services utilization plan ought to include a plan for handling wait lists and such.

For example, if an immunization clinic is being held, the services utilization plan ought to balance the anticipated number of individuals seeking immunizations against the rate at which individuals can be processed for the immunization, the length of time needed to give the immunization, and the number of program staff available to implement the immunization clinic. An imbalance will result in either people waiting for long periods or staff not having work.

Because the particulars of studying queues can be complex, large health programs—and particularly those that are ongoing—may find it valuable to hire an operations specialist to study the issue of queuing. Consultation with such experts can ensure that the health program is provided in the most timely and efficient manner possible.

Intervention Delivery

The fact that the discussion of intervention delivery appears halfway through this text is no accident. The actual delivery of the intervention, though it takes the most effort (see Exhibit 8.1), is relatively easy if the planning has been well done and the process theory has been thoroughly thought out.

Delivery of the intervention ought to follow the protocols and procedures developed specifically for the health program. Such adherence to the plan ensures that the intervention is delivered in a standardized and consistent manner. The level of detail included in the protocols and procedures will vary across programs, of course. For example, if the health program intervention involves secondary prevention of breast cancer with mammography screening, then the intervention protocol will include considerable details about the procedure for doing the actual mammogram, the taking of a history before the mammogram is performed, and notification and referral of those screened. In contrast, if the health program is a metropolitan-wide mass-media awareness campaign about the value of adult immunizations, then the intervention protocol will need to allow for flexibility in accessing and communicating with media contacts while providing guidance in who to approach, which topics to address and to avoid, and which products (e.g., public service announcements, video clips, flyers) to distribute to which media sources.

If the program focuses on an evidence-based intervention, it may be necessary to provide the intervention in a variety of settings. For example, Nix, Pinderhughes, Bierman, Maples, and Conduct Problems Prevention Research Group (2005) used established intervention strategies for children with behavior problems and their families, but provided those interventions in three ways: (1) at the school during the school day, (2) at the school not during school hours, and (3) at home visits. They considered this plan to entail multiple forms of service delivery. During the development of the services delivery plan, program planners have the opportunity to revisit the intervention and determine the best venue or location for the services.

One aspect of the intervention that makes common sense, but is often neglected, is pilot-testing the program. Prior to full program implementation, the program may be pretested, with the program developers paying attention to the various program components. Pretesting can take many different forms, such as having focus groups review materials and make comments, providing the program for free to a small group, or having experts comment on the program design and materials. In particular, marketing materials and media messages ought to be pretested. Characteristics to be assessed include the materials' attractiveness, comprehension, acceptability, and persuasion. Any materials that will be read by program participants should also be tested for readability. Word processing software typically includes features that will determine the reading difficulty and the grade at which the material is written. The rule of thumb is the lower the level, the better. No one wants to struggle with technical language, complex sentences, or large words. For example, this paragraph contains 188 words and is written at a twelfth-grade level. Generally, an eighth-grade reading level is recommended for materials. Exhibit 8.4 has this paragraph written at an eighth-grade level.

Pretesting of the interventions ought to include pretesting of the evaluation instruments that will be used during the program and after the program has been completed. As more health programs are required by funding agencies to

---

Exhibit 8.4   Paragraph Rewritten at an Eighth-Grade Reading Level

---

It makes common sense to try out a program before it begins, but this is often not done. Before starting a program, try out the handouts and the program parts. There are many ways to see if the people in the program will understand the handouts and program. One way is to have a focus group look over the materials and make comments. Another way is give the program to a small group of people for free and see if there are any problems. Also, experts can help by making comments on the program and the handouts. Advertisements and media messages need to be tried out before they are used, too. Look at how attractive they look, how easy it is for people to understand them, whether people will accept the message, and how good the messages are at convincing people. Also, handouts need to be checked for how easy they are to read. Today, word processing software can check them and show the grade level it is written at. The rule of thumb is that lower grade levels are better because no one wants to work at reading words, long sentences, or large words. For example, this paragraph has 217 words and is written a little below the eighth-grade level.

---

document their success, the evaluation is becoming more integral to the actual intervention and overall program delivery.

SERVICES UTILIZATION PLAN OUTPUTS

Outputs of the services utilization plan include the number of units of service provided and the quantity of service completions. *Units of service* is a term used to refer the agency- or program-specific quantification of what was provided, such as hours per client, number of inpatient visits, number of educational sessions, or number of hours of client contact. Because what constitutes a unit of service can vary widely, each health program must specify what it considers a unit of service. Another service utilization output is the number of services that have been completed. For health programs, this might be the number of immunization clinics held, the number of completed referrals for medical follow-up, or the number of health educational courses provided.

Ensuring that a mechanism is in place to track the service plan outputs is a critical managerial responsibility. Table 8.4 is a template for tracking the interventions and the units of service outputs. Fuller et al. (2007) used this format to show the amount of reach across different target populations.

One other services utilization output exists as well: the materials developed and produced as part of the effort to provide the health program, such as public service announcements, educational videos, annual reports, or curricula. Another

Table 8.4   Table for Tracking Services Utilization Outputs Using Example Interventions and Hypothetical Activities

Intervention Component	Target Audience A: Persons with Health Problem	Target Audience B: Clinics	Target Audience C: City
Individual education	100 persons at risk	76 providers visited	
Individual screening	600 persons	30 providers	1000 persons screened at health fairs
Group education	15 groups at hospital	8 groups at 3 clinics	15 groups at library; 6 groups at school
Population education	2000 flyers; 600 stickers	50 posters	25 public service announcements (PSAs); 10 health fairs
Individual support for behavior	125 persons at risk in 22 groups	32 providers in 8 groups	

key output is the work flow—that is, the extent to which program staff have work over a given time period or that work is done in a coordinated manner.

As the health program is implemented, keeping a record of the various outputs is essential, because they are a major component of the subsequent process evaluation of activities focused on program implementation. These evaluation activities are discussed in detail in Chapter 9.

Summary: Elements of Organizational and Services Utilization Plans

This chapter has explained the elements of the organizational plan and services utilization plan, which collectively make up the process theory. In designing and planning for a health program, attention to the process theory becomes a reality check that the needed resources and processes are in place to initiate the program.

For example, continuing with the Layetteville example, Figure 8.3 gives a possible process theory for a neural tube defect prevention program. However, the process theory needs to correspond and to support the intervention theory. When the process theory is combined with the effect theory, a comprehensive view of the program becomes possible (Figure 8.4). Having a diagram such as Figure 8.4 allows planners to determine what might be missing as part of the effort to address the health problem and to deliver the intervention, as well as what has been added that might not be essential to achieving the desired program effect.

PROGRAM THEORY AS A LOGIC MODEL

A *logic model*, as a tool for program planning and evaluation, is a diagram that shows the relationship of inputs and activities to outputs, immediate outcomes, and long-term outcomes. Since their introduction in the late 1980s, logic models have become ubiquitous and are frequently required by funding agencies. Even the Centers for Disease Control and Prevention (CDC) has engaged in the process of developing logic models for its programs, such as the Research Prevention Center (Wright et al., 2008). A logic model is one-page tabular summary of the program theory. Table 8.5 is an example of a logic model for the neural tube defect health problem and the interventions chosen to address the problem.

Comparing the process and effect theories for congenital anomalies health problem (Figure 8.4) with the logic model for the same problem (Table 8.5), the differences and areas of overlap become clear. The logic model has more details about activities, but does not draw a strong distinction between intervention activities and supportive activities that are clear in the process theory. The process theory, because it focuses only on aspects of implementation, does not include the outcomes or impacts. The connection between the process theory and outcomes would be included in the overall program theory and highly specific intervention theory. Each of these approaches is best thought of as a tool to help anticipate needs and gaps, to engage in thinking about the entire program, and to ultimately have a plan of what the program encompasses that can be used to guide process and effect evaluations.

Kaplan and Garrett (2005) drew upon experience with three comprehensive, multisite programs when they reviewed the corresponding logic models to identify the value of logic models. They found that development of a logic model not only fostered collaboration for already strong coalitions, but also proved challenging for diverse and under-resourced organizations or coalitions. The logic models they reviewed did reveal assumptions that led to changes in staffing for the program, but more often the assumptions were unstated or

Figure 8.3   Process Theory for Neural Tube Defects and Congenital Anomalies Health Problem

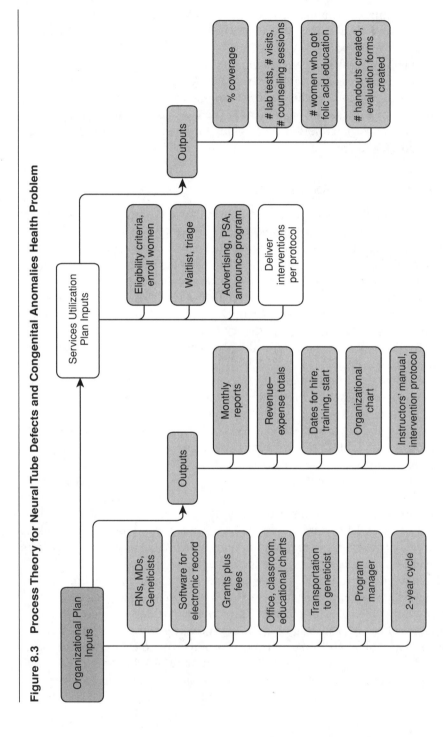

Figure 8.4 Effect and Process Theory for Neural Tube Defect Prevention Program

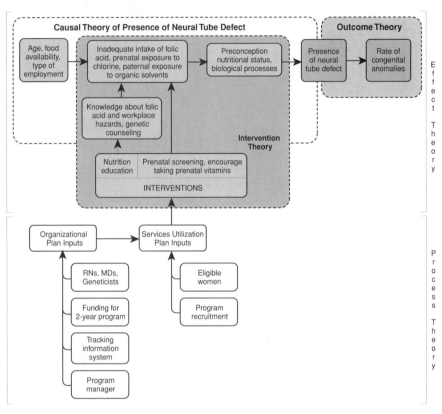

unrealistic. These authors also found that the lack of attention to the rationale for the program—in other words, the intervention theory—was related to the heavy emphasis that the logic model put on activities and outcomes. A key benefit of the logic model was that it facilitated communication with internal and external stakeholders, including funders. Kaplan and Garrett's research is a poignant reminder that no tool is without both benefits and drawbacks.

PROGRAM THEORY AS A BUSINESS PLAN

A *business plan* is a document that summarizes the analyses behind the development of a product, service, or program; substantiates the development of a program based on a wide range of crucial considerations; and provides

Table 8.5 Hypothetical Logic Model of Program for Reducing Congenital Anomalies

Assumptions	Inputs	Activities	Outputs	Immediate Outcome	Long-Term Outcome
Health problem is important to community of providers and residents	Program personnel: RNs, primary care MDs, geneticists	Create a time line and tracking system	Number of educational materials; program manual; number of staff trained	Improved knowledge of folic acid	Rate of congenital anomalies
Residents have access to health care and food sources	Funding for 2 years; information system for tracking participants	Conduct staff training Create program protocol and manual; create PSAs and recruitment materials	Number of women screened for type of employment and serum folic acid; percentage of women who start folic acid preconception	Percentage of births with neural tube defects (anencephaly, spina bifida), cleft lip, or palate	

details for implementation of the program. Business plans, in contrast to the diagrammatic layout of the process theory and logic models, are written documents. Nevertheless, as with the process theory diagram and logic models, the overriding intent is to communicate the details of the program and to provide evidence that the details have been thoroughly thought out and actions are well planned and coordinated.

Research has shown that business plans do facilitate decision making, as well as accelerate development of the product or service (Delmar & Shane, 2003). The use of business plans is advocated in medicine (Cohn & Schwartz, 2002), nursing (Fralic & Morjikian, 2006), and public health (Orton, Umble, Zelt, Porter, & Johnson, 2007). Mostly, however, business plans are used for entrepreneurial endeavors (Hindle & Mainprize, 2006). Although development of health programs is rarely thought of as an entrepreneurial activity, the development of health services is very appropriately viewed from this perspective. For example, Adams and Crow (2005) developed a business plan for a new nurse case management service for rural hospitals. Their business plan detailed contained the financial aspects, reviewed trends within the rural healthcare industry, a marketing plan, and reviewed legal risks.

Table 8.6 lists the basic elements of a business plan, along with the corresponding elements of the organizational plan, services utilization plan, and logic model. As Table 8.6 makes clear, the business plan, because it is a written document, has greater detail in many areas. By comparison, logic models provide the least amount of information and the least specific information. More detail, particularly on the financial characteristics of the proposed program, is often needed to effectively and convincingly communicate the need for the proposed health program.

ACROSS THE PYRAMID

At the direct services level of the public health pyramid, implementation of a health program will be very similar to the implementation of other health services. However, particular attention ought to focus on tailoring the human resources to the programmatic intervention. The social marketing plan will also be targeted to individuals and individual behaviors.

Likewise, at the enabling services level, a match between providers and the health program intervention is necessary. If the program intervention is an enabling service, the providers (human resources) are more likely to have a background or expertise in social services. Enabling service programs are also more likely to use volunteers, a decision that has implications for the managerial resources needed. The social marketing plan will also need to be tailored to the aggregate targeted by the program. Because many enabling services either require a referral or are accessed via a referral, the social marketing of

Table 8.6   **Generic Elements of a Business Plan, with Their Purpose and Corresponding Element of the Process Theory and Logic Model**

Business Plan Format	Purpose	Process Theory Element	Logic Model Element
Title/cover page	Gives a first impression		
Executive summary	Gives a first impression		
Business concept	Describes the program design, with goals and objectives	Entire program theory	Entire logic model
Market analysis	Analyzes the demand, need, competition, and effect on existing services and health status	Community needs assessment	
Financial analysis	Projects revenues and expenses, states the fiscal assumptions used in analyses	Organizational plan inputs: monetary resources, budget	
Risk and competitive analysis	Discloses the sources and types of possible failures with alternatives to avoid those failures; balances failure risks with merits of the program		
Operational plan	Shows how personnel, management, space, and equipment come together for the program; delineates resource requirements	Organizational plan inputs: human, informational, physical, managerial, time resources, transportation	Inputs, activities
Marketing plan	Describes strategy to reach the target audience, branding, distribution, price, promotion	Service utilization plan: social marketing, participants	Activities
Milestones	Gives time frame for accomplishment of key tasks and outcomes	Process and outcome objectives	Immediate and long-term outcomes

the program may focus as much on the providers making the referrals as on the target audience of clients.

At the population services level, as at the other levels of the public health pyramid, a match must exist between the abilities and skills of the providers and the health program intervention. Social marketing to a population will have a broad base of appeal and will almost certainly use mass media.

This chapter has dealt mostly with the infrastructure level of the public health pyramid. Having a highly specified, comprehensive organizational plan and services utilization plan provides a strong foundation for implementing an effective health program. Also, having the necessary and appropriate resources for the health program is an indicator of the quality of the infrastructure. Even the most creative ideas and the most scientifically sound programs will fail if they lack an adequate infrastructure. Too often attention is focused on the health program interventions and clients, without the prerequisite attention and effort being devoted to developing and maintaining the programmatic infrastructure. For this reason, the organizational plan must identify resources for the infrastructure as well as resources for the services utilization plan activities. In addition, if the health program is intended to increase the capacity of the infrastructure—for example, to improve workforce capacity—an organizational plan and services utilization plan for such a program is still warranted as a step to ensure the success of the program.

DISCUSSION QUESTIONS AND ACTIVITIES

1. In what ways might each type of accountability be affected by or related to social marketing?

2. How do the outputs of the organizational plan and the services utilization plan relate to the process theory objectives?

3. For a health program at the direct services level, the enabling services level, and the population services level of the public health pyramid, speculate on how fixed and variable costs might change. Discuss the implications of these changes on the results of a break-even analysis.

4. Imagine that you are serving on a committee to establish an information management system for a new health program. Which factors would you argue to be included, and what would be your rationale for their inclusion?

5. In what ways might you write or develop objectives to minimize underinclusion or overinclusion in a health program?

INTERNET RESOURCES

There is a wealth of resources on developing various types of logic models and program theory models. The following list represents the diverse perspectives and approaches.

Kellogg Foundation Evaluation Manual

This text, which is available as a pdf-format file, is a comprehensive textbook on evaluation. Chapter 5 (http://www.wkkf.org/Pubs/Tools/Evaluation/Pub770.pdf) relates to the development of program theory.

ReCAPP BDI Logic Model Course

For an audio experience, cruise through the highly recommended "course" on logic models found at http://www.etr.org/recapp/logicmodelcourse/. The material is presented in a Power-Point presentation.

Centers for Disease Control and Prevention

The CDC has meta-site for logic models with some good links; find it at http://www.cdc.gov/eval/resources.htm#logic%20model. The CDC also provides scholarly papers on marketing at http://www.cdc.gov/healthmarketing.

Break-Even Analysis

There are no more excuses for not doing a break-even analysis with either of these online calculators. The calculator offered by KJE Computer Solutions (http://dinkytown.com/java/BreakEven.html) gives a nice graph based on totals that you input, whereas the one presented by Deluca (http://legacy.ncsu.edu/classes/ted430/java/mecon.html) allows for more refined analysis with variable inputs. Both include definitions of terms.

Tools of Change

The Canadian website at http://www.toolsofchange.com/English/firstsplit.asp has links to social marketing as well as a wealth of examples of programs using various techniques for motivation.

Social Marketing Institute

Working papers and published articles at the Social Marketing Institute website (http://www.social-marketing.org/papers.html) are a scholarly resource.

Business Plans

Numerous resources on developing business plans can be found on the Internet, including some sites that provide "how to" guides and templates. Entrepreneur.com has an entire section dedicated to developing business plans at http://www.entrepreneur.com/businessplan/. The nonprofit My Own Business offers an entire online course about developing a business; the section on business plans (http://www.myownbusiness.org/s2/) includes basics, formatting, examples, and templates.

REFERENCES

Adams, M. H., & Crow, C. S. (2005). Development of a nurse case management service: A proposed business plan for rural hospitals. *Lippincott's Case Management, 10,* 148–158.

Bazerman, M. H. (2005). *Judgment in managerial decision making* (6th ed.) New York: John Wiley & Sons.

Bluthenthal, R. N., Heinzerling, K. G., Anderson, R., Flynn, N. M., & Kral, A. H. (2008). Approval for syringe exchange programs in California: Results from a local approach to HIV prevention. *American Journal of Public Health, 98*(2), 278–283.

Bowen, D. J., Kuniyuki, A., Shattuck, A., Nixon, D. W., & Sponzo, R. W. (2000). Results of a volunteer program to conduct dietary intervention research for women. *Annals of Behavioral Medicine, 22*, 94–100.

Centers for Disease Control and Prevention (CDC). (2008). *Health marketing*. Retrieved March 26, 2008, from http://www.cdc.gov/healthmarketing

Cohn, K. H., & Schwartz, R. W. (2002). Business plan writing for physicians. *American Journal of Surgery, 184*, 114–120.

Delmar, F., & Shane, S. (2003). Does business planning facilitate the development of new ventures? *Strategic Management Journal, 24*, 1165–1185.

Ferrari, J. R., Luhrs, T., & Lyman, V. (2007). Eldercare volunteers and employees: Predicting caregiver experiences from service motives and sense of community. *Journal of Primary Prevention, 28*, 467–479.

Finkler, S. A., Ward, D. M., & Baker, J. J. (2007). *Essentials of cost accounting for health care organizations* (3rd ed). Sudbury, MA: Jones and Bartlett.

Foster, E. M., Johnson-Shelton, D., & Taylor, T. K. (2007). Measuring time costs in interventions designed to reduce behavior problems among children and youth. *American Journal of Community Psychology, 40*, 64–81.

Fralic, M. F., & Morjikian, R. L. (2006). The RWJ executive nurse fellows program, part 3: Making the business case. *Journal of Nursing Administration, 36*, 96–102.

Freeze, R. D., & Kulkami, U. (2007). Knowledge management capacity: Defining knowledge assets. *Journal of Knowledge Management, 11*(6), 94–109.

Fuller, C. M., Galea, S., Caceres, W., Blaney, S., Sisco, S., & Vlahov, D. (2007). Multilevel community-based intervention to increase access to sterile syringes among injection drug users through pharmacy sales in New York City. *American Journal of Public Health, 97*, 117–124.

Hindle, K., & Mainprize, B. (2006). A systematic approach to writing and rating entrepreneurial business plans. *Journal of Private Equity, 9(3)*, 7–20.

Hintgen, T. L., Radichel, T. J., Clark, M. B., Sather, T. W., & Johnson, K. L. (2000). Volunteers, communication, and relationships: Synergistic possibilities. *Topics in Stroke Rehabilitation, 7*(2), 1–9.

Kaplan, S. A., & Garrett, K. E. (2005). The use of logic models by community-based initiatives. *Evaluation and Program Planning, 28*, 167–172.

Kettner, P. M., Moroney, R. M., & Martin, L. L. (1999). *Designing and managing programs: An effectiveness based approach* (2nd ed.). Thousand Oaks, CA: Sage Publications.

Kotler, P., & Zaltman, G. (1971). Social marketing: an approach to planned social change. *Journal of Marketing, 35*, 3–12.

Landis, K. L., & Loar, C. W. (2007). Project New Hope: Volunteers caring for children in need. *AORN Journal, 86*, 769–779.

Morrow-Howell, N., Kinnevy, S., & Mann, M. (1999). The perceived benefits of participating in volunteer and educational activities. *Journal of Gerontological Social Work, 32*(2), 65–80.

Nix, R. L., Pinderhughes, E. E., Bierman, K. L., Maples, J. J., & Conduct Problems Prevention Research Group. (2005). Decoupling the relation between risk factors for conduct problems and the receipt of intervention services: Participation across multiple components of a prevention program. *American Journal of Community Psychology, 36*, 307–325.

Orton, S., Umble, K., Zelt, S., Porter, J., & Johnson, J. (2007). Management Academy for Public Health: Creating entrepreneurial managers. *American Journal of Public Health, 97*, 601–605.

Orzano, A. J., Tallia, A. F., McInerney, C. R., McDaniel, R. R. Jr., & Crabtree, B. F. (2007). Strategies for developing a knowledge-driven culture in your practice. *Family Practice Management, 14*, 32–36.

Pazoki, R., Nabipour, I., Seyednezami, N., & Imami, S. R. (2007). Effects of a community-based healthy heart program on women's physical activity: A randomized controlled trial guided by community-based participatory research (CBPR). *BMC Public Health, 7*(147), 216.

Posner, B. Z. (1995). What it takes to be a good manager. In J. R. Meredith & S. J. Mantel, *Project management: A managerial approach* (3rd ed., pp. 146–149). New York: John Wiley & Sons.

Roessler, A., Carter, H., Campbell, L., & MacLeod, R. (1999). Diversity among hospice volunteers: A challenge for the development of a responsive volunteer program. *American Journal of Hospice and Palliative Care, 16*, 656–664.

Rossi, P. H., & Freeman, H. E. (1993). *Evaluation: A systematic approach.* (5th ed.). Thousand Oaks, CA: Sage Publications.

Schafer, E., Vogel, M. K., Viegas, S., & Hausafus, C. (1998). Volunteer peer counselors increase breast feeding duration among rural low-income women. *Birth, 25*, 101–106.

Tousman, S., Arnold, D., Helland, W., Roth, R., Heshelman, N., Castaneda, O. et al. (2007). Evaluation of a hand washing program for 2nd-graders. *Journal of School Nursing, 23*, 342–348.

Trettin, L., & Musham, C. (2000). Using focus groups to design a community health program: What roles should volunteers play? *Journal of Health Care for the Poor and Underserved, 11*, 444–455.

Turnock, B. J. (2009). *Public health: What it is and how it works* (4th ed.) Sudbury, MA: Jones and Bartlett.

Walsh, D. C., Rudd, R. E., Moeykens, B. A., & Moloney, T. W. (1993, Summer). Social marketing for public health. *Health Affairs*, 104–119.

Wright, D. S., Anderson, L. A., Brownson, R. C., Gwaltney, M. K., Scherer, J., Cross, A. W., et al. (2008). Engaging partners to initiate evaluation efforts: Tactics used and lessons learned from the prevention research centers program. *Preventing Chronic Disease, 5*, A21. Retrieved May 23, 2008, from http://www.cdc.gov/pcd/issues/2008/jan/06_0127.htm

CHAPTER 9

Process Evaluation:
Measuring Inputs and Outputs

Once the health program has started, stakeholders, funding agencies, and program staff all want to know if the program is being or was implemented successfully and as planned. Answering this question becomes possible by devoting attention to the implementation. This chapter covers techniques and issues related to documenting, monitoring, and evaluating the implementation of the program. These topics are addressed in relationship to the components of the program theory, including the process of creating data that can be used to assess the achievement of the process objectives established during the planning phase. Documenting and assessing the extent to which the process objectives have been achieved, and at what cost, are important aspects of providing a program. Maintaining a focus on the quality and quantity of implementation helps identify gaps between program accomplishments and process objective targets. As with the development of the program interventions and plan, input from recipients and stakeholders while gathering and interpreting data enriches the understanding about the health program implementation.

ASSESSING THE IMPLEMENTATION

Questions that focus on elements of the organizational and service utilization plans are essentially questions about implementation, rather than about effects of the program. These questions tend to fall into one of three levels of sophistication in regard to program implementation. Although slightly different in focus and emphasis, all three categories of questions are concerned with assessing the elements of the process theory portion of the program theory (Figure 9.1). Accordingly, the measures and data collection for each are likely to be quite similar—in fact, depending on the programmatic circumstances, they may even be the same. Therefore, this chapter covers these three types of questions in an integrated manner.

Figure 9.1   Elements of the Process Theory Included in a Process Evaluation

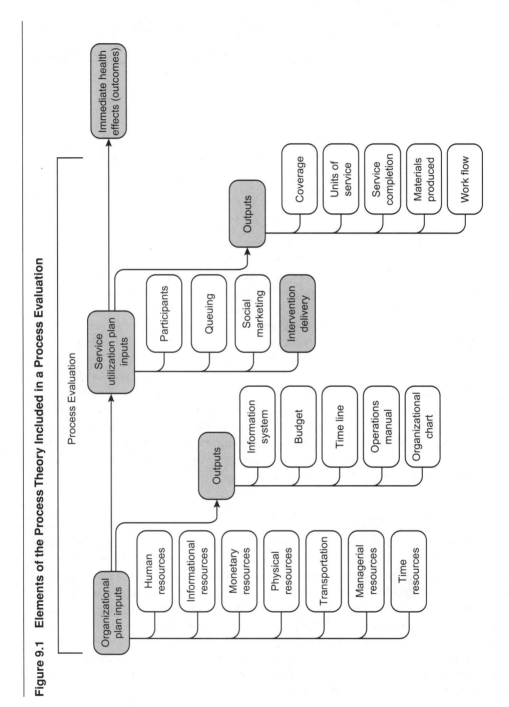

Unfortunately, terms describing implementation-focused questions are not used consistently in the literature. The following description of the three levels of questions provides a framework for understanding the various terms, such as process monitoring, program monitoring, process evaluation, and implementation monitoring.

Implementation Documentation

Implementation documentation refers to the simple tallying of activities and processes carried out as implementation activities of the program. Questions of this sort represent the simplest level of sophistication. As simple documentation, this line of questioning does not lead to subsequent interpretations of what was documented and, therefore, does not prompt program managers to take actions to change or improve the program.

Implementation documentation certainly involves collecting the data specified in the process objectives. Accurate, complete, and timely implementation documentation is the foundation for the next levels of questions about implementation. In other words, although implementation documentation is necessary, it is not sufficient.

Implementation documentation is carried out, in part, to meet the requirements of funding agencies—specifically, to demonstrate the extent of program implementation. Required reporting often entails a predetermined set of data that will need to be collected and used in the report to the funding agency. Thus not all aspects of implementation documentation are under the control of the program administration or evaluators. Ideally, the data collection requested by the funding agency will be consistent with and built into the process objectives.

Implementation Assessment

The next level of sophistication focuses on implementation assessment. *Implementation assessment* is the ongoing, nearly real-time activity of collecting data about the implementation of the program for the purpose of making timely corrections or modifications to the implementation through changes to elements of the process theory. Implementation assessment is called either program monitoring or process monitoring.

Process monitoring, the term used in this textbook to refer to this level of implementation assessment, is the ongoing, real-time assessment of the implementation of the program. It is integrated into the implementation of the program as a managerial or oversight tool to ensure that the program is being delivered within the parameters established during the planning stage. Ideally, process monitoring could lead to a favorable subsequent implementation evaluation.

Program monitoring is concerned with the elements described in this chapter. In addition, some of its aspects are similar to quality improvement techniques, which are discussed in Chapter 10. Each program is associated with a set of process objectives, and the implementation assessment activities are focused on achieving those objectives. This linkage between the implementation assessment activities and the process objectives keeps the monitoring activities reasonable in scope and focused on key or critical processes for having a successful program.

One purpose of implementation assessment is to provide managerial guidance and oversight of the implementation of the program. Program monitoring, like the quality improvement methodologies discussed in Chapter 10, can provide data on which to base changes or corrections in the delivery of the program. The interactive and iterative nature of planning and implementing a health program inevitably requires some degree of flexibility, particularly for programs that are continuous, ongoing, or repeated. This state of flux may be why Chalmers and colleagues (2003) found that over a five-year period, the monitoring system for a community coalition program needed to be modified.

The process monitoring information can inform decision making regarding which aspects of the organizational plan or the service utilization plan are ineffective in accomplishing the process objectives. The actualization of this flexibility and the willingness to make changes amount to corrective managerial practice. Through such actions, program managers address issues of accountability and quality. Additionally, process monitoring can function as a warning system for problems in delivery of the program and can provide a basis for modifying the process theory for subsequent revisions of the program.

Implementation Evaluation

The most sophisticated level of questioning comprises implementation evaluation. *Implementation evaluation* is a comprehensive, retrospective determination of the extent to which the program was delivered as designed and whether the variations might have had significant or important implications for the program effects. Implementation evaluation is generally called process evaluation. *Process evaluation* entails systematic research to assess the extent to which the program was delivered as intended. It is, therefore, the systematic examination of programmatic coverage and delivery. Patton (1997, p. 196) defined process evaluation as "finding out if the program has all its parts, if the parts are functional, operating as they are supposed to be operating." Although the term is not used consistently in the literature, process evaluation is used in this text to refer to implementation evaluation.

Process evaluation has at least two purposes. One purpose is to gather data about the delivery of the program so that the results of an effect evaluation can be interpreted within the context of the program delivery. That is, if the intervention does not have effects on the health problem, it will be important to verify that the program was, in fact, delivered, and to quantify the degree of intensity and faithfulness to the program design. Process evaluations are intended to demonstrate that program specifications are met and, as such, are useful for ensuring that the work being done by program staff is consistent with the program's process objectives and plan. Process evaluations help identify whether the implementation of the program contributed to the program's failure, as distinct from whether the effect theory was incorrect (Figure 9.2).

The second purpose of process evaluations relates to the dissemination or replication of the health program. Put simply, the process evaluation provides comprehensive operational information to the new sites so that the program can be successfully replicated.

EFFICACY, EFFECTIVENESS, AND EFFICIENCY

In evaluating programs, one concern is often whether the program was efficacious, effective, and efficient. These three terms are often used as synonyms, with minimal attention being paid to the important differences among the concepts. In fact, these differences have implications for the role of the process evaluation, and reveal the underlying reasons for the different evaluation activities needed to quantify each.

Figure 9.2   Roots of Program Failure

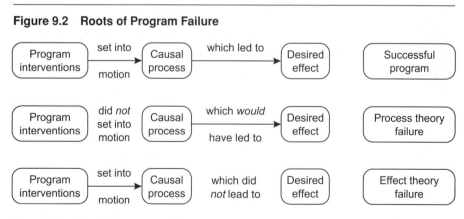

Source: Weiss, Carol H. *Evaluation*, Second Edition, © 1998. Reprinted by permission of Pearson Education, Inc., Upper Saddle River, NJ.

Of the three terms, efficacy is probably the one most likely to be misused, usually instead of effectiveness. *Efficacy* is the maximum potential effect under ideal conditions. Because ideal conditions are difficult to create, the efficacy of an intervention is determined through rigorous studies—usually clinical trials, especially randomized clinical trials. Randomized clinical trials, by controlling many of the potential influences, provide a context in which the greatest possible effect of a treatment or intervention can be directly attributed to that treatment or intervention. Because of the costs and ethical considerations involved in clinical trials, efficacy evaluations of health programs are seldom done unless they are performed as part of evaluation research. In efficacy studies, the role of a process evaluation is to establish that the health program intervention is being carried out precisely according to the intervention protocol.

Effectiveness is the realistic potential for achieving the desired outcome when a treatment or intervention is used in real life. The degree of effectiveness of an intervention reflects what can be expected given the normally messy situations that occur when health programs are delivered to real-world clients. Data from outcome assessments and outcome evaluations, as well as from evaluation research, provide practical experience with the anticipated level of intervention effectiveness. The degree of effectiveness may be reflected in several different statistics, depending on the evaluation design and methods. Any statistic that denotes the degree of difference related to having received the programmatic intervention—whether a difference score, a correlation coefficient, or an odds ratio—provides information on the degree of effectiveness. In this way, existing studies of the effectiveness of interventions provide a benchmark against which to gauge the success of subsequent or similar programs. As a consequence, such studies have value beyond their specific findings. The role of a process evaluation in effectiveness studies is not only to ensure that the program is being provided according to protocol, but also to document situations, events, and circumstances that influenced the delivery of the intervention.

Efficiency is, generically, the relationship between the amount of output and the amount of input, with higher outputs that are achieved with fewer inputs being deemed more efficient. With regard to health programs, efficiency is generally thought of in terms of the amount of effect from the program intervention—that is, the ultimate output—compared to the amount of inputs that went into providing the intervention. Data are collected as part of implementation documentation on the expenditures for all types of inputs into the program as well as on the outputs from the organizational and service utilization plans. Efficiency is then calculated as the cost per unit of output, where the unit of output is selected from the various outputs of the program. Using this basic notion of cost per output, efficiency could also be calculated per process objective.

DATA COLLECTION METHODS

Along with the question of what to measure is the question of how to collect data. At least seven categories of methods of data collection are appropriate for process evaluations: activity logs, organizational records, client records, observation, questionnaires, interviews, and case studies (Table 9.1). This list of data collection methods does not preclude disciplined creativity in developing and using data collection methods or tools that are uniquely tailored to the program, including checklists (Simbar, Dibazari, Saeidi, & Majd, 2005). The use of activity logs, whether paper and pencil or web based (Turner, Yorkston, Hart, Drew, & McClure, 2006) and organizational records tends to be more specific to process evaluation. Chapter 3 provides information on developing questionnaires and client records (as secondary data), and Chapter 15 describes techniques for interviewing, observation, and developing case studies.

The choice of a method of data collection needs to be congruent with the indicators in the process objectives and the best method for arriving at a conclusion about whether the process objective target was reached. Each method has its own advantages and disadvantages, and these need to be carefully considered when choosing a data collection method.

For all data collection methods, high standards must be met in terms of the quality of the data collected, the reliability of the tools, and the accuracy of data entry. The need for reliability extends to assessing and establishing an acceptable degree of inter-rater reliability in the use of checklists and activity logs. Having a reliable means of assessing delivery of the intervention is especially important when the consistency of intervention delivery is problematic or when the program is a pilot that is being evaluated as an experiment.

QUANTIFYING INPUTS TO THE ORGANIZATIONAL PLAN

During program development, specific organizational resources are identified as being key to implementing the health program. Both inputs and outputs of the organizational plan are included in an implementation evaluation (Figure 9.3), which determines the extent to which those inputs were available and used and the quantity of outputs. Although every input could be monitored, tracking all of them would be neither prudent nor feasible. Each program will have a set of concerns and interests with regard to the organizational plan inputs, as reflected in organizational plan process objectives. Thus the choice of which organizational plan inputs are evaluated is influenced by the earlier work of the program planners and the current concerns of program staff.

Table 9.1   Methods of Collecting Process Evaluation Data

Method	When to Use	Examples of Measures	Pros	Cons
Activity log	Have list of actions that are discrete, and a common understanding exists for what those are; need quantitative data	Number of sessions, number of participants, time received inquiry phone calls, date of press release	Can tailor log to the program activities, easy to use, easy to analyze data, applicable across pyramid levels	May become too long, may not be completed on a regular basis, easy to falsify
Checklist	Have a list of actions or behaviors that can be observed	Yes or no: Set up room for session, gave supportive comments, distributed program materials	Simple to use, can be developed to include a time frame, data entry is straightforward, applicable across pyramid levels	Difficult to narrow list items, challenging to write items for consistent interpretation, reliability needs to be established
Organizational records	Have existing records that capture information needed and can legally access those records; need quantitative data	Length of time on waiting list, number of computers bought or upgraded, number of hours worked	Accessibility to the information, applicable across pyramid levels	Need a data abstraction form, records may not include what is needed, may require complex data linking and data analysis
Client records	Have existing records that capture information needed and can legally access those records; need quantitative data	Program attendance, client compliance with program elements	Accessibility to the information	Need a data abstraction form, records may not include what is needed, may require complex data linking and data analysis

Method	When to Use	Examples of Measures	Pros	Cons
Observation	Need to have data on interpersonal interactions or sequences of events	Number staff-participant interactions	Data may reveal unexpected results, naturalistic, can quantify observations	Time intensive, need observation checklist, complex data analysis
Questionnaire	Need to quickly collect data from reliable respondents and have a reliable and valid questionnaire; need quantitative data	Degree of satisfaction with program, degree of compliance with program interventions	Can collect pencil-and-paper version for many programs, applicable across pyramid levels	Respondent must have good reading skills and motivation to complete the questionnaire, will gather useless data if not well written, can be expensive for population-level programs
Interview	Have time and need qualitative data or have respondents for whom questionnaire is not appropriate	Commitment of staff to program and intervention	Able to get detailed descriptions during one-on-one interview, possibly new insights	Time intensive, need private place for the interview, need interview question and format, more complex data analysis
Case study	Need to understand the full set of interactions around the program and the context in which it is functioning	Degree to which managerial personnel make changes to ensure fidelity of intervention	Gives very thorough picture of program and provides new insights	Extremely complex because it uses multiple methods over period of time, time intensive, very complex data analysis

Figure 9.3   Examples of Organizational Plan Inputs and Outputs That Can Be Measured

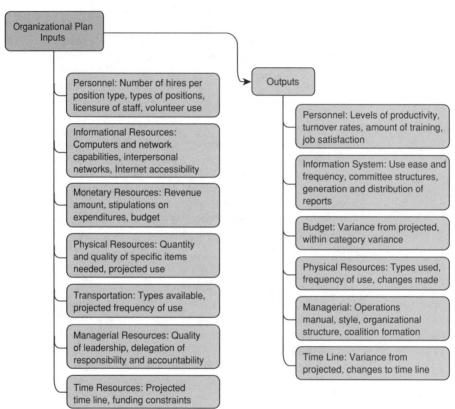

A variety of measures can be used to measure each organizational plan input and output (Table 9.2), although the specific measures will depend on the program and its objectives. At a minimum, the human resources and physical resources devoted to and utilized by the program must be monitored. These two organizational plan inputs are used as examples of considerations that would be involved in monitoring inputs. These discussions are not intended to be definitive, but rather illustrative of how to approach the development of a process evaluation plan.

Human Resources

Both the quantity and the quality of the human resources used by the health program ought to be assessed, given that human resources often constitute the

Table 9.2   Example of Measures of Inputs and Outputs of the Organizational Plan

Input	Measures of Input	Measures of Output
Human resources	Number of full-time equivalents (FTEs), number of new hires, number of volunteers, percentage of licensed personnel, percentage of personnel with certification, educational level of staff, hours of training and orientation	Number of hours worked, staff-to-recipient ratio, hours per client contact per staff, degree of job satisfaction of staff and volunteers, degree commitment of staff to program and intervention
Informational resources	Number of computers bought or upgraded, number of program recruitment efforts, availability of communication hardware and software, ease of process data entry and retrieval, ease of impact data entry and retrieval	Degree to which computer and telecommunication systems facilitate delivery of the intervention, availability and accessibility of personnel, budget, operating, meeting, or other reports
Monetary resources	Amount of grant monies and donations, amount of indirect costs deducted from the program, number of proposals submitted for program funding	Dollars or percent variance from budgeted per line item, number of grants awarded, profit or loss
Physical resources	Number and type of capital equipment, number and type of office or clinical equipment, square footage of office space	Extent to which changes are made to physical resources needed for intervention delivery, replacement of aged equipment
Transportation	Parking fees, total mileage per month, number of bus passes used, program vehicle expenses	Mileage per staff, number of clients receiving transportation assistance, transportation cost per staff or per program participant
Managerial resources	Place in organizational chart, years of experience, educational level, degree of ability to clearly and persuasively communicate	Extent to which managers are viewed by staff as controlling or delegating, degree to which managerial personnel make changes to ensure fidelity of intervention
Time resources	Time line developed, presence of deadline dates	Number of days delayed, percentage of deadlines met, number of repeated requests

largest cost component of a program budget. The importance of tracking the staffing levels of a program is reflected in the results of a study carried out by Rosenheck and Seibyl (2005). Using five years of data on staffing levels, these authors were able to find an association between higher staffing levels and better outcomes for program participants. This section does not present a definitive list of measures of human resource inputs, but rather is meant to provide some guidance and ideas for monitoring related to human resources.

Not only is the quantity of personnel relevant, but those individuals' level of commitment to the program, their competencies in terms of knowledge and skills, and their attitudes are also critical considerations. The degree of commitment to the program is important to assess, given that program staff who lose commitment to the health program are less likely to fully implement the program as designed. A change in commitment levels may reflect unanticipated challenges to the delivery of the program. For example, the program staff may develop lower levels of commitment because of obvious failures of the intervention or because of undesirable side effects of the program. Thus monitoring the program staff's commitment to the program and to the interventions is one avenue for gaining insights into program implementation.

The extent to which program personnel are competent to deliver the program also provides information on the extent of program implementation. If licensed health professionals are required to deliver the intervention, but the program managers have insufficient fiscal resources to hire such individuals, then the program is not likely to be implemented as planned. Thus the extent to which the credentials of program staff match the competencies needed for program implementation provides more evidence of the extent to which the designed interventions are delivered. This statement is not meant to imply that unlicensed personnel are not qualified. Indeed, many types of interventions and health programs rely heavily and appropriately on a wide range of qualifications for program staff. Rather, the issue is the extent to which the program staff's qualifications actually match what is required to fully implement the program so as to gain the maximum effect for program participants.

As the health program evolves over iterations of implementation, the qualifications needed by program staff might change as well. These changing needs in relation to staff qualifications ought to be uncovered and noted through an implementation assessment or evaluation. The observed change may lead to a revision of the process theory for the program.

The participation of stakeholders continues into the process evaluation. The inclusion of volunteers and stakeholders as human resources in the organizational plan is intended to serve as a continual reminder that these individuals and groups need to be actively engaged in the various stages of the health program. Ideas from program staff about ways to improve the program can be part of the process evaluation. Their ideas may help increase the effectiveness and efficiency of the program without compromising the integrity of the intervention as conceptualized. Their ideas may also provide insights into which aspects of the intervention were not implemented as intended. For example, staff members are very likely to pick up on and articulate the difference between what they were asked to do and what they are actually able to do with the given resources.

Another human resources input into many public health programs is the membership of a community consortium, coalition, or advisory board. The rationale for using community coalitions or consortia is based on the belief that the inclusion of such groups of individuals from the target population not only fosters the development of culturally appropriate health programs, but also influences the context of the program in ways that enhance the service utilization plan. Determining the extent to which this human resource was utilized may be mandated by various federal funding agencies. For example, as part of a Centers for Disease Control and Prevention (CDC) initiative to reduce racial and ethnic disparities across five health conditions, each grantee was required to have and to report on the status of its community coalition. Similarly, as part of a Maternal and Child Health Bureau program to reduce infant mortality, grantees had to have a community consortium and report on the functioning of that consortium.

Attendance records for community consortia or advisory board meetings are indicators of the amount of input of that type of human resource. The positions and organizations represented by the membership of the consortia or advisory board is another indicator of the human resources capability and diversity. Process monitoring data related to coalitions can reveal difficulties in mobilizing the community as a whole and elucidate the preferential interests of various groups. Process evaluation data help assess whether coalition activities have contributed any program effect. For example, Hays, Hays, DeVille, and Mulhall (2000) found that the structural characteristics of a coalition—particularly membership diversity and sectoral representation—were differentially related to community effects of the health program. Such process information can be important for future coalition development.

Whereas commitment to and belief in the program and passion for the health problem are viewed as human resource inputs, job satisfaction is viewed as an output of the program. This distinction is important as a way to differentiate whether the correct inputs were obtained—namely, motivated individuals—from whether the human resources inputs were converted to satisfied staff. The effort to screen and hire volunteers and staff might also be important in this regard.

The preceding discussion hints that a wide variety of measures might be appropriate to document, monitor, and evaluate human resources. The number of staff members per job category, the number of full-time equivalent (FTE) workers per job category, and the number of staff members with licensure and certifications are the absolute minimum data to be collected.

Physical Resources

Documenting the extent to which facilities are adequate in terms of the types of rooms needed to provide the health program or the accessibility of equipment can be particularly relevant for some health programs, especially if specific physical resources are essential for the success of the program. Lack of or failure to use the necessary physical resources may indicate that the program was not fully implemented. For example, if a health promotion program includes both an educational component requiring only a classroom and a cooking demonstration component requiring a kitchen, then the process monitoring needs to include documentation of the use of both facilities. If no kitchen facilities were used for the program, then only the educational component of the program was implemented. Knowing that facility limitations were an issue such that only one component of the program was implemented provides an explanation for a weak program effect on the stated health outcomes.

The simplest measure of physical facilities would be a dichotomous variable (i.e., yes/no) as to whether the facilities or equipment specified in the process objective were used. However, for physical resources such as a classroom, it may also be useful for process monitoring purposes to collect data on whether the room was heated, well lit, and so forth. Similarly, if physical resources include items such as blood pressure cuffs or supplies for vaccination, then it may be informative to document or monitor their placement, adequacy, expiration dates, disposal safety, and such. These seemingly mundane aspects of the physical resources can influence whether program staff utilize those resources as intended.

QUANTIFYING OUTPUTS OF THE ORGANIZATIONAL PLAN

Just as only key organizational plan inputs are evaluated, so only key organizational outputs can realistically be evaluated. Those outputs associated with process objectives are the minimum to be included in the evaluation. For some programs it may important to understand the organizational structure, such as where in the organizational hierarchy the health program director is located. The program director's position in the organizational chart can indicate the relative importance of the health program and, hence, the ability of the program manager to garner resources for the program. Here, two organizational plan outputs—information systems and budgets—are used as examples of different approaches to the measurement of organizational plan outputs.

Information Systems

Computerized systems enable program managers to collect data in the same format from all program staff, thereby enabling easier aggregation of those data across staff members and analysis at the program level. The ability to process data and generate needed reports is an output of the information systems. Given the increasingly central role played by information systems in acquiring program funds and documenting program implementation and effects, mechanisms ought to exist for monitoring the extent to which the computer hardware and software are capable and programmed to generate the needed reports. These strategies may range from a quarterly report generated by the information systems department to a simple tally of the number of computers with specific software. Tracking the number of problems, requests, and complaints would be another approach to measuring the information system outputs.

Information systems and computerized databases have become critical for capturing and maintaining data related to processes and participant outcomes. If the process evaluation is well thought through and thoroughly developed before the program begins, then the information system and database can be set up and ready to accept data at the start of the program. Achieving this level of preparation requires knowing which data elements will be needed. If program staff are expected to contribute process evaluation data through the computerized system, staff training on how to use the computerized system will be necessary. The importance of correctly entering data in a timely manner must be explained in terms of personnel's role in ensuring that the data are reliable and, therefore, useful for all concerned. Testing the system, including the personnel involved in using or maintaining the information system, involves checking that relevant data are collected and stored, that the data can be manipulated to provide answers to programmatic questions, and that those inputting the data are doing so reliably.

Of course, the same information system (or a comparable one) will likely be used for evaluating the effect of the program. As a consequence, part of the process evaluation may include an assessment of the system's capacity to handle data from the effect evaluation.

Measures of the information system output will include items such as staff perception of ease of use, frequency of using critical databases, amount of time clients are on hold, number of calls waiting to be answered, number and frequency of reports generated, and perceived usefulness of the reports generated. Information systems also include the use of inter- and intra-organizational communication. Measures of interpersonal information systems include the number of active committees, the number of community meetings attended by staff, the perceived accuracy and timeliness of information received, and the number and types of modes of intra-organizational communication used, such as email, memos, listservs, and meetings.

Monetary Resources: Budget Variance

On an ongoing and regular basis (usually monthly), the program manager ought to determine the extent to which current expenditures exceed (or not) the projected program expenditures. The difference between the budgeted and actual expenditures or income is called the *budget variance.*

The variance is calculated for each category or line item as a simple subtraction of expenditures from the budgeted amount, which can be easily calculated with the use of spreadsheets. When the program budget is developed during the planning stage, it would be wise to have the spreadsheet set up in a way that makes it easy to include columns for variance. Because of delays associated with billing, timing of organizational fiscal reports, and the various dates selected by the organization at the beginning of a fiscal year, the actual expenses and income will always be based only on what is available at any given time. As bills are posted and income recorded, the expenditures and income must be updated.

Severe negative variances can occur because of over-expenditures or inadequate income, whereas severe positive variances can arise due to under-expenditures or greatly increased income. Either way, the presence of a significant variance alerts program managers that the program may not be delivered as planned and that some aspect of the program may need further scrutiny and modification.

Although it is not a daily activity for most programs, weekly updating of the budget variance may be required for some programs. This would be especially true near the end of a grant-funded program, at which time the balance needs to be near zero. During the program implementation, the overall variance ought to be no more than 10% to 20% of the projected budget. Some funding agencies will specify the degree of budget variance that is acceptable and indicate at what point the budget needs to be renegotiated with the funding agency. Program managers, by monitoring the budget variance on at least a monthly basis, can make needed adjustments to spending throughout the fiscal year, so that the year-end variance is within an acceptable range.

QUANTIFYING INPUTS TO THE SERVICES UTILIZATION PLAN

Process evaluation typically is equated with elements that are included in an evaluation of the services utilization plan—namely, data on the participants and program delivery (Figure 9.4). As mentioned earlier in regard to evaluating the organizational plan, the process objectives serve as a guide as to which possible inputs and outputs are crucial to evaluate. Table 9.3 provides some examples of measures that are useful for service utilization plan monitoring.

Participants and Recipients

The most basic data about participants is a simple count of how many or inquired about the program were served. However, other types of data about program participants are reasonable to collect.

A simple, straightforward documentation of demographic characteristics— whether through interviews, self-report questionnaires, or clinic records—is

Figure 9.4   Examples of Services Utilization Inputs and Outputs That Can Be Measured

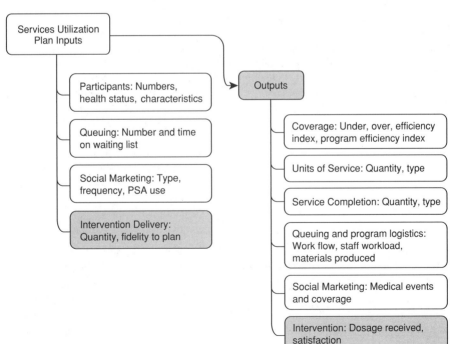

Table 9.3   Examples of Measures of Inputs and Outputs of the Services Utilization Plan

Element	Measures of Input	Measures of Output
Program reach	Number of requests for program	Percent under-coverage, percent over-coverage
Participants	Number of recipients/participants, number of persons denied program or not qualified for program	Efficiency index, program efficiency index, degree of satisfaction with program
Queuing and program logistics	Number on waiting list, presence of system to move individuals from waiting list to program or alternative programs	Length of time on waiting list, evenness of work among staff and across time (work flow), number and types of materials produced
Social marketing	Type of social marketing, quality of marketing, extent of social marketing analysis	Number of advertising events, number of requests for program based on social marketing efforts
Intervention	Number of meetings to standardize program, extent of revisions based on previous cycle of intervention delivery, extent of revisions based on new research evidence	Fidelity to intervention plan, number of sessions, hours of program delivery, number of participants completing intervention (service completion), number of requests for additional program delivery, use of materials produced

one means to collect this type of data. Demographic data are necessary for determining the extent to which the target audience has been reached and whether the social marketing approaches were effective. These data can be readily collected during program sign-in or intake procedures, especially for direct and enabling services. Demographic data on recipients of population-focused programs may be more difficult to obtain directly, given that population-based health programs do not require recipients to be physically present at a given location. For example, it would be very difficult to determine the number of recipients of health messages delivered via billboards.

Some basic information about the health status of participants can be collected and prove important for later analyses of program effect. Measures of health status information can range from the simple, such as a single question rating of overall health, to a checklist of diagnoses, to findings from a detailed medical history and physical examination. The complexity of the health measure will correspond to the level of the public health pyramid at which the program is aimed and the target audience characteristics.

Intervention Delivery and Fidelity

Intervention fidelity indicates whether the intervention was provided as designed and planned; that is, it comprises the alignment of the intervention activities with the elements of the intervention theory. The concept of intervention fidelity applies to single, one-time programs as well as to standardized interventions adopted by numerous organizations. Unless high intervention fidelity is achieved, the program may fail to reach the desired outcomes. Mihalic, Fagan, and Argamaso (2008) acknowledged that achieving high implementation fidelity can be difficult for community-based organizations to achieve, but is critical for clinical trials (Spillane et al., 2007). Adequate and ongoing process monitoring can help prevent the program failure due to inadequate program implementation by detecting the source of the failure to have full intervention fidelity.

Intervention fidelity may be compromised in three ways. First, an intervention can fail because of the lack of a program (nonprogram, no treatment), meaning that the program was not provided. If the intervention requires a sophisticated delivery system, it may not be delivered. For example, a program that involves coordinating services among a variety of health professionals employed by different agencies can easily result in no program. An alternative way for no treatment to occur is that the delivery of the intervention in some way negates the intervention. Having program personnel who are not supportive, encouraging, or empathetic would negate intended program interventions that require such qualities in staff. Similarly, physical resources—for example, a building with limited and difficult access—might negate interventions for persons with disabilities.

The second way that an intervention can fail is if an intervention other than the one designed and planned is provided, or if the dosage is drastically reduced. If an educational program is designed to cover five topics but only one topic is covered despite holding the classes for the designated number of hours, the program will be dramatically diluted, possibly to the point of having no effect on participants. The process objectives that specify the program content and quantity can be used to assess whether the strength (dosage) of the intervention was delivered as intended. It is also possible that the intervention theory was flawed; if so, although the actual program may be delivered as planned, the inadequacy of the intervention as conceptualized will lead to intervention failure.

The third way that an intervention can fail is if the intervention is provided in an inconsistent manner, resulting in a nonstandardized treatment across time or across recipients. A standardized intervention is necessary to ensure that the intervention is responsible for the outcomes. If program personnel use their own discretion to alter the intervention, there is no assurance that the intervention as planned is responsible for the health effects found in an outcome evaluation. One approach to minimize this potential source of program failure is to incorporate the program theory in the training of program personnel, thereby ensuring that they appreciate the need to follow the guidelines for delivery of the program. Of course, the organizational plan outputs of policies, procedures, and standardized materials need to be in place and used as tools to help standardize the program.

Inconsistency in intervention delivery can also have a more insidious and hidden cause. Both program participants and program staff have their own working explanations or theories of how a program affects participants. As described in Chapter 6, the espoused theory is the stated or espoused explanation for how things happen (Argyris, 1992). In a properly functioning program, the effect theory becomes known and understood by program staff; therefore, it also ought to be the espoused theory. Of course, staff inevitably know what they are supposed to say about the program interventions, regardless of whether they believe it or whether their actions match their espoused theory.

The actions that staff take to achieve the ends constitute their theory-in-use—that is, the working theory that staff actually use. One key aspect of process monitoring is to observe the theory-in-use, as it provides insights into which intervention was provided to recipients, and then compare it to the intervention theory developed during the planning stage. It is especially important to observe the theory-in-use during the process monitoring and to compare it to the program intervention theory.

Naturally, some programs will be more prone to inconsistency than other programs. For example, the espoused theory and the theory-in-use among staff in immunization clinics are likely to be quite congruent. In contrast, staff in gun violence prevention programs are more likely to demonstrate incongruence between the two theories because such a program entails complex interpersonal interactions and addresses socially sensitive problems.

Without standardized interventions, it will be difficult to connect the health effects of the program to the program interventions. For this reason, the process evaluation of the intervention needs to take into account the possible sources of inconsistency in how the program intervention is delivered.

Findings from the program evaluation may be confusing or misleading if the espoused theory and the theory-in-use are incongruent. Implementation of the program may be inconsistent, with some staff providing the program according to the espoused theory and other personnel delivering the program based on their theory-in-use.

The inconsistencies among the three theories (intervention theory, espoused theory, and theory-in-use) can be a source of *decision drift*. Although a decision may be made as a milestone in the planning process, over time the decision can evolve in unexpected ways among planners and program staff. Decision drift is a natural process in long-term health programs, but it can also occur within short spans of time—even within single meetings. Decision drift is detrimental only if it results in a program that lacks coherence or that no longer addresses the health problem. Through process evaluation, the extent to which decision drift has occurred can be assessed and the specific areas in which it occurred can be pinpointed. Recognizing that decision drift has occurred provides a basis for either revising the decisions or modifying the program elements and objectives to bring them more in line with the current decisions. Which action to take will depend on whether the decision drift has resulted in a more or less efficient and effective health program.

QUANTIFYING OUTPUTS OF THE SERVICES UTILIZATION PLAN

During a process evaluation of each of the services utilization plan outputs, one of the first decisions to be made is which time frame will be used. Because many health programs are vulnerable to seasonal fluctuations, the time frame used is often highly significant. For some programs, annual measures will be more reasonable; for other, shorter programs, the end of the program will be sufficient. Ideally, the evaluation of the services utilization plan outputs should occur as close to "real time" as possible, rather than being retrospective, to ensure that programmatic changes are made in a timely fashion.

The service utilization plan outputs discussed here are coverage, units of service, service completion, work flow, and materials produced. These outputs are assessed with regard to the extent that corresponding process objectives have been achieved.

Coverage as Program Reach

The extent to which the program reached its intended audience is called *coverage*, but may also be referred to as *reach*. Studies of programs have identified attention to coverage as important to understanding why the programs did not have the expected effects (Gottfredson et al., 2006) and for determining which program effects were associated with coverage (Macinko, de Souza, Guanais, & Simoes, 2007). Means used to track program coverage have included documentation, monitoring, and evaluation. If the coverage rates are less than expected or predicted, then it is important to identify the barriers to accessing the program, which may entail a qualitative approach (Sobo, Seid, & Gelhard, 2006). There are several ways to quantify and interpret coverage.

Measures of Coverage

Monitoring the degree of participation in a health program is a basic aspect of process evaluation. All funding agencies and program managers want assurances that the program had participants. The mechanism for tracking the number of individuals served by the program must be in place before the process evaluation begins. Measures of coverage require having accurate data on the number of program participants within a given time period. Collecting data on a frequent or periodic basis allows for ongoing monitoring and still makes possible the aggregation of the numbers to get totals for a given time period. For example, if immunization clinics are offered three times per month, managers may count the number of participants per clinic, and then add the totals for all three clinics to obtain a total number of persons served per month.

Coverage is assessed with regard to under-coverage and over-coverage. Data from the needs assessment are required regarding the numbers of individuals in need and not in need of the program. These data, along with the actual number of individuals served by the program, form a matrix of under-coverage, ideal coverage, and over-coverage (Table 9.4). The number crunching involved in calculating the different measures of coverage is simple, yet can yield a great deal of information about which program component needs attention due to under-coverage. Exhibit 9.1 lists the formulas for coverage measures. A

Table 9.4   Matrix of Under-Coverage, Ideal Coverage, and Over-Coverage

	Persons Not Served by the Program	**Persons Served by the Program**
Persons Not in Need of Program	Ideal coverage	*Over-coverage*
Persons in Need of Program	*Under-coverage*	Ideal coverage

Exhibit 9.1   Formulas for Measures of Coverage

Percentage of over-coverage $= \dfrac{\text{number not in need but served}}{\text{number served}}$

Percentage of under-coverage $= \dfrac{\text{number in need and served}}{\text{number in need}}$

Coverage efficiency $=$ (number served $-$ number over-coverage) / number in need

Efficiency index $= \dfrac{\text{(number in need and served / number in need)} \times 100}{\text{standard stated in objectives}}$

Program efficiency index $= \dfrac{\text{sum of efficiency indices}}{\text{number of components in the program}}$

---

narrative example of coverage measures is shown in Exhibit 9.2, with the corresponding data in a spreadsheet (Excel) being shown in Exhibit 9.3.

Under-coverage is measured as the number of individuals who are in need of the service and actually received the service divided by the number of individuals who are in need. It occurs when the program is not delivered to a large portion of the target audience. On the other side of the coin, *over-coverage* occurs when the program is being used by individuals not in the target audience. It is calculated as the number of individuals who are not in need of the service but who receive the service divided by the number who receive the service. Assessments of under- and over-coverage can be used to determine how to improve a program (Miller & Robles, 1996).

A more telling indicator is coverage efficiency. *Coverage efficiency* is calculated as the number served minus the over-coverage divided by the number in need. If there is no under- or over-coverage, then the coverage efficiency will be 100%. As can be seen in Exhibit 9.3, it is difficult to reach that level of coverage efficiency.

The coverage efficiency index can be applied to the program to create the program efficiency index. The *program coverage efficiency index* is calculated by summing the efficiency indices for each program component and then dividing this sum by the number of program components.

Although these measures of coverage provide information about the extent to which the program is reaching the target audience, they do not provide information on the extent to which the program is meeting its objectives. To make this determination, another calculation is needed. That is, the percentage

---

**Exhibit 9.2   Example of Coverage and Dosage Measures,
Narrative Background**

Last year Bowe County funded programs that address the top five health problems in Layetteville. The community needs assessment data revealed the number of individuals or families in need of each program. Of the 1000 persons on whom assessment data were collected, 300 were at risk for diabetes, 200 were in need of adult immunizations, 600 adolescents were at risk for violence, 250 women were at risk for congenital anomalies, and 250 adolescent girls were sexually active. The county requires that each program provide annual reports on its coverage efficiency and weighted program dosage average. The grant contract also stipulates that the programs must meet at least 75% of their coverage efficiency target, and the program intervention dosage must average at least 80%.

Each program set a target for its coverage efficiency objective. The Diabetes Prevention Program chose 90%. The Adult Immunization Program set its target at 98%, and the Adolescent Violence Prevention Program estimated it could achieve 70% coverage. The Adult Immunization Program considered full dosage to have received three vaccines; the program had 200 persons receive the first vaccine, 190 persons receive the second vaccine, and 160 persons receive all three vaccines. The Congenital Anomalies Prevention Program set its coverage efficiency at 85%; that program served 200 women, of whom 100 were at risk and needed the program, and an additional 100 women who were at risk did not receive the program.

Using the formulas in Exhibit 9.1, three of the programs provided the coverage information as shown in Exhibit 9.3, and one program provided the intervention dosage information shown in Exhibit 9.4 (later in this chapter). The county is reviewing the data provided by these programs, and it intends to use the data to make recommendations to neighboring counties that have expressed interest in funding similar programs.

---

of coverage efficiency achieved can be compared to the percentage coverage efficiency specified as the objective target (see Exhibit 9.3). This calculation uses the numbers from the under- and over-coverage matrix and the target value set in the objective. It represents another way for program managers and staff to determine whether the program is reaching its objectives.

High coverage results indicate that the program has achieved good marketing and program recruitment. Taken as a set, coverage measures indicate the extent to which efforts to enroll individuals in the program are effective and the target audience is being reached. They also indicate areas warranting managerial action and further tailoring of the program.

Exhibit 9.3   Examples of Coverage Measures Using an Excel Spreadsheet

	A	B	C	D	E	F	G	H	I	J
1										
2	Diabetes Prevention Program									
3		Not in Program	In Program	Total		Coverage Efficiency Objective, Target %:		90		Formulas for Calculating Coverage
4	Already diagnosed	650	50	700		Over-coverage		20%		C4/C6
5	At high risk	100	200	300		Under-coverage		33%		B5/D5
6	Total	750	250	1000		Coverage Efficiency		67%		(C6-C4)/D5
7						% Coverage Efficiency		74%		(C5/D5)/H3 *100
8						Target Achieved				
9	Adult Immunization Program									
10		No Vaccine	Got Vaccine	Total		Coverage Efficiency Objective, Target %:		98		
11	Not need vaccine	790	10	800		Over-coverage		5%		C11/C13
12	Need vaccine	10	190	200		Under-coverage		5%		B12/D12
13	Total	800	200	1000		Coverage Efficiency		95%		(C13-C11)/D12
14						% Coverage Efficiency		97%		(C12/D12)/H10 * 100
15						Target Achieved				
16	Adolescent Violence Prevention Program									
17		Non-participant	In Program	Total		Coverage Efficiency Objective, Target %:		70		
18	Low risk, no need	150	250	400		Over-coverage		50%		C18/C20
19	High risk, has need	350	250	600		Under-coverage		58%		B19/D19
20	Total	500	500	1000		Coverage Efficiency		42%		(C20-C18)/D19
21						% Coverage Efficiency		60%		(C19/D19)/H17 *100
22						Target Achieved				

When thinking about the sources of data needed to measure participation, one must think in terms of target populations and recipients. The number of individuals in need of the program—specifically, the size of target population—ought to have been determined through the community assessment. If the community needs assessment data do not include some estimation of the size of the target audience, it becomes virtually impossible to determine whether the program is dealing with under-coverage or over-coverage. At best, the level of coverage can be estimated only from alternative data sources.

Units of Service

For some programs, it will be important to distinguish between the number of program participants and the number of contacts. Outreach programs may be quite successful in making a high number of contacts with potential program participants, but the number of individuals who actually show up for the program may be a small fraction of that number. In this case, a decision must be made about whether the number of individuals contacted is equivalent to the number of outreach recipients. This is a gray area and each program will have a slightly different answer to this question. The key is to make clear the item being counted and the definition on which it is based. In particular, the process objective should specify what is being counted.

The unit of service must be clearly defined and articulated before the count can begin. A *unit of service* (UOS) is a predetermined unit, such as number of contact hours, number of individual clients seen, number of educational sessions offered, or size of caseload. This measure is primarily used for programs at the direct or enabling services levels of the public health pyramid. For some programs, the UOS is specified by the funding agency, in which case data for that UOS become a minimum of what is included in the process evaluation of services delivered.

Participant-Related Issues

Dosage Measurement

Of the five dosage elements (frequency, duration, strength, route of administration, and administration credibility), frequency and duration have the greatest relevance for ongoing monitoring. Frequency of the intervention—whether hourly, daily, weekly, or monthly—and duration of the intervention—whether one session, eight weeks of classes, or six months of exposure—are the elements of dosage that may vary from the objectives laid out in the plan because of either program or participant factors. Thus, to ensure that the planned dosage was received by the participants, it will be important to determine the degree to which program participants completed the health program—in other words, *service completion*. The inverse of service completion is the dropout rate of the program.

One-shot programs, such as screening clinics, are likely to have different completion rates than programs with longer-term involvement with the participants, such as substance abuse counseling, Meals on Wheels, or exercise classes. For some enabling services, service completion is the achievement of the service plan or care plan. Counting the number of participants who have completed their service plan provides different information on the extent to which the intervention was implemented and the dosage received by the average participant. Service plan completion can be estimated only if staff members keep good records of enrollment and record participant attendance on an individual basis.

Drastic changes in completion rates may signal problems with program staff or with the design of the program. The process objectives should include a threshold for what is an acceptable program completion rate.

Level of participation is a corollary of service completion. If the intervention or impact theories are predicated on a certain level of participation, then data on the level of participation need to be collected as a means of determining whether participants received the appropriate "dose" of the intervention. For some health programs, level of participation might be a simple yes/no on attendance at, say, an immunization clinic, or it might comprise a weighted calculation of the percentage of time during a set of sessions in which the participant was actively engaged with the group. The measure chosen will depend on the nature of the program and the target and indicator specified in the process objective. A low level of participation can result if program personnel are not skilled in engaging participants (a managerial issue) or if the intervention is not appealing to the participants (a process theory issue).

The dosage received by a program participant can be calculated if accurate and complete data have been collected on each participant and the quantity of intervention received. Continuing with the congenital anomalies prevention program in Layetteville, Exhibit 9.4 shows the dosage for three women. Suppose that the program has four components—screening, prenatal counseling, use of prenatal vitamins, and a cooking class—and each component has a different planned amount specified in the intervention theory and the corresponding process objectives. If the amount of each component received by each woman is recorded, then the program dosage can be calculated for each woman. Using the program average dosage for each component, a weighted average dosage can then be calculated. The advantage of calculating the weighted average dosage is that it takes into account any variation in planned dosage for components.

The main challenge in calculating the dosage is the collection of data in a manner that enables its calculation. If they know the program average per program component, the program manager and planners can make more informed

Exhibit 9.4 Examples of Calculating Dosage for the Congenital Anomalies Prevention Program Using Excel

	A	B	C	D	E	F
1		Program Component	Unit	Planned	Amount	Percentage
2				Amount	Received	Received
3	Participant A	Screening	Session	2	2	100%
4		Prenatal counseling	Session	4	4	100%
5		Prenatal vitamins	Weeks	52	43	83%
6		Cooking class	Hours	8	7	88%
7						
8	Participant B	Screening	Session	2	2	100%
9		Prenatal counseling	Session	4	3	75%
10		Prenatal vitamins	Weeks	52	32	62%
11		Cooking class	Hours	8	4	50%
12						
13	Participant C	Screening	Session	2	1	50%
14		Prenatal counseling	Session	4	2	50%
15		Prenatal vitamins	Weeks	52	20	38%
16		Cooking class	Hours	8	1	13%
17						
18					Average Amount	Avg Percent
19	Program	Screening	Session	2	1.7	83%
20	Average	Prenatal counseling	Session	4	3.0	75%
21		Prenatal vitamins	Weeks	52	31.7	61%
22		Cooking class	Hours	8	4.0	50%
23		Weighted average dosage				84.2%
24						
25	Formulas for Calculating Program Average, Based on 3 Participants	Screening	Session	2	(e3+e8+e13)/3	(f3+f8+f13)/3
26		Prenatal counseling	Session	4	(e4+e9+e14)/3	(f4+f9+f14)/3
27		Prenatal vitamins	Weeks	52	(e5+e10+e15)/3	(f5+f10+f15)/3
28		Cooking class	Hours	8	(e6+e11+e16)/3	(f6+f11+f16)/3
29		Weighted average dosage (assuming all participants have the same planned amount)				(((F19*D19) + (F20*D20) + (F21*D21) + (F22*D22)) / D19 +
30						D20 + D21 + D22) /100

decisions about program modifications and changes, such as which components need revision or additional support.

Satisfaction Measurement

Participant satisfaction with the program is an element of process evaluation and not a health outcome of the program. This perspective stands in contrast to the general vernacular of classifying satisfaction as an outcome. The rationale for thinking of satisfaction as a process output stems from the definition of *satisfaction*: the degree to which participants receive what they expect to receive and the extent to which their expectations are met with regard to how they are treated (Parasuraman, Zeithaml, & Berry, 1985). What is received, what is expected, and how one is treated are all elements of the service utilization plan, rather than parts of the effect theory of how the intervention leads to health changes.

Satisfaction with health services functions in interesting ways. For example, Franciosi and colleagues (2004) found that lower satisfaction with providers was related to more severe clinical conditions and lower levels of psychological adaptation to diabetes. In mental health, Morris and colleagues (2005) found that increased satisfaction with care in a sample of patients with bipolar disorder was associated with a decreased sense of hopelessness. Satisfaction of clients and patients has also been found to be related to program effects, such as adherence to medication regimens (Horne, Hankins, & Jenkins, 2001). Satisfaction with services has received considerable attention in the health services field, with questionnaires having been developed for use in specific settings, such as primary healthcare settings; for specific programs, such as the Neonatal Screening Program (Mazlan, Hickson, & Driscoll, 2006); and for specific health conditions. This level of specificity for the patient or consumer satisfaction questionnaire is reflective of the need to have rigorous measures of satisfaction.

Most funding agencies are interested in knowing the satisfaction level of participants in the programs they are funding. Most participants, clients, and patients report being somewhere in the range "satisfied to very satisfied" in regard to the services they receive, perhaps because it is difficult to measure satisfaction in a way that does not lead to a ceiling effect. A *ceiling effect* occurs when the measurement tool is constructed so that respondents do not have an opportunity to distinguish among levels at the high end of the scale. It becomes apparent when the item has a high mean value and very low standard deviation. In other words, the distribution becomes highly skewed to one side. For example, if the satisfaction scale is a five-point Likert-type scale, the difference between 4 ("somewhat satisfied") and 5 ("very satisfied") will lead to 5 being chosen more often than 4. One remedy for avoiding the ceiling effect is to use a scale of 1 to 10, which then allows respondents to distinguish among 7, 8, 9, and 10 as levels of satisfaction.

Other difficulties exist in developing a measure of satisfaction. One challenge is to create a measure that is culturally sensitive and appropriate to subgroups of participants. Fongwa, Hays, Gutierrez, and Stewart (2006) specifically created a measure for African Americans but caution that the measure needs testing with other ethnic groups.

Another challenge is that self-report responses on a questionnaire may not be the same as responses in an interview. Marcinowicz, Chlabicz, and Grebowski (2007) found a discrepancy in this regard, with more negative responses being offered by patients when interviewed compared to their questionnaire responses.

Yet another difficulty stems from the conceptual definition of satisfaction, which entails a match between expectations and experience. Developing a measure that captures both expectations and actual experience will be longer, more complex to complete, and more challenging to analyze. For these reasons, the use of an existing satisfaction measure is highly recommended.

The last difficulty in measuring satisfaction concerns the scope of what is important in terms of satisfaction. For example, inpatient satisfaction questionnaires generally include items about parking and food service alongside items about the courtesy of staff (Gesell, 2001; Mostyn, Race, Seibert, & Johnson, 2000). If such items are included, their relevance to the organizational and service utilization plans should be explicit.

Program Logistics

Work Flow

Interaction inevitably occurs between the procedures used for managing waiting participants and the amount of work done by program staff. Measures of work flow are one indicator of the amount of work done by the program staff and the queuing of participants. Examples of work flow measures include minutes that participants wait to be seen, number of days between signing up for the program and beginning the program, number of days between being referred to the program and being accepted into the health program, and amount of time required for program staff to complete a specific task. Of course, the amount of work done by program staff is influenced by the volume of program participants and the rate at which they participate in the program. For direct services health programs, the volume and queuing will greatly affect the work flow of program staff. For population-based programs, the level of cooperation from others, such as media representatives, may affect the work flow of program staff, such as in delivery of a mass media campaign.

Data related to both volume of participants and work flow come from a variety of sources. Observations of program staff, participant records, appointment logs, class sign-in sheets, and billing statements are common sources of these data. For some programs, planners may decide to develop specific data collection forms. If this step is taken, the program staff should be involved in the process, as using an empowerment approach to planning increases the likelihood that optimal measures will be developed and used by program staff.

Materials Produced

Both the quantity and the quality of the materials produced for the health program need to be considered in the process evaluation. Having data about the materials provides insights into the work done by staff and the extent to which the intervention was delivered in the manner planned. One managerial insight that has emerged from studies tracking the production of materials is that resources are sometimes directed more toward the materials than toward implementation of the intervention. Data about production of materials can be difficult to obtain and will be very program specific.

ACROSS THE PYRAMID

Across the public health pyramid, process monitoring and evaluation focus on the inputs and outputs of the organizational and service utilization plans—albeit tailored to the specific program, of course (Table 9.5). For programs at the direct services level, data will measure units of service such as number of individuals served and number of contact hours with individuals. Such measures are consistent with the nature of health programs designed for the direct services level of the pyramid. At the enabling services level, process monitoring and evaluation indicators are likely to be similar to those used at the direct services level, but modified to reflect the specific program and the use of different sources of data.

At the population-based services level of the public health pyramid, as at the direct services and enabling services levels, program process evaluations and monitoring efforts ought to address inputs and outputs of the organizational and service utilization plans. This is true if the program is implemented at the community level. For example, Glick, Prelip, Myerson, and Eilers (2008) focused on documenting the extent to which a fetal alcohol syndrome prevention campaign reached the intended audience. The units of service measured at this level of the pyramid could include number of individuals served, number of agencies involved, or number of households reached.

At the infrastructure level, process monitoring and process evaluation focus on the program infrastructure. If the health program is designed for one of the other levels of the pyramid, then the infrastructure becomes the source of the inputs and outputs of the organizational and service utilization plans. Of course, a program may be designed and intended to actually change the infrastructure. For example, Pearson, Wu, Schaefer, Bonomi, Shortell, and Mendel (2005) conducted a process evaluation of the implementation of the chronic care model across 42 organizations, focusing on the changes made at the sites to implement the program. Infrastructure units of service could comprise the number of employees involved, and outputs might consist of the number of policy or procedure updates and job satisfaction, especially if the employees are considered inputs into the program.

Table 9.5   Examples of Process Evaluation Measures Across the Public Health Pyramid

	Direct Services	Enabling Services	Population Services	Infrastructure
Organizational Plan Input	Provider credentials, location	Provider credentials, physical resources (e.g., cars)	Provider credentials, managerial resources	Personnel qualifications, managerial resources, fiscal resources
Organizational Plan Output	Protocols and procedures for service delivery, data about individual participants	Protocols and procedures for service delivery, data about participants	Protocols and procedures for service delivery	Budget variance, fiscal accountability, data and management information systems
Service Utilization Plan Input	Wait times, characteristics of participants	Wait times, characteristics of participants	Characteristics of the population	Characteristics of the workforce
Service Utilization Plan Output	Measures of coverage	Measures of coverage	Measures of coverage	Materials produced, number of participants

---

DISCUSSION QUESTIONS AND ACTIVITIES

1. Involvement of community coalitions and consortia in the implementation of health programs has become widespread. What would be possible and appropriate measures or indicators of having implemented community coalitions or consortia as part of the program delivery?

2. What would you suggest as methods and techniques to avoid the failure of interventions? Justify your ideas in terms of the various ways that interventions can fail.

3. To obtain accurate measures of coverage, which information systems and data collection methods need to be in place? Which steps can ensure that these elements are put in place in a timely manner?

4. Process monitoring and process evaluation data are useful only when they are interpreted correctly and subsequently used to make program changes. Outline a plan, with actions and stakeholders, for increasing the likelihood that the process data will contribute to accurate and responsible program delivery.

5. Using the information in Exhibit 9.2, calculate the measures of coverage for the Congenital Anomalies Prevention Program, specifically the percent over-coverage, percent under-coverage, coverage efficiency, and the percent coverage efficiency target achieved. Of the various programs for which coverage data are available, which programs seem to be most efficient?

6. Using the information in Exhibit 9.2, calculate the dosage for the Adult Immunization Program for 150 needed and received the full vaccination.

INTERNET RESOURCES

Workbook for Designing a Process Evaluation

This workbook has some nice tools and a simple presentation: http://health.state.ga.us/pdfs/ppe/Workbook%20for%20Designing%20a%20Process%20Evaluation.pdf.

UNICEF

UNICEF has created a one-page tool that includes key questions to ask as part of a process evaluation: http://www.unicef.org/lifeskills/index_10489.html#Process%20indicators%20for%20the%20programme.

CYFERnet

North Carolina State University's CYFERnet includes a resource page specific to process evaluation, including links to CDC and WHO documents on process evaluations. Find it at http://cyfernet.ces.ncsu.edu/cyfres/browse_3.php?cat_id=851&category_name=Process+Evaluation&search=Evaluation&subcat=Evaluation+Tools+and+Instruments&search_type=browse.

REFERENCES

Argyris, C. (1992). *On organizational learning*. Cambridge, MA: Blackwell Publishers.

Chalmers, M. L., Housemann, R. A., Wiggs, I., Newcomb-Hagood, L., Malone, B., & Brownson, R. C. (2003). Process evaluation of a monitoring log system for community coalition activities: Five-year results and lessons learned. *American Journal of Health Promotion, 17,* 190–196.

Fongwa, M. N., Hays, R. D., Gutierrez, P. R., & Stewart, A. L. (2006). Psychometric characteristics of a patient satisfaction instrument tailored to the concerns of African Americans. *Ethnicity & Disease, 16*, 948–955.

Franciosi, M., Pellegrini, F., De Berardis, G., Belfiglio, M., Di Nardo, B., Greenfield, S., et al. (2004). The QuED Study Group: Quality of care and outcomes in type 2 diabetes. *Diabetes Research and Clinical Practice, 66*(3), 277–286.

Gesell, S. B. (2001). A measure of satisfaction for the assisted-living industry. *Journal of Healthcare Quality: Promoting Excellence in Healthcare, 23*, 16–25.

Glick, D., Prelip, M., Myerson, A., & Eilers, K. (2008). Fetal alcohol syndrome prevention using community-based narrowcasting campaigns. *Health Promotion Practice, 9*, 93–103.

Gottfredson, D., Kumpfer, K., Polizzi-Fox, D., Wilson, D., Puryear, V., Beatty, P., et al. (2006). The Strengthening Washington D.C. Families Project: A randomized effectiveness trial of family-based prevention. *Prevention Science, 7*, 57–74.

Hays, C. E., Hays, S. P., DeVille, J. O., & Mulhall, P. F. (2000). Capacity for effectiveness: The relationship between coalition structure and community impact. *Evaluation and Program Planning, 23*, 373–379.

Horne, R., Hankins, M., & Jenkins, R. (2001). The Satisfaction with Information about Medicines Scale (SIMS): A new measurement tool for audit and research. *Quality in Health Care, 10*, 135–140.

Macinko, J., de Souza, M., Guanais, F. C., & Simoes, C. (2007). Going to scale with community-based primary care: An analysis of the family health program and infant mortality in Brazil, 1999–2004. *Social Science and Medicine, 65*, 2070–2080.

Marcinowicz, L., Chlabicz, S., & Grebowski, R. (2007). Open-ended questions in surveys of patients' satisfaction with family doctors. *Journal of Health Services Research and Policy, 12*, 86–89.

Mazlan, R., Hickson, L., & Driscoll, C. (2006). Measuring parent satisfaction with a neonatal hearing screening program. *Journal of the American Academy of Audiology, 14*, 253–264.

Mihalic, S. F., Fagan, A. A., & Argamaso, S. (2008). Implementing the LifeSkills Training drug prevention program: Factors related to implementation fidelity. *Implementation Science, 3*, 5.

Miller, A. B., & Robles, S. C. (1996). Workshop on screening for cancer of the uterine cervix in Central America. *Bulletin of the Pan American Health Organization, 30*, 397–408.

Morris, C. D., Miklowitz, D. J., Wisniewski, S. R., Giese, A. A., Thomas, M. R., & Allen, M. H. (2005). Care satisfaction, hope, and life functioning among adults with bipolar disorder: Data from the first 1000 participants in the Systematic Treatment Enhancement Program. *Comprehensive Psychiatry, 4*, 98–104.

Mostyn, M. M., Race, K. E., Seibert, J. H., & Johnson, M. (2000). Quality assurance in nursing home facilities: Measuring customer satisfaction. *American Journal of Medical Quality, 15*, 54–61.

Parasuraman, A., Zeithaml, V. A., & Berry, L. L. (1985). A conceptual model of service quality and its implications for future research. *Journal of Marketing, 49*, 41–50.

Patton, M. Q. (1997). *Utilization-focused evaluation* (3rd ed.). Thousand Oaks, CA: Sage Publications.

Pearson, M. L., Wu, S., Schaefer, J., Bonomi, A. E., Shortell, S. M., & Mendel, P. (2005). Assessing the implementation of the chronic care model in quality improvement collaboratives. *Health Services Research, 40*, 978–996.

Rosenheck, R. A., & Seibyl, C. L. (2005). A longitudinal perspective on monitoring outcomes of an innovative program. *Psychiatric Services, 56,* 301–307.

Simbar, M., Dibazari, Z. A., Saeidi, J. A., & Majd, H. A. (2005). Assessment of quality of care in postpartum wards of Shaheed Beheshti Medical Science University hospitals, 2004. *International Journal of Health Care Quality Assurance, 18,* 333–342.

Sobo, E. J., Seid, M., & Gelhard, L. R. (2006). Parent-identified barriers to pediatric health care: A process-oriented model. *Health Services Research, 4,* 148–171.

Spillane, V., Byrne, M. C., Byrne, M., Leathem, C. S., O'Malley, M., & Cupples, M. E. (2007). Monitoring treatment fidelity in a randomized controlled trial of a complex intervention. *Journal of Advanced Nursing, 60,* 343–352.

Turner, C., Yorkston, E., Hart, K., Drew, L., & McClure, R. (2006). Simplifying data collection for process evaluation of community coalition activities: An electronic web-based application. *Health Promotion Journal of Australia, 17,* 48–53.

CHAPTER 10

Program Quality and Fidelity: Managerial and Contextual Considerations

This chapter reviews the current trends and approaches to managing healthcare organizations that collectively form the context within which a health program must function. The trends and approaches described here are important for the influences they exert on healthcare organizations. The assumption is that health programs are based in a wide range of types of healthcare organizations, such as federal agencies, state and local health departments, not-for-profit and for-profit health systems, community-based not-for-profit organizations, church-affiliated organizations, and international relief and assistance organizations. Commonalities exist across these organizations, with many being subject to the same legal constraints and obligations. Most healthcare organizations experience similar pressures to ensure and document the quality of health care provided, and all face a growing need for electronic information systems. The content of this chapter is intended to illuminate that broader healthcare environment as a contextual influence that managers and planners of health programs must navigate to achieve high program quality and intervention fidelity.

Of primary importance is accountability—thus the chapter begins with a discussion of this topic. That discussion is followed by a review and synthesis of the currently pervasive approaches being used by healthcare organizations to achieve and maintain healthcare quality. Most health programs need to fit within the broader quality system being used by the healthcare organization. Processes dealing with ensuring a desired level of quality can lead to change efforts intended to remedy a quality problem or enhance the existing quality of the program. Whether on a small or large scale, managers and directors of health programs will need to draw upon their knowledge of and skills at facilitating group change. For this reason, the chapter includes a review of key group process concepts as related to making changes happen.

THE ACCOUNTABILITY CONTEXT

Accountability and responsibility are cornerstones for program implementation. *Accountability* means being held answerable for actions taken and the subsequent success or failure of the program. *Responsibility* means having the charge to ensure that things are done, and done within the specified parameters. Program managers are generally both accountable for the program and responsible for seeing that the program is carried out. Accountability with regard to program implementation fits within the twin realms of program accountability and professional accountability.

Program Accountability

Program managers are accountable for the program in six areas (Rossi, Freeman, & Lipsey, 1999), as summarized in Table 10.1. Each area of accountability requires some thought, planning, and oversight. In other words, through careful attention to the organizational plan and the services utilization plan, each type of accountability can be achieved.

Three types of accountability relate to the organizational plan: fiscal, legal, and efficiency. *Fiscal accountability* refers to the need for sound accounting, careful documentation of expenses, and tracking of revenues. *Legal accountability* encompasses staff acting in accordance with local, state, and federal laws and within their professional licensure limits. *Efficiency accountability* means that the program is delivered with efficient use of the resources.

Two types of accountability relate to the services utilization plan: coverage and service delivery. *Coverage accountability* relates to the program reaching the intended recipients; it is documented with the calculation procedures described in Chapter 9. *Service delivery accountability* comprises the extent to which the intervention is provided as planned. It is indicated by not only the number of units of service provided, but also the number of times that the program intervention protocol was not followed or the number of changes made to the intervention.

Finally, one type of accountability relates to the effect theory: impact accountability. *Impact accountability* is concerned with the program having an outcome and impact on the target audience and recipients. The indicators for impact accountability are highly tailored to reflect the effect theory of the program.

Professional Accountability

Professional accountability refers to an individual from a health profession being bound by the corresponding professional norms and codes, including the moral and ethical codes related to serving the public interest. As discussed in Chapter 8, members of the multidisciplinary team may be licensed and

Table 10.1   Types of Program Accountability, with Definitions and Examples of Process Evaluation Indicators

Accountability Type	Definition: The Extent to Which	Examples of Indicators
Organizational Plan Related		
Efficiency	Resources are utilized without waste or redundancy	Dollars spent on the program, cost per client served, cost per unit of outcome
Fiscal	Resources are managed according to the budget	Existence of receipts and bills paid, number of errors found during annual audit, percent variance from budget
Legal	Legal, regulatory, and ethical standards are met	Number of malpractice suits, number of investigations, number of personnel with current licensure
Service Utilization Plan Related		
Coverage	The target population is reached	Coverage efficiency, efficiency index, percent coverage efficiency target achieved
Service delivery	The intervention is provided as planned	Number of units of service provided, number of breaches of intervention protocol, number of modifications to intervention
Effect Theory Related		
Impact	Participants change or are changed because of the intervention	Very program-specific health and behavior indicators

required by law to practice within those boundaries. These professional ethics and norms generally provide a broader, more encompassing, and less well-codified set of rules to guide professional behavior. Professional accountability becomes important to programs in a variety of ways that can influence the program planning or implementation, with its concerns typically falling into the realm of either personal professional accountability or generic public health professional accountability.

Personal professional accountability encompasses situations in which an individual is not performing according to professional standards and norms. This mandate creates the need for managerial support and possible supervision to ensure that professionals are held accountable for meeting their professional standards. Ideally, failure to perform according to professional standards will be rare among the program staff. However, if it does occur, a program manager ought to seek help from the human resources department to resolve the issue.

The more complex concept of generic public health professional accountability is concerned with the extent to which the program addresses social justice and disparity problems. Given that program budgets are always tight, with correspondingly specific program eligibility criteria usually being established, some individuals in need of the program and who would participate may potentially not be accepted into the program. This situation has the potential to create an ethical dilemma that puts professional accountability at odds with the program limitations. In other words, public health professionals who have social justice as an element of their professional accountability may view the program as being at odds with their professional accountability. The take-away message is that wise program planners and managers never lose sight of the relevance of professional accountability in their program and take that issue into consideration during the planning stages.

PERFORMANCE AND QUALITY: NAVIGATING THE INTERFACE

Health programs exist within the complex and constantly evolving healthcare system, which is changed by fads and managerial fashions as much as by new scientific evidence. One fad that has become standard fare is attention to quality through a variety of now well-established procedures and approaches.

The focus on ways to improve the quality of health care and health services began with Donabedian's work in 1966 (Donabedian, 1966). Donabedian (1980) was the first in health care to suggest taking a systems approach by investigating structure, processes, and outcomes. His approach focused attention on organizational processes involved in providing care, which have no standardized reporting in contrast to the standardized reporting of diagnoses. Over time, however, well-developed approaches to studying processes became accepted as a means of improving organizational efficiency and effectiveness. The more widely known and used approaches are summarized here, and their relevance to managing health programs is discussed in some depth.

The quality improvement approaches discussed in this section are distinct from the older, yet still very important field of quality assurance. *Quality assurance* entails using the minimum acceptable requirements for processes and standards for outputs as the criteria for taking corrective action. For example, laboratory tests must be conducted within strict parameters that ensure accuracy of testing. The laboratory processes' and tests' accuracy are regularly assessed against those standards and requirements. Quality assurance can be an important element of ensuring that program interventions are delivered as planned and according to the program standards. In other words, quality assurance teams typically seek to identify errors and bring processes into compliance. The corrective managerial actions generated from quality assurance programs tend to stress following procedures, rather than identifying larger, more systemwide program process improvements. This relatively narrow focus explains why quality assurance does not foster or result in overall improvement but rather serves to maintain a minimum standard.

Quality Improvement Approaches

Continuous quality improvement (CQI) (Juran, 1989) and total quality management (TQM) (Deming, 1982) were adopted by healthcare organizations as tools to reduce costs while improving the quality of services. By the 1990s, both approaches had become popular means of enhancing organizational effectiveness and were commonplace in healthcare organizations (Shortell et al., 2000). CQI and TQM are based on the premise that problems are best addressed through attention to the system as a whole and that employees are the best source of possible solutions. For the most part, these approaches focus on examining organizational processes using statistical and other scientific tools.

Although CQI and TQM initially had different emphases, both targeted processes were based on systems theory and relied on engineering and operations management tools to analyze the situation. Over time, they have evolved into more generic ongoing processes for assessing the inputs into key organizational processes that influence the use of resources and of patient outcomes. As ongoing organizational processes, quality improvement efforts are conducted by standing quality improvement committees that include employees who are directly involved in the processes being addressed.

The tools used by improvement committees rely on statistical analyses and graphic displays of the statistical information. Seven basic tools are used to statistically control the processes (Figure 10.1). These tools are easy to use and require minimal statistical knowledge, which probably accounts for their wide application. The creation of the displays and the data displayed both contribute to insights for process improvement.

Figure 10.1   List of Quality Improvement Tools with Graphic Examples*

Tools	What the Tool Does	Visual Example
Cause-and-effect diagram, Ishikawa or Fishbone chart	Identifies many possible causes for an effect or problem, sorts contributing causes into sequenced and useful categories	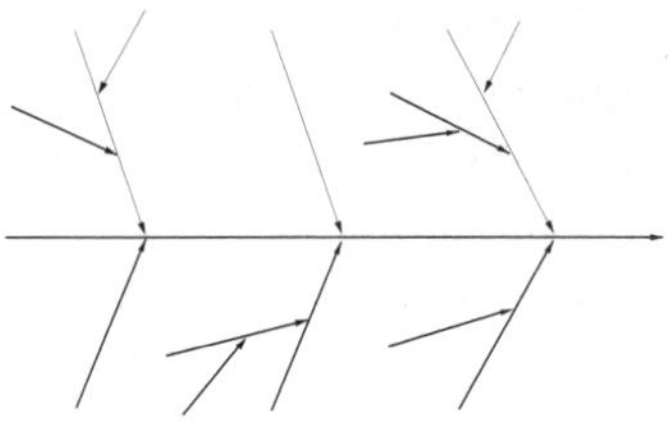
Check sheet	Form for collecting and analyzing data	**Check Data to Be Reviewed and Analyzed** ☐ Name recorded ☐ Age recorded ☐ Visit at recommended interval ☐ Attended health promotion class
Control charts	Graph shows values relative to upper and lower control limits set at 3 sigma (standard deviations) for one variable either across individuals as shown or across time (not shown)	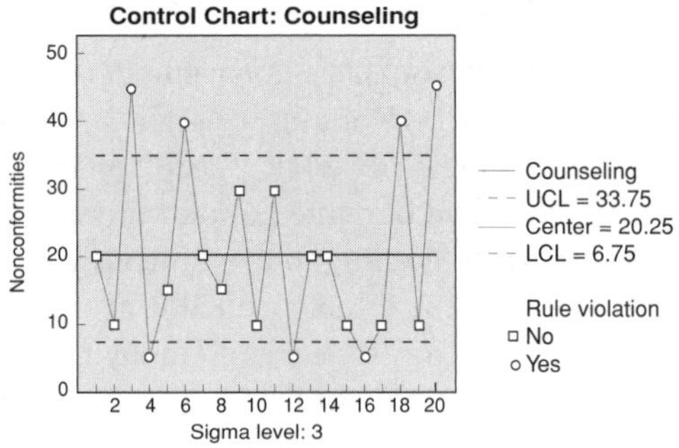
Histogram	Shows frequency distributions for one variable (used age of 20 women in the NTD prevention program)	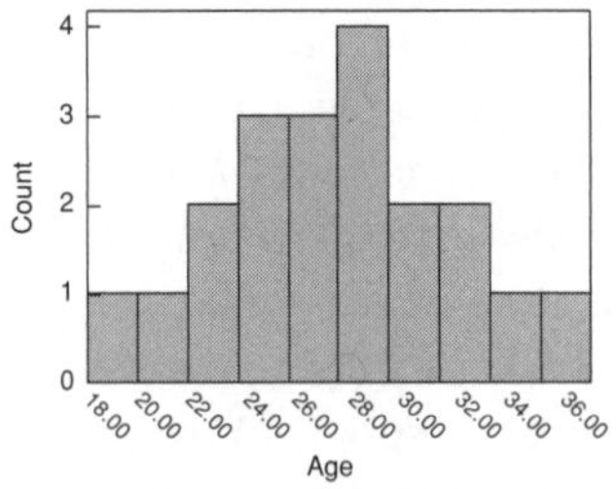

Figure 10.1   List of Quality Improvement Tools with Graphic Examples*

Tools	What the Tool Does	Visual Example
Pareto chart	Bar graph to help identify the few "problem" individuals or variables that create the majority of the non-conformity to the process (used 0 = no screening, 1 = yes screened to understand who exceeds the recommended 20 minutes, numbers above bars represent numbers of persons)	
Scatter diagram	Graph shows relationship between pairs of numerical data with one variable on each axis (used age and number of minutes of counseling, dots represent individuals)	
Flowchart	Shows separate process steps in sequential order, with connections between processes and end points	

* The control chart, historgram, Pareto chart, and scatter diagram were author created using SPSS© v.15 (http://www.spss.com/), whereas the fishbone and flowchart were developed using Chartist © v.4 (http://www.novagraph.com/)

PERT charts diagram the sequence of events against a specific time line, thereby showing when tasks need to be accomplished. *Fishbone diagrams,* or cause diagrams, are representations of sequential events and major factors at play at each stage. *Control charts* show an average, with upper and lower confidence limits and standard deviations. They indicate whether a variable is within the acceptable parameters, and they result in a heavy focus on setting and staying within control limits and parameters for a select set of outcome indicators. *Histograms* are simple bar graphs showing the frequency of a value for one variable. *Pareto charts* are bit more complicated—they use a bar graph to identify the major source of a problem. *Scatter diagrams* show the relationship between two variables by using the data from each individual. They make it easy to see the direction of the relationship. *Flowcharts* diagram the sequence of activities from start to outcome.

CQI/TQM methodologies are constantly being updated by popular, albeit similar, approaches. For example, Six Sigma is a process to reduce variation in clinical and business processes (Lazarus & Neely, 2003). All of the quality improvement approaches use a data-driven approach to analyze process variations as the basis for taking corrective actions to control the degree of variation in the process. These variations are attributed to actions that deviate from the specified protocol product.

Another widely adopted approach is the Balanced Scorecard (BSC). BSC was developed by Kaplan and Norton (1992, 1996) as a tool for businesses that integrates financial performance measures with measures of customer satisfaction, internal processes, and organizational learning. Although initially developed for for-profit businesses, the BSC approach has since been adapted for use in the not-for-profit sector (Urrutia & Eriksen, 2005) as well as the British National Health Service (Radnor & Lovell, 2003).

Relevance to Health Programs

Evaluations can be affected by the presence of CQI/TQM in several ways. Mark and Pines (1995) suggest that the evaluation will be influenced by whether an organization is engaged in CQI/TQM because employees will already be sensitized to the use of data, will have had an introduction to data analysis methods, and will be accustomed to participating in analytic and change activities. Staff, because of their participation in CQI/TQM teams, may expect to be involved in the development of a program and its evaluation. For all these reasons, involving program staff may be slightly easier in organizations using CQI/TQM.

It also may be easier to develop program theory in organizations that practice CQI/TQM because staff will already have training and knowledge of techniques that can be very useful in program planning, especially PERT charts, fishbone diagrams, and control charts. These skills help personnel articulate and then construct diagrams of underlying processes, especially when program planners are developing the process theory. They also make the CQI/TQM way of thinking and methods useful in designing and conducting process monitoring evaluations. In particular, familiarity with CQI/TQM methods facilitates the identification of problems related to the implementation of the service utilization plan and deficiencies in the organizational plan.

Even organizations with strong process improvement processes need program evaluations, however—especially outcome or impact evaluations. When they were originally implemented, the quality improvement approaches emphasized a strict focus on processes as they affect outputs. More recently, improvement approaches have begun encompassing consideration of outcomes. Evaluators and program planners working in healthcare organizations will inevitably experience the continual introduction of new approaches to improve the processes and outcomes of those organizations. Because such methodologies direct attention toward solving problems, program evaluators need to be sensitive to how current process improvement approaches might influence program development and implementation and, hence, the evaluation. Organizational process improvement approaches differ from evaluation with regard to the underlying philosophy, the purposes, the personnel who carry out the activity, and the methods used (Table 10.2).

Performance Measurement

As with most terms in evaluation, there is no consensus on the definition of "performance measures," but the following generic definition gives a sense of what they are. *Performance measures* are indicators of process, output, or outcomes that have been developed to be used as standardized indicators by health programs, initiatives, practitioners, or organizations.

The passage of the Government Performance Results Act of 1993 placed a new and stronger emphasis on performance measures. The Act requires that the each federal governmental agency "express the performance goals for a particular program activity in an objective, quantifiable, and measurable form" (Office of Management and Budget, n.d.). This mandate has led federal agencies that fund health programs, whether as research projects or national infrastructure building, to develop and implement performance measures to which they hold their grantees accountable. The trend toward performance measures continued with the No Child Left Behind Act of 2001. As Berry and Eddy (2008) point out, the emphasis on standardized testing and use of evidence in education is affecting the practice of evaluation.

Table 10.2   Comparison of Improvement Methodologies and Program Process Evaluation

	Process Improvement Methodologies	Program Process Evaluation
Philosophy	Organizations can be more effective if they use staff expertise to improve services and products	Programs need to be justified in terms of their effect on participants
Purpose	Systems analysis and improvement focus on identified problem areas from the point of view of customer needs	Evaluators determine whether a program was provided as planned and if it made a difference to the participants (customers)
Approach	Team-based approach to identifying and analyzing the problem	Evaluator-driven approach to data collection and analysis
Who does it	Staff–employees from any or all departments, mid-level managers, top-level executives	Evaluators and program managers, with or without the participation of employees or stakeholders
Methods	Engineering approaches to systems analysis	Scientific research methods

The criteria for good performance measures include the following characteristics (Krumholz et al., 2006). Performance measures must be useful in improving patient outcomes by being evidence based. They must also be interpretable by practitioners and actionable by improvement committees. The measures must utilize rigorous measurement design that includes validity and reliability. Because many performance measures are also rates, they must specify who is included in the denominators and numerators. Lastly, measurement implementation to obtain the performance measures data must feasible.

Table 10.3 shows the key elements generally used in performance measures. Performance measures, including those approved by the federal Office of Management and Budget (OMB), will have these highly specific characteristics. In addition, performance measures vary across accrediting bodies and the various performance measurement systems (Table 10.4).

The assumption is that the necessity of reporting on performance measures forces program managers to pay attention to what is measured, and subsequently to undertake improvement efforts for performance measures not achieved or reached. In reality, the evidence in support of this premise is equivocal. For

Table 10.3   Definitions of Terms Used in Performance Measurement

Performance Measurement Element	Definition
Measure type	Broad health status that the performance measure is intended to describe.
Measure	Statement in measurable terms of the desired health status or behavior, as it relates to the measurement type.
Numerator	Definition by which to assign individuals into the numerator so as to quantify the measure.
Denominator	Definition by which to assign individuals into the denominator so as to quantify the measure.
Rationale for measure	Brief explanation of relationship of the measure to the measurement type. Includes reference to the appropriate *Healthy People 2010* objective.
Limitations of measure	Statement of which key factors might contribute to the potential failure of program, which would be captured in the measure.
Use of measure	Suggestions for how the measure might be used in program development or policy making.
Data resources	List of relevant sources of data for estimating the measure.
Limitations of data	Brief statement of those factors that may contribute to inaccurate, not valid, or not reliable data from the data resource listed.

Table 10.4   Partial List of Existing Performance Measurement Systems Used by Healthcare Organizations, with Their Websites

Name (Acronym)	Sponsoring Organization(s)	Website
Capacity Assessment for Title V (CAST-5)	Association of Maternal and Child Health Programs and Johns Hopkins University	http://www.amchp.org/topics/a-g/cast.php
Consumer Assessment of Health Plans (CAHPS®)	Agency for Healthcare Research and Quality	https://www.cahps.ahrq.gov/default.asp
Healthcare Effectiveness Data and Information Set (HEDIS)	National Commission on Quality Assurance	http://www.ncqa.org/tabid/59/Default.aspx
Joint Commission	Joint Commission on Accreditation of Healthcare Organizations (JACHO)	http://www.jointcommission.org/
National Public Health Performance Standards (NPHPS)	CDC and a variety of public health organizations	http://www.cdc.gov/od/ocphp/nphpsp/index.htm

example, Bradley and colleagues (2006) found only a small correlation between performance on a set of performance measures related to acute myocardial infarct care and patient outcomes. Nonetheless, even the marginal or small improvements in outcomes that result from attention to performance measurement may cumulatively or over time contribute to a clinically significant improvement in health outcomes.

Relevance to Health Programs

The list of performance measure characteristics described earlier reveals that performance measures are fairly similar to program objectives, in terms of both intent and content. Thus, when developing process and outcome objectives, it may be important to align the objectives with the performance measures or to have objectives that are the performance measures on which the program needs to report. Achieving such cohesion, of course, requires that program planners, managers, and evaluators communicate and share full information on the performance measures being required by funding agencies. In addition, it will be incumbent upon the evaluator to explain the connection between performance measures and the program evaluation, as well as to help reduce redundancies in what is being tracked and measured.

Informatics and Information Technology

The importance of informatics and information technology to developing, managing, and evaluating a health program cannot be understated. Information technology ranges from electronic medical records, data warehousing, web-based patient education, wireless applications, and telemedicine to biometrics and handheld technology. During the development of the organizational plan, the appropriate information technology for the program ought to have been carefully considered and chosen. Nevertheless, having the technology is only of value if the data collected first are turned into information and then knowledge. It is in this spirit that the topic is revisited here as it relates to program quality and intervention fidelity.

One potential advantage of having a health information system in place is that it contains and makes available very current data. Most health information systems perform nearly real-time data collection. If program managers or evaluators have access to this information, then they can obtain very current data on the implementation of the program interventions. Timely access to process data can be used on a regular basis to monitor for any deviations from the intervention as well as for the program's closeness to the targets specified in the process objectives. Naturally, an organization's ability to maximize its access to this type of very useful information will depend on program planners having included the key variables in the data being collected and on having negotiated for access to or reports from the database.

Another potential advantage can be derived from implementation of an effective health information system. It is possible that data needed for process monitoring or effects evaluation are already being collected. This is especially likely if the health program is being implemented by a health system or plan. The vast majority of health systems and plans already collect key indicators of care and service quality through the Healthcare Effectiveness Data and Information Set (HEDIS) and performance measures for the Joint Commission on Accreditation of Healthcare Organizations (JCAHO). Most healthcare organizations have established electronic information systems that are designed to gather data on the performance indicators for these two systems. Knowing whether the program organization collects these data can help the program planner and manager.

For example, consider the Bowe County program to increase adult immunizations. One of the HEDIS measures is the percentage of adults older than age 65 who have received influenza immunizations. Thus, if one process objective addresses physician ordering of immunizations, then it would be possible to collaborate with the health systems in Bowe County to receive quarterly reports on this HEDIS measure.

CREATING CHANGE FOR QUALITY AND FIDELITY

The purpose of collecting, analyzing, and reviewing process data is to create a feedback loop within the program that both leads to improvements that strengthen the program implementation and maintains the optimally functioning elements of the program. The feedback loop consists of first interpreting the process data, then formulating and implementing corrective managerial or programmatic actions. In other words, changes are made to ensure program quality and fidelity.

Interpreting Implementation Data

Before any actions are taken to modify the program processes, data from the process evaluation need be converted into information. Implementation data collected about the program processes become information when the data are given meaning.

Giving the data meaning begins by comparing the data from the process monitoring with the targets stated in the process objectives. Ideally, each objective dealing with the organizational plan and service utilization plan will be compared with actual program accomplishments as documented in the process evaluation. Calculating the efficiency index (described in Chapter 9) is one way to determine the extent to which process objectives were met. An alternative is to use a simple tally of the number of process objectives met, exceeded, or not met. Both approaches summarize the process data in a way that allows the program evaluator, manager, staff, and stakeholders to make sense of the program's accomplishments and shortfalls. Part of the process of making sense of these data is to determine the sources of gaps between targets and actual performance.

Attention to coverage is a critical area for interpretation because of its importance in determining the cause of program failure, should the effect evaluation reveal no programmatic effect on the participants. If the program is delivered to individuals who are not in the target group, and hence would not benefit from the program, then the intervention will appear to have no effect. Understanding the reasons for under- or over-coverage is tricky. The data will reveal whether a programwide problem exists; if so, a qualitative investigation could then be conducted to understand what occurred. Such an inquiry into the perceptions of participants (especially those not in need of the program who are participants) and of program staff would provide additional data as a basis for interpretation. Also, the interpretation may suggest that the extent to which the objectives were met was a function of the objective targets not being realistic, in terms of being either too high or too low.

Program staff ought to be included in discussions about the degree of congruence found between the objectives and the program's actual accomplishments. Their insights can provide plausible explanations for gaps and reveal the need to collect other information related to the cause of the gap between desired and actual program implementation.

Over-coverage is equally likely to result from poor program administration as from the program inadvertently addressing an unrecognized need. When over-coverage occurs, recruitment, screening, or enrollment procedures may be faulty or inadequate. These administrative issues can be addressed with staff training and revisions of the procedures. Over-coverage resulting from an unrecognized need is more difficult to assess and may require further study.

Consider an immunization clinic for school-age children. If many children are brought for immunizations when those children are already fully immunized, then over-coverage exists. In fact, the unrecognized need in this case may be parental confusion regarding school immunizations or lack of a centralized immunization tracking system.

Another example of over-coverage would be more than the expected number of senior citizens attending a free lunch program. The unrecognized need may be for socialization opportunities for the seniors of the community, or perhaps the free ride to and from the luncheon site is the only way for the seniors to get to a nearby mall. In this case, over-coverage can be thought of as a form of expressed needs. Thus the reason for over-coverage, if not administrative, may lead to new programs.

Under-coverage is also a possibility. In such a case, barriers to access, availability, acceptability, and affordability are the most likely causes of the problem. Under-coverage also results if marketing about the program is inadequate. One other possible cause of under-coverage stems from a faulty community assessment that overestimated the number in need of the program.

Another consideration is the extent to which program components are provided. This is especially important for complex programs that incorporate interdependent program components. Using the Layetteville program for violence prevention as an example, program components include education, parental support, and policing. If any one of these components is lacking, the other components might fail to show any effects because the components were designed to have synergistic effects. The process data that reveal a missing component challenge program planners and managers to interpret that information in terms of feasibility, the degree to which the objectives were realistic, and events in the context of the program.

Maintaining Program Process Quality and Fidelity

The analysis and interpretation of the implementation evaluation data ought to lead to identification of actions that can be taken to maintain or improve the program processes. Of course, process data are valuable only if they are used in a timely manner to make alterations in the program implementation. In this regard, implementation monitoring is similar to the various improvement approaches and methodologies already discussed. Once the areas of deficit or weakness or the unachieved objectives have been identified, action is required. Findings from process evaluations may lead program managers to take one of two possible avenues of action.

Implementation-Focused Actions

One set of actions comprises managerial actions focused on the day-to-day implementation processes and activities related to the organizational plan or the services utilization plan. Actions may, for example, address the coverage aspect of the service utilization plan. Suppose under-coverage results from a small program that attempts to tackle a big problem. In this instance, documentation of the under-coverage, along with documentation of program success in achieving the desired effects, can be used to seek funds to expand the program. If serious under-coverage is found in the process evaluation, then the social marketing plan that was implemented ought to be reviewed and perhaps revised based on the available process evaluation data about the participants. In addition, attention may need to be directed toward reviewing the cultural acceptability of the program.

If the program has been ongoing for several years and the indices of efficiency are declining, then it may be time to fine-tune the program (Rossi & Freeman, 1993). This might entail updating the needs assessment to have more current and accurate numbers for the population in need, revising program objectives to reflect current practice and situations, altering the marketing strategy, or adjusting elements of the organizational plan. The specific fine-tuning would depend on the process data and the interpretations made in regard to those data.

A report with a description of how the process data were collected and an outline of the connections between the data and the program objectives is usually a product or output of the process evaluation. The report ought to address organizational plan objectives and achievements, as well as service utilization plan objectives and achievements. The report, or appropriate portions of it, can be shared with program staff, funding agencies, and other stakeholders. A periodic process evaluation that is shared with program staff can be used to identify factors that contribute to the "success" or "poor performance" of the program. Findings from the process evaluation can be shared in ways that maintain individual confidentiality but allow staff members to see their productivity in comparison to that of other staff. Reasons for higher and lower productivity that are amenable to managerial intervention might be identified. In addition, sharing the process evaluation data with staff provides an opportunity for personnel to express their concerns, point out challenges in complying with intervention specifications, and demonstrate their overall morale as it relates to the project.

Process Theory–Focused Actions

The other set of actions that can be taken in response to an evaluation focuses on revising or modifying aspects of the process theory, excluding the interventions themselves. The interventions, which are part of the effect theory, are excluded from revision until sufficient effect data are available to determine whether the types and dosage of interventions are actually contributing to the desired health outcomes. However, the quality and fidelity of delivery or provision of the interventions are appropriately the focus of actions.

This fine distinction can be seen in the following example. Suppose that adult immunization clinics are scheduled for Mondays in the early afternoon, but the attendance records indicate poor attendance. Some informally collected qualitative data indicate that the seniors go for free lunches at that time. Then, in interpreting the low percentage of reach and managing the program to achieve its target objectives, it would be reasonable to change the dates for the clinic and increase the social marketing efforts, without changing the immunizations provided or the eligibility criteria. This example shows the extent to which much of the revision to the process theory is just common sense. Although a change in the day of the immunization clinic is a simple solution, it may not be simple to implement because of other constraints and organizational factors. In some cases, a simple solution may require considerable effort to make the change.

Managing Group Processes for Quality and Fidelity

Identifying the aspects of the process implementation that are in need of modification, refinement, or change is useful only to the extent that the program staff can then be motivated to make the changes. Managerial capabilities—an organizational plan input—become important at this juncture. Two considerations are the natural individual and group negative reactions to being evaluated and the corresponding skills needed to address such reactions.

The natural inclination upon being evaluated, especially on work performance, is to become defensive. When the program manager and evaluators bring to the program staff a set of recommendations for change, staff may interpret this action as them receiving a poor performance evaluation. Also, the program staff reaction is likely to be defensive. The approach used to gain support from the program staff for the proposed modifications can determine the success or failure of making the needed modifications, so managers need to utilize skills related to managing groups (specifically, the program staff) as part of this approach.

Group process skills include communicating, motivating, identifying a purpose and direction setting, setting group norms, understanding stages of group formation, cooperation building, and providing guidance but not control. This partial list of group skills hints at the potential complexity of steering a group toward a desired set of actions and processes. The program manager may use a wide range of strategies to ensure the quality and fidelity of the program implementation. Drawing on network theory, he or she may choose to win over a central and well-connected staff member as a way to influence the broader net of staff. Alternatively, the program manager may draw upon the theory of group formation (forming, storming, norming, performing) if a new program has brought together a new team to implement the health program. If the program staff are highly motivated and professional, the program manager may instead choose to rely on the self-organization principle of complexity theory and allow the staff to evolve in ways that enhance the quality and fidelity of the program. Whichever approach is employed, the program manager should consciously choose an action path that fits with the program and the degree of change needed.

When and What Not to Change

For all the talk about making changes to ensure the quality of the program and fidelity of the intervention, sometimes it is not advisable to make changes. The obvious time not to make changes is when activities and objectives are on track, on target, and on time. For some programs, circumstances may make it imprudent to implement changes, such as when critical stakeholders are resistant, there are insufficient funds to complete a change, or the process data are ambiguous and open to widely divergent interpretations.

If a program is based on a tried-and-true theory or is a replication of an existing successful program, then it would be best not to modify the actual intervention until sufficient outcome data are available to determine the program's effectiveness. A change to the intervention should be postponed until sufficient outcome data substantiate that the intervention is causing adverse, undesirable, or dangerous side effects or that it is not at all effective. Making a change to the actual intervention, rather than the processes, requires revising the effect theory as well as any corresponding portions of the process theory.

FORMATIVE EVALUATIONS

A *formative evaluation* is an assessment during the initial stages of the implementation process and preliminary outcomes. It is performed if a program is new or experimental and is under some type of political scrutiny. The term "formative" suggests that the evaluation is conducted as the program is forming or in its early stages of implementation.

Formative evaluations, because they are conducted before the full implementation of a program, can be thought of as diagnostic of early problems with the program process theory. For such evaluations to be useful, program managers need to have at least some preliminary data on whether the intervention is the "right" intervention. This may require collecting some very rudimentary but salient health outcome data. Formative evaluations also frequently entail the use of multiple methods, employing both quantitative methods and qualitative approaches. The qualitative approaches, such as focus groups and interviews, can be helpful in understanding problems from the perspective of either the program staff or the program participants. The other requirement for a useful formative evaluation is that it is done in a timely manner and with strong feedback and reporting to the program manger. This approach ensures that corrective modifications can be made early in the program implementation.

ACROSS THE PYRAMID

At the direct services level of the public health pyramid, accountability and attention to quality are most readily seen in the vast array of accrediting bodies and certifications for both individual practitioners and healthcare organizations that provide direct services. Depending on the health program, the quality assurance and fidelity issues are likely to be related to individual providers or to the program staff in general. The source of program infidelity will influence the action plans and the interpersonal communication needed to achieve high program quality.

At the enabling services level, accrediting bodies for enabling services and programs are also likely to hold the program managers accountable for the quality of the program. The challenges facing these program managers and evaluators will be similar to the challenges faced by their counterparts at the direct services level. The nature of enabling services, such as being more community based and group focused, may make it more challenging to initiate corrective actions, should process monitoring reveal poor program fidelity.

At the population services level, it can be difficult to monitor the implementation in a timely manner, making it difficult to have a quality improvement process. This challenge does not negate the importance of maintaining the quality and fidelity of population-level interventions. The other issue at the population services level is the fact that programs may be decentralized. For example, immunization clinics are run by local health departments and large healthcare systems. But if the program is essentially a state health program, with state financial support, then the state immunization program manager will be accountable for the quality of the decentralized system.

At the infrastructure level, the management of the health program is an infrastructure element. Naturally, managers of programs targeted at the health workforce also must be held accountable for the quality of the implementation. Most of the quality improvement approaches mentioned earlier are intended to lead to changes in the infrastructure of personnel deployment, resource distribution, and process modification. The BSC might be particularly relevant as an infrastructure tool, because it addresses the organization's ability to learn.

DISCUSSION QUESTIONS

1. Imagine that you need to explain to a community of stakeholders the difference between a quality improvement approach and a process evaluation approach. What would you summarize as being unique to each approach, and what are the similarities between the two approaches?

2. Construct a hypothetical flowchart for Bowe County and Layetteville's program to increase the rates of immunizations for adults, beginning with recruitment and proceeding through complete immunization.

3. Look at the scatter diagram, Pareto chart, and control chart in Figure 10.1, which were based on data from 20 women in the Congenital Anomalies Prevention Program in Layetteville. For each one, write one statement that describes the key information conveyed in that chart. Based on these three statements, what would you recommend to the program manager in terms of quality improvement?

4. Of the different types of accountability, which do you view as most important, most difficult to achieve, and of most value to stakeholders? Justify and explain your choices.

INTERNET RESOURCES

Many organizations focus specifically on quality improvement in health care.

National Committee on Quality Assurance

NCQA is the organization that has established the HEDIS measures. Information about HEDIS is available at http://www.ncqa.org/.

American Society for Quality

The American Society for Quality (http://www.asq.org/index.html) has a variety of resources that are accessible from its website.

Total Quality Management Glossary

A list of terms used in CQI/TQM is given at this website: http://www.quality.org/TQM-MSI/TQM-glossary.html.

National Quality Forum

An interesting report, *The National Voluntary Consensus Standards for Hospital Care: An Initial Performance Measure Set* (2003), is available at http://www.qualityforum.org/pdf/reports/hospital_measures.pdf.

Agency for Healthcare Research and Quality

AHRQ has published an excellent online book about performance measurement; find it at http://www.ahrq.gov/chtoolbx/index.htm. Although this book is geared toward child groups, the content is applicable to other populations as well.

Ohio Department of Health

The Ohio Department of Health is collecting six measures endorsed by the Joint Commission, the Centers for Medicare and Medicaid Services, and the National Quality Forum regarding heart attacks, heart failure, and pneumonia. It is also collecting five patient safety indicators created by the Agency for Healthcare Research and Quality regarding surgical procedures. These measures can be found at http://www.odh.ohio.gov/healthStats/hlthserv/hospitaldata/hospperf.aspx. The Ohio example shows how much data are already being collected that may be useful for monitoring program implementation and effects.

Government Accountability Office

The GAO produced a fascinating report following the Hurricane Katrina disaster focusing on the alignment of CDC and HRSA performance measures regarding preparedness. Find it at http://www.gao.gov/new.items/d07485r.pdf.

Government Performance Results Act of 1993

Here is the official webpage describing the GPRA: http://www.whitehouse.gov/omb/mgmt-gpra/gplaw2m.html.

University of Washington, Turning Point Program

This organization has published a book on performance measurement. Find it online at http://www.turningpointprogram.org/Pages/pdfs/perform_manage/pmc_guide.pdf.

REFERENCES

Berry, T., & Eddy, R. M. (2008). Consequences of No Child Left Behind for educational evaluation. *New Directions for Evaluation, 117,* 21–36.

Bradley, E. H., Herrin, J., Elbel, B., McNamara, R. L., Magid, D. J., Nallamothu, B. K., et al. (2006). Hospital quality for acute myocardial infarction: Correlation among process measures with relationship with short-term mortality. *Journal of the American Medical Association, 296,* 72–78.

Deming, W. E. (1982). *Quality, productivity, and competitive position.* Cambridge, MA: MIT Press.

Donabedian, A. (1966). Evaluating the quality of medical care. *Milbank Memorial Fund Quarterly, 44*(3, Part 2), 166–206.

Donabedian, A. (1980). *Explorations in quality assessment and monitoring. Volume 1: The definition of quality and approaches to its assessment.* Ann Arbor, MI: Health Administration Press.

Juran, J. M. (1989). *Juran on leadership for quality: An executive handbook.* New York: Free Press.

Kaplan, R. S., & Norton, D. P. (1992). The Balanced Scorecard: Measures that drive performance. *Harvard Business Review, 70,* 71–79.

Kaplan, R. S., & Norton, D. P. (1996). *The balanced scorecard: Translating strategy into action.* Boston: Harvard Business School Press.

Krumholz, H. M., Anderson, J. L., Brooks, N. H., Fesmire, F. M., Lambrew, C. T., Landrum, M. B., et al. (2006). ACC/AHA clinical performance measures for adults with ST-elevation and non-ST-elevation myocardial infarction: A report of the American College of Cardiology/American Heart Association Task Force on Performance Measures (Writing Committee to Develop Performance Measures). *Journal of the American College of Cardiology, 4,* 236–265.

Lazarus, I. R., & Neely, C. (2003). Six Sigma: Raising the bar. *Managed Healthcare Executive, 13,* 31–33.

Mark, M. M., & Pines, E. (1995). Implications of continuous quality improvement for program evaluation and evaluators. *Evaluation Practice, 16,* 131–139.

Office of Management and Budget. (n.d.). *Government Performance Act of 1993.* Retrieved May 15, 2008, from http://www. whitehouse.gov/omb/mgmt-gpra/gplaw2m.html

Radnor, Z., & Lovell, B. (2003). Success factors for implementation of the Balanced Scorecard in the public sector. *Journal of Corporate Real Estate, 6*(1), 99–108.

Rossi, P. H., & Freeman, H. E. (1993). *Evaluation: A systematic approach* (5th ed.). Thousand Oaks, CA: Sage Publications.

Rossi, P. H., Freeman, H. E., & Lipsey, M. L. (1999). *Evaluation: A systematic approach* (6th ed.). Thousand Oaks, CA: Sage Publications.

Shortell, S. M., Jones, R. H., Rademaker, A. W., Gilles, R. R., Dranove, D. S., Hughes, E. F. X., et al. (2000). Assessing the impact of total quality management and organizational culture on multiple outcomes of patient care for coronary artery bypass graft surgery patients. *Medical Care, 38,* 207–217.

Urrutia, I., & Eriksen, S. D. (2005). Application of the Balanced Scorecard in Spanish private health-care management. *Measuring Business Excellence, 9*(4), 16–26.

Outcome and Impact Evaluation of Health Programs

CHAPTER 11

Planning the Intervention Effects Evaluation

In the daily work of implementing a program, evaluation of intervention effects can seem like a luxury. The reality is that conducting an evaluation whose purpose is to identify whether the intervention had an effect requires considerable forethought regarding a broad range of issues, each of which has the potential to seriously detract from the credibility of the evaluation.

The intervention effect evaluation deserves the same degree of attention during program planning as does development of the program interventions; ideally, it should be designed concurrently with the program. All too often, only after the goals and objectives are finalized and the program is up and running is attention then focused on developing the evaluation. Well-articulated program outcome goals and outcome objectives facilitate development of the evaluation, but insights about the program process can be gained from developing an evaluation plan.

Given these considerations, the placement of this book's chapters on intervention effects evaluation after the chapters on program development and monitoring ought not to be interpreted as when planning the intervention effect evaluation is done. As highlighted in the planning and evaluation cycle (Figure 11.1), the planning and decisions about the effect evaluation ought to occur as the program is being developed.

The contents of this chapter address the broad areas of data collection and evaluation rigor, within the context of the program theory and feasibility considerations. The information presented in this and the next chapters on designs and sampling is not intended to duplicate the extensive treatment of research methods and statistics provided in research textbooks. Instead, basic research content is presented as the background for the problems commonly encountered in conducting a health program evaluation, and practical suggestions are provided for minimizing those problems. Because the focus here is on practical solutions to real problems, the suggestions offered in this chapter

Figure 11.1   Planning and Evaluation Cycle, with Effect Evaluation Highlighted

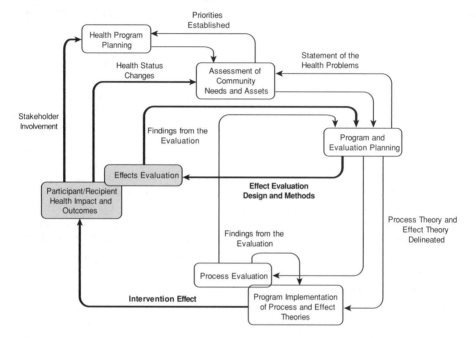

may differ from those usually found in research and statistics textbooks. Nonetheless, good research methods and statistics textbooks are invaluable resources and references that ought to be on the bookshelf of every program evaluator.

Planning the evaluation begins with selecting the evaluation questions and then proceeds to developing the details of the evaluation implementation plan, similar to the details of the program organization plan. Aspects of the evaluation plan related to data collection are discussed next—namely, levels of measurement and levels of analysis, as well as techniques to collect data. A review of designs that can be used to conduct the evaluation and issues related to sampling are discussed in Chapters 11 and 12. These elements of evaluations are closely aligned with research methodology, and achieving scientific rigor is the first yardstick used when planning the intervention effects evaluation.

DEVELOPING THE EVALUATION QUESTIONS

The first step in planning the evaluation is deciding which questions the effect evaluation must be able to answer. The first place to start in developing the evaluation questions is with the logic model, the effect theory, and the outcome objectives—they ought to be the basis for decisions about the focus and purpose of the intervention evaluation. The effect theory draws attention to the specific aspects of the health problem that are being addressed by the program. Many aspects of the health problem and possible health outcomes of the program could potentially be addressed by an evaluation, and novice evaluators and enthusiastic program supporters will be sorely tempted to include as much as possible in the evaluation. Succumbing to this temptation will lead to higher evaluation costs, produce an overwhelming amount of data to analyze and interpret, and distract from the essence of the program. Thus staying focused on key outcome objectives minimizes the chance that the evaluation will become a fishing expedition. In other words, designing an evaluation can quickly lead to the development of a creative "wish list" of statements such as "if only we knew x about the recipients and y about their health." The outcome objectives serve as a sounding board against which to determine whether that "if only we knew" statement has relevance and importance to understanding whether the program was effective.

Why an evaluation is done and what is expected from the evaluation must be considered early in the evaluation planning. The obvious reason for doing an evaluation is to determine the effect of the program on recipients. Patton (1997) has argued that the usefulness of evaluation information ought to be a major reason for doing the evaluation. Nevertheless, evaluations may be conducted for other reasons, such as to fulfill requirements of funding agencies. The need to respond to funding agency requirements can be an opportunity to engage program stakeholders and elicit their interests with regard to why an evaluation should be performed. Information that stakeholders want from an evaluation, once made explicit, then can be incorporated into the evaluation.

A key aspect of the "why do an evaluation" question is the determination of who cares whether the evaluation is done and what it might find. There might also be a desire to "prove" that the program was the source of some beneficial change. Evaluations that attempt to answer causal questions are the most difficult type to perform, but causality testing provides the richest information for understanding the validity of the effect theory.

Characteristics of the Right Question

Evaluations ought to be useful, as well as scientifically sound and based on the program objectives (Patton, 1978, 1997). From the perspective of being useful, the "right" evaluation question has three characteristics (Patton, 1978), and evaluation questions with all of these characteristics will lead to useful and feasible evaluations.

One characteristic is that relevant data can be collected. Relevant data may not be easily accessible, and their successful collection may require negotiation and reliance on the effect theory, as the following true story reveals. A community agency wanted to know if its program was having an effect on the substance abuse rates among school-age children. The stakeholders did not believe that data collected several years prior to the program's implementation from across the state were relevant to their community. Yet data could not be collected from children in grades six through eight regarding their use of illegal drugs (an intermediate program outcome) because the school board refused to allow the evaluators into the schools. Thus the evaluation question of whether the substance abuse prevention intervention changed the behavior of these children could not be answered. Eventually, the program staff restated the question to focus on whether children who had received the substance abuse prevention program had learned about the negative health effects of illegal substances (a direct program outcome). The school board was willing to allow data on this question to be collected from children.

Another characteristic of the right evaluation question is that more than one answer is possible. While this characteristic may seem counterintuitive, allowing for the possibility of multiple answers shows less bias on the part of the evaluator for arriving at the desired answer. Evaluations that are flexible and inclusive may yield multiple answers that may reveal subtle differences among participants or program components that were not anticipated. Compare the evaluation question of "Did the program make a difference to participants?" with the evaluation question of "Which types of changes did participants experience?" The second question makes it possible to identify not only changes that were anticipated based on the effect theory, but also other changes that may not have been anticipated.

A third consideration is that the right evaluation question produces information that decision makers want and feel they need. Stakeholders also ought to want the information from the evaluation and be interested in the answer to the evaluation question. Ultimately, the right question will produce information that decision makers *can* use, regardless of whether it actually *is* used in decision making. The test of usefulness of the information generated by the evaluation will help avoid the fishing expedition problem and, more importantly, could be a point at which developing the evaluation provides feedback relevant to the design of the intervention.

As these three characteristics suggest, having a clear purpose for the evaluation and knowing what is needed as an end product of the evaluation are the critical first steps in developing the evaluation question. The nature of the effect evaluation will be influenced by the skill and sophistication of those persons doing the evaluation as well as the purpose of evaluation. The key factor in stating the intervention effect evaluation question is the degree to which the evaluation must document or explain health changes in program participants.

Outcome Documentation, Outcome Assessment, and Outcome Evaluation

Evaluation of the effect of the intervention can range from the simple to the highly complex. At minimum, it ought to document the effect of the program in terms of reaching the stated outcome and impact objectives. An *outcome documentation evaluation* asks the question, "To what extent were the outcome objectives met?" To answer this question, an outcome documentation evaluation will use data collection methods that are very closely related to the objectives. In this way, the outcome objectives that flowed from the effect theory become the cornerstone of an outcome documentation evaluation.

The next level of complexity is an *outcome assessment evaluation*, which seeks to answer the question, "To what extent is any noticeable change or difference in participants related to having received the program interventions?" An outcome assessment goes beyond merely documenting that the objectives were met by quantifying the extent to which the interventions seem related to changes observed or measured among program recipients. With this type of effect evaluation, the data collection may need to be more complex and better able to detect smaller and more specific changes in program participants. Note that the outcome assessment addresses the existence of a relationship between those persons who received the program and the presence of a change, but does not attempt to determine whether the change was caused by the program. This subtle linguistic difference, which is often not recognized by stakeholders, is actually an enormous difference from the point of view of the evaluation design.

The most complex and difficult question to answer is "Were the changes or differences due to participants having received the program and nothing else?" To answer this question, an *outcome evaluation* is needed. Because this type of effect evaluation seeks to attribute changes in program participants to the interventions, and nothing else, the data collection and sample selection must be able to detect changes due to the program and other potentially influential factors that are not part of the program. This highly rigorous requirement makes an outcome evaluation the most like basic research (especially clinical trials) into the causes of health problems and the efficacy of interventions.

Thinking of the three levels of program effects evaluation (Table 11.1) as outcome documentation, outcome assessment, and outcome evaluation helps delineate the level of complexity needed in data collection, the degree of

Table 11.1   Three Levels of Intervention Effects Evaluations

	Outcome Documentation	Outcome Assessment	Outcome Evaluation
Purpose	Show that outcome and impact objectives were met	Determine whether participants in the program experienced any change/benefit	Determine whether participating in the program caused a change or benefit for recipients
Relationship to program effect theory	Confirms reaching benchmarks set in the objectives that were based on program effect theory	Supports program effect theory	Verifies program effect theory
Level of rigor required	Minimal	Moderate	Maximum
Data collection	Data type and collection timing based on objectives being measured	Data type based on program effect theory; timing based on feasibility	Data type based on program effect theory; baseline or pre-intervention data required as well as post-intervention data

scientific rigor required, and the design of the evaluation. Design of the evaluation is discussed in detail in Chapter 12.

Evaluation and Research

The distinction between evaluation and research can be ambiguous and is often blurred in the minds of stakeholders. Nonetheless, fundamental differences do exist (Table 11.2), particularly with regard to purpose and audiences for the final report. Much less distinction is made with regard to methods and designs—both draw heavily from methodologies used in behavioral and health sciences.

The differences between research and evaluation are important to appreciate for two reasons. First, communicating the differences to stakeholders and

Table 11.2   Differences Between Evaluation and Research

Characteristic	Research	Evaluation
Goal or purpose	Generation of new knowledge for prediction	Social accountability and program or policy decision making
Questions addressed	Scientist's own questions	Questions derived from program goals and impact objectives
Nature of problem addressed	Areas where knowledge is lacking	Outcomes and impacts related to program
Guiding theory	Theory used as basis for hypothesis testing	Theory underlying the program interventions, theory of evaluation
Appropriate techniques	Sampling, statistics, hypothesis testing, and so on	Whichever research techniques fit with the problem
Setting	Anywhere that is appropriate to the question	Any setting where evaluators can access the program recipients and nonrecipient controls
Dissemination	Scientific journals	Internal and externally viewed program reports, scientific journals
Allegiance	Scientific community	Funding source, policy preference, scientific community

program staff helps establish realistic expectations about implementing the evaluation and about the findings of the evaluation. As a consequence, it will be easier to gain their cooperation and feedback on the feasibility of the evaluation. Second, understanding the differences can allay anxieties about spending undue amounts of time "doing research," which will take time away from providing the program, the primary concern of program staff.

Research, in a pure sense, is done for the purpose of generating knowledge, whereas program *evaluation* is done for the purpose of understanding the extent to which the intervention was effective. These need not be mutually exclusive purposes. That is, a good program evaluation can advance knowledge, just as knowledge from research can be used in program development. *Evaluation research* is performed for the purpose of generating knowledge about the effectiveness of a program and, as such, represents the blending of research and evaluation.

While these three terms are often used interchangeably or ambiguously, it is easiest to think of evaluation research as research done by professional evaluators, following standards for evaluation and using research methods and designs. Evaluation research is most often an outcome assessment or an outcome evaluation. In this regard, it tends to be more complex, to be costly, and to require more evaluation skill than most program staff have. This discussion is not meant to imply that simpler outcome documentation is not valuable. The value always lies in the evaluation addressing the right question for the program.

Rigor in Evaluation

Rigor is important in evaluation, as in research, because there is a need to have confidence that the findings and results are as true a representation as possible of what happened. The playing cards are often stacked against finding any difference from a program because of programmatic reasons, such as having a weak or ineffective intervention, and because of evaluation research methods reasons, such as having measures with low validity or reliability. Rigor results from minimizing the natural flaws associated with doing evaluation, which might otherwise diminish the evaluators' ability to identify the amount of effect of the program. The net effects are those that are attributable only to the program, whereas the total change includes effects from the intervention as well as effects that are artifacts of the evaluation design (Figure 11.2), such as history, maturation of the participants, or societal changes. The purpose of the effect evaluation is to identify the net effects, so rigor is used to minimize the inclusion of non-intervention effects and design effects.

VARIABLES FROM THE PROGRAM EFFECT THEORY

Based on the effect theory, the health program planner should have developed outcome and impact objectives that focus on what the program ought to achieve. Just as process objectives are useful in developing the program monitoring evaluation, so the effect theory and the outcome and impact objectives

Figure 11.2   Diagram of Net Effects to Which Measures Need to Be Sensitive

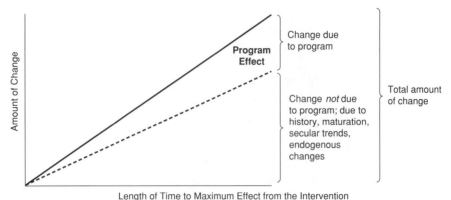

serve as cornerstones that guide decisions regarding what to measure in the intervention effect evaluation.

The effect theory is composed of three theories, as explained in Chapter 5 the causal theory explains the relationships among the existing factors, the main causal factors of the health problem, the moderating and mediating factors, and the health outcome. The intervention theory specifies how the programmatic interventions change the main causal factors of the health problem, as well as the moderating and mediating factors. The impact theory explains how the immediate health outcomes become the longer-term health impacts. The effect evaluation uses these theories as the basis for deciding what to measure, specifically with regard to the main causal factors of the health problem and the health outcomes. At minimum, the causal factors and health outcomes specified in the theories need to be measured.

Program evaluators use the nomenclature convention used in research and statistics. The outcome and impact variables are designated as y, the dependent variable, and the variables that precede the impact are designated as x, independent variables. Strictly speaking, any antecedent existing, causal, moderating, or mediating factor is an independent variable, as is the intervention. This nomenclature is shown in Figure 11.3. Labeling the variables as x and y at this stage of planning will help later, during data analysis.

Outcome and Impact Dependent Variables

The heart of any evaluation is *what*—that is, which health or behavioral characteristic—is assessed for a change or outcome. The "what" question

Figure 11.3   Using the Effect Theory to Identify Effect Evaluation Variables

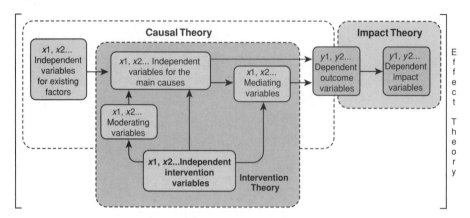

ought to be answered directly from the "what" aspect of the outcome objective, which in turn comes from the "risk of x" portion of the community health statement. For example, for the Bowe County diagnosis regarding African Americans older than age 40 being at high risk for developing type 2 diabetes and its associated comorbidities, the evaluation measures the outcome in the form of diabetes incidence. The choice in this situation revolves around which laboratory test or indicator of a new diagnosis of diabetes to use—not whether to measure incidence or knowledge about diabetes.

The outcome variable, called the dependent variable (y), is the same as was specified in the outcome objectives. Similarly, the long-term health impact variable is also a dependent variable, as specified in the outcome objectives. The difference between these two dependent variables is a matter of what the evaluation question is. In the newborn health example, the outcome as a dependent variable would be used for questions such as "Was the rate of neural tube defects lower among program participants?" In contrast, the impact variable, the rate of birth defects, would be used for a question such as "Was having a state folic acid promotion program related to a decrease in birth defects?"

Typically, health program evaluations assess the effect of programs in the six domains of well-being or physical health: knowledge, lifestyle behaviors, cognitive processes, mental health, social health, and resources. These domains of health and well-being can also be related to the existing, causal, moderating, and mediating factors of the health problem of concern. During development of the program effect theory and logic model, the health program planners should have determined the role of those domains on the health problem.

In planning the evaluation, it will be crucial to refer back to those discussions and decisions as a means of deciding whether the health domain is the dependent variable or an independent variable in the intervention evaluation. At this juncture, during the discussion of what exactly is the dependent variable, program staff and stakeholders might potentially gain new insights into their program and want to modify the effect or intervention theory. This discussion, if it occurs before the program is implemented, can then become one of the feedback loops to program development or improvement. In any event, the outcome objectives provide direct guidance and ought to specify which indicators, and subsequently which measures, to use in the evaluation. If the outcome objectives fail to be helpful, this is another point at which developing the evaluation can provide refinement to the program development effort.

If the program planners were enthusiastic, energetic, and perhaps overly ambitious, the list of outcome objectives may have become extensive. The program evaluators then face a choice between measuring everything on the laundry list or selecting key outcome objectives for measurement. Attempting to measure many outcomes is another form of going on a fishing expedition. Remember, there is a 5% probability that something will be statistically significant (i.e., $p < .05$) just by chance alone. Therefore, evaluators would be wise to work with program planners and stakeholders to narrow the field from all possible outcomes to only those outcomes about which having information is critical. Also, just because an outcome can be evaluated does not translate into it being worth evaluating—don't evaluate the obvious (Patton, 1997). For example, there is no benefit to evaluating the antibody status of the adults who attended an immunization clinic and had received the recommended adult vaccines.

For programs with multiple intervention components and multiple health outcomes, at least one health outcome per program component needs to be measured. For this reason, it may be difficult to construct a short list of dependent variables, especially if different outcomes are expected for each component. The intervention theory related to that component will help identify those variables that are key or common across program components or are central to achieving overall program success. Those dependent outcome or impact variables need to be measured.

Who is included in the evaluation is derived from the "among [target population]" portion of the community health statement and the "who" in the outcome objectives. The delineation of "who" leads to consideration of the sample and of the appropriate sampling frame given the program's target population. At minimum, the "who" includes program recipients who are assessed for degree of program effect. However, if the health program has the potential to reach and affect an audience beyond known recipients, such as might happen with a mass media educational campaign, then the issue of who to assess becomes more complex. This decision also leads to consideration of the use of a comparison group whose members did not receive the program. The task of deciding who ought to be in the comparison group is discussed in detail with regard to sampling in Chapter 13.

Causal Factors as Independent Variables

Evaluators may be tempted to include in the evaluation measures of various existing factors and causal factors to the health problem. Because the list of these factors can be extensive, decisions need to be made as to which factors are crucial in explaining the health outcomes of the program. For outcome documentation, these factors need not be measured; instead, only the outcomes as stated in the objectives are measured. For outcome assessment and especially for outcome evaluation, however, key antecedent factors and causal factors will be important to measure. The program effect theory can help identify the specific variables in each category that should be included in the evaluation.

The causal factors are considered a set of independent variables because they are independent relative to the health outcome that is the true dependent variable. Whether these independent variables will be measured before and after the program, or in both participant and control groups, is a design decision that is made based on available resources and the level of scientific rigor needed in the evaluation. Causal factors, as key independent variables, are the first variables to be considered for measurement. Having data on the presence and strength of the causal factors of the health problem can provide extremely useful information that helps program planners and managers understand how the intervention effect was manifested. For example, descriptive data on causal factors can reveal patterns of intervention effects among different groups of participants and identify whether the interventions were mismatched to the causal factors found among the actual program participants.

Antecedent, Moderating, and Mediating Factors as Variables

Other factors can influence the effectiveness of interventions, such as moderating and mediating variables. Recall that a *moderating variable* affects the strength or direction of the relationship between two other variables, whereas a *mediating variable*, sometimes called an intervening variable, is necessary for the relationship between two other variables to exist (Donaldson, 2001). The difference between these two types of variables is based on their role in the relationship between the independent and dependent variables (Donaldson, 2001). The value in distinguishing whether a factor functions as a moderating or mediating variable comes in deciding whether it is important to measure and, especially later, when conducting data analysis and making interpretations. Critical to the program evaluation is the idea that the intervention theory is correct—in other words, that the interventions actually lead to the desired change in the causes of the health problem, given the antecedent, moderating, and mediating factors.

The importance of identifying and including moderators and mediators in evaluations is stressed by Bauman and colleagues (Bauman, Sallis, Dzewaltowski, & Owen, 2002), who focused on understanding influences on the success of physical activity interventions. Inclusion of moderating and mediating variables facilitates understanding which factors influence the effectiveness of an intervention. For example, Foshee and colleagues (2005) found that prior experience with violence moderated the violence prevention program effects, whereas changes in community norms mediated the effectiveness of the program's interventions. Perhaps not surprisingly, Burke, Beilin, Cutt, Mansour, and Mori (2007) found that gender moderated the effect of an exercise program such that the program had a large effect among women. These authors also found that self-efficacy was a mediator of changes in diet. These studies demonstrate how having information on moderating and mediating variables provides more specific information about program effectiveness.

Figure 11.4 depicts the effect theory for reducing congenital anomalies in Bowe County. It shows that the factors identified through the needs assessment become variables in the effect evaluation.

MEASUREMENT CONSIDERATIONS

Units of Observation

The unit that is observed or measured in the evaluation must match the level at which the program is targeted and delivered. For example, the violence prevention program interventions in Layetteville are targeted at schools and neighborhoods, as well as at high-risk adolescents. Consequently, the effect evaluation should take place at the individual, school, and neighborhood levels. The evaluation seeking to determine the degree of change within the neighborhood might use a questionnaire that asks community members about their neighborood. With the congenital anomalies prevention program, the intervention component is aimed at families. If the questionnaire is given to only one individual within the family and asks questions about that individual's perceptions or behaviors, then there is a mismatch between the level targeted by the intervention (family) and the unit on which evaluation data are

Figure 11.4   Effect Theory of Reducing Congenital Anomalies Showing Variables

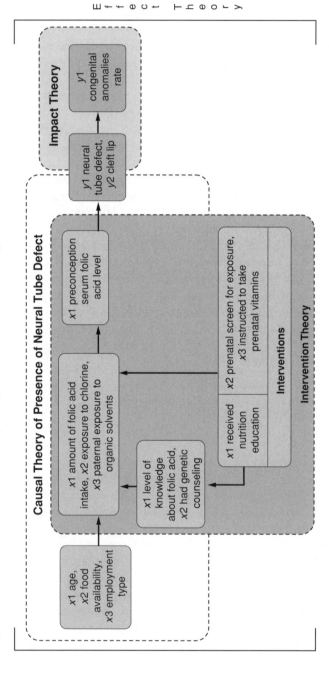

collected (individual). The same rationale applies to evaluating community- or neighborhood-level interventions (Best, Brown, Cameron, Smith, & MacDonald, 1989). As these examples demonstrate, the unit and level of observation are important in terms of ensuring that the effect evaluation data are collected in a way that maximizes the potential to find the intervention effects. A levels mismatch decreases that possibility.

Types of Variables (Levels of Measurement)

Another factor to consider is which type of variable to use in the evaluation, meaning how complex is the information gathered by each variable. Variables are classified according to the level of complexity of information, and each level has its own advantages and disadvantages (Table 11.3).

Nominal variables are the simplest, in that the information indicates only yes/no, absent/present, or a name. Nominal variables that give only yes/no type of information are also called dichotomous; variables that have simple categories, such as job title or medical diagnosis, are called categorical.

Table 11.3   Advantages and Disadvantages of Using Each Type of Variable

Type	Examples	Advantage	Disadvantage
Nominal, categorical	ZIP code, race, yes/no	Easy to understand	Limited information from the data
Ordinal, rank	Social class, Likert-type scale, "top ten" list (worst to best)	Gives considerable information, can collapse into nominal categories	Sometimes statistically treated as a nominal variable, ranking can be a difficult task for respondents
Interval, continuous	Temperature, IQ, distances, dollars, inches, dates of birth	Gives most information; can collapse into nominal or ordinal categories; used as a continuous variable	Can be difficult to construct valid and reliable interval variables

Ordinal variables provide slightly more information by indicating an order, a sequence, or a rank. The most common ordinal variabes are generated from a Likert-type scale, such as good, fair, and poor. The task of giving a list of items a rank can be a difficult task for respondents and creates challenges for data entry and analysis.

The most complex, rich, and complete information is provided by *interval* variables, in which the intervals between the values are equal on an absolute scale. Generally, interval variables are continuous with no practical starting or ending points to the values, like the number of DNA base pairs. As a consequence, they are also called continuous variables. However, some interval variables do have limits, such as the lab values for HgbAlc, a measure of blood sugar, or the number of hospital admissions for gunshot wounds. These items are considered discrete interval variables. In terms of statistical tests, whether a variable is an interval variable is less important than whether zero can be a starting point. In health care, the issue of having a starting point, or zero value, is often quite relevant and can affect the subsequent statistical analysis. For example, the number of days hospitalized is an interval variable with a valid zero value as the starting point for the variable.

For each domain of health and well-being, variables can be constructed at each of the three levels (Table 11.4). Careful attention to the level of the measurement is crucial for several reasons. One reason is that the measurement level directly relates to the statistical tests that can be used with that level of measurement (as will be further discussed in Chapter 14). Basically, a higher level of measurement (interval) enables use of a greater variety of statistics. Another reason is that the level of measurement influences whether clinically meaningful information is contained in the variable. In addition, the level of measurement must be sufficiently sensitive so that a distinction can be found among participants with regard to program effects (Green & Lewis, 1986).

Timing

"When," or the timing of the evaluation, is guided by the "by when" portion of the outcome objectives. The "by when" determination ought to have been made based on the intervention theory and the causal theory, which indicate the duration of the intervention effects and the amount of time needed to achieve a noticeable effect. The "by when" consideration thus provides guidance as to three aspects of the intervention effects: the earliest time at which an intervention effect ought to be found, the time at which the maximum intervention effect is expected to occur, and the rate at which change in the health domain is expected to occur. All of this information is used in

Table 11.4   Examples of Nominal, Ordinal, and Continuous Variables for Different Health Domains

Dependent Outcome Variable	Nominal, Categorical	Ordinal	Interval, Continuous
Physiological Health Domain			
Childhood immunization	Yes/no up-to-date	None required, one immunization required, more than one immunization required	Rubella titer
Physical abuse	Yes/no have experienced physical abuse; type of abuse	Level of abuse is same, more, or less than last month	Rate of physical abuse in a county; number of times abused in past 6 months
Workplace injury	ICD-10cm for injury	Level of severity of injury	Number of disability days per year in construction industry
Knowledge Domain			
Understand how alcohol affects judgment	Agree/disagree	Three most common ways alcohol affects judgment	Score on test of knowledge about effects of alcohol
Behavioral Domain			
Breastfeeding	Yes/no breastfed	Category for how long breastfed: 2 weeks, 3–6 weeks, more than 6 weeks	Number of days breastfed
Smoking	Yes/no smoke	Light, moderate, or heavy smoker	Nicotine levels

Table 11.4   Examples of Nominal, Ordinal, and Continuous Variables for Different Health Domains *(Continued)*

Dependent Outcome Variable	Nominal, Categorical	Ordinal	Interval, Continuous
Readiness of change	Yes/no likely to change next week	Stage of change in terms of readiness	How likely (on 100-point scale) will change in next week
Cognitive Process Domain			
Legally competent	Yes/no; *DSM-IV* code for mental illness	Level of mental incapacity	Score on standardized competency questionnaire
Mental Health Domain			
Depression	Above/below clinical cut-off on score for depression	Rank of depression on list of prevalence of mental health problems	Score on standardized depression scale, such as CES-D or Beck Depression Inventory
Social Health Domain			
Social support network	Yes/no have friends	Degree of support in network (low, medium, high)	Number of people in social support network
Resources Domain			
Housing situation	Homeless or not	Housing autonomy (own, rent monthly, rent weekly, homeless)	Number of days living at current residence

choosing methods, specifically with regard to when to collect data. An additional consideration with regard to "when" is whether baseline or pre-intervention data are needed as part of the evaluation plan. If baseline data are needed, then decisions will center on how far in advance of receiving the program it is reasonable and feasible to collect data

The outcome objectives, because they focus on the program participants, may not have taken into account programmatic timing. For example, if a program involves cycles, as with a series of classes, then the evaluation ought to occur after at least one group has received the full intervention. For this type of information, the process objectives need to be reviewed, along with the findings from the process evaluation, because at minimum the outcome evaluation ought to be done after the program is sufficiently well implemented.

Maticka-Tyndale, Wildish, and Gichuru (2007) created a time line table that shows both intervention activities and evaluation activities. Table 11.5 provides a generic example of such a time line. A time line of intervention activities and data collection, although not standard practice, is extremely valuable, especially for complex, multi-component interventions.

Sensitivity of Measures

An interplay exists between the nature of the factor being measured and the measure itself. Of concern is that the measure be sensitive enough to variations and fluctuations in the factor that even minor changes can be detected. *Measure sensitivity* is the extent to which the difference among or within individuals can be detected. Fluctuations can occur because of individual variations, changes over time, or the influence of other factors. Given these possibilities, evaluators need to choose the measure used to collect data on the factor carefully. For many of the measures used in health care and health programs, publications exist of evaluations or research on the measure or studies that used the measure. Such reports provide information as to which measures will be sensitive enough to meet the needs of the evaluation.

An example helps to illustrate this point. If one outcome objective of the health program is to reduce anemia in pregnant women, then some blood samples are used to determine anemia. Different tests can be used, depending on the program's focus. If the program is focused on overall rates of anemia, measuring hematocrit is sufficient. If the program is focused on a specific cause of anemia, such as folic acid deficiency, a more sensitive measure of anemia is needed.

Sensitivity concerns have prompted the development of almost innumerable measures, some of which have been compiled in books, such as Cohen, Underwood, and Gottlieb's (2000) compilation of social support measures or Bowling's (1997) review of quality-of-life measurement scales. These and similar compendia are helpful in selecting a measure that matches the program outcome objectives. Naturally, literature searches will also yield current research on instruments and tests that have validity and reliability.

Table 11.5   Example Time Line Showing the Sequence of Intervention and Evaluation Activities

Date	Intervention Activity	Evaluation Activity
Month 1	Pilot intervention with small group	Conduct focus group to refine intervention acceptability and element of services utilization plan
Month 2	Recruit into program, screen for eligibility	Randomly assign to program or wait list, collect data for baseline and comparison • Participants: $n = 150$ • Nonparticipant controls (from wait list): $n = 150$
Month 3	Provide intervention (i.e., group sessions, counseling, media messages) to first group of participants	Analyze baseline pre-intervention data
Month 4	Recruit participants into program, screen for eligibility	Collect post-intervention data • Participants (time 1) who completed program: $n = 125$ • New nonparticipant controls (from wait list): $n = 130$
Month 5	Repeat intervention (i.e., group sessions, counseling, media messages) for those on the wait list	Analyze data
Month 6		Collect post-intervention data • Current program participants (time 1): $n = 120$ • Previous program participants (time 2): $n = 95$ • Current nonparticipant controls: $n = 110$ Analyze data

THREATS TO DATA QUALITY

No matter how good the planning or the amount of effort put into generating the best possible data, some problems are guaranteed to exist that will affect the overall quality of the data available for analysis.

Missing Data

A very common problem is missing data. Data can be missing on single items in a survey or variables in existing records. It is important to anticipate possible reasons for the missing data. For example, survey data could be missing because of a sensitive question, a page skipped, no response category to capture a possible valid response, or an answer that is not known to the participant. Similarly, data can be missing if medical information is to be abstracted from medical records, but the data were not recorded by the provider, the provider did not gather the data, or laboratory reports are missing. Part of planning the evaluation is to imagine the worst-case scenarios in terms of data collection and to have plans to prevent those situations from occurring. Once the data have been collected, it is highly unlikely that any missing data can be retrieved. Being proactive about training data collectors, surveyors, and data abstractors and making the measurement tools as fail-safe as possible are the best steps to minimize the problem posed by missing data.

After the data have been collected, evaluators should review the data for missing items before undertaking the analysis of those data. If the missing data follow a haphazard pattern, rather than occurring in a systemic pattern, then the occasionally missed item will not dramatically affect the analysis and subsequent findings. Conversely, if there is a systematic pattern to the missing data, then decisions will need to be made regarding the analysis plan. Systematic skips or extensive missing data will have a consistent effect on results of analyses involving that item or variable.

Reliability Concerns

One potential threat to data quality is shortcomings in the reliability of the data. *Reliability* refers to the extent to which the data are free of errors. Several sources of errors can diminish the reliability of the data. For example, the instrument, tool, measure, or test used to collect the data may be flawed. Another factor that can lower instrument reliability is lack of age appropriateness when children are the respondents (Hennessy, 1999). The reliability of the instrument can be statistically assessed as the alpha coefficient or the half-split coefficient (Pedhazur & Schmelkin, 1991), which can be calculated using statistical packages and spreadsheets (Black, 1999). The extent to which the instrument consistently measures what was intended can be affected by the wording of the questions.

Another source of data error is the person providing the data—in other words, the test taker. An individual may vary from day to day in terms of his or her responses, mood, knowledge, or physiological parameters. To assess the likelihood of this type of data error, the reliability of the instrument, regardless of such influences, can be statistically tested using the test–retest approach in which the same group of individuals are measured twice. Higher correlations between those two scores indicate that the instrument was constructed so that data collected are not affected by minor fluctuations within individuals.

An instrument also can be affected by differences across individuals. In such cases, the degree to which the individuals agree is assessed with the *inter-rater agreement*, sometimes referred to as inter-observer agreement. It is particularly important to establish high inter-rater agreement, meaning between individuals, when abstracting data from medical or other records. Interpretations of what is being abstracted and what needs to be abstracted can vary across individuals if they are not given specific training on the data abstraction task. Having a high degree of inter-rater agreement increases the confidence that the data collected across abstractors is highly comparable. The simplest approach to calculating inter-rater agreement is a percent agreement, where the denominator is the number of items to be coded and the numerator is the number of items for which both raters had "correct" agreement. Alternatively, a statistical approach is to calculate the kappa statistic (Cohen, 1960), a measure of agreement that takes into account not only the observed agreements, but also the expected agreements. Kappa values can be calculated using statistical software packages.

Another aspect of data reliability is the quality of the data entry into the statistical software. Data need to be reliably entered. The problem of low data entry reliability can be minimized greatly by training those doing the data entry and by performing data entry verification. To estimate the data entry accuracy, evaluators may select a portion of the data to be double-entered by a second data entry person, and then keep track of the percentage of data entered for which there was a discrepancy. At least a 95% accuracy rate is needed. On one research project that involved a large survey, female inmates from the state prison entered survey data into a database. Being skeptical, the researchers performed data verification on 10% of the surveys. The data entry accuracy rate was found to be 99.8%—much better than the minimum 95% accuracy rate.

Validity of Measures

The *validity* of a measure is the degree to which the tool captures what it purports to measure—in other words, the extent to which the tool measures what it is intended to measure. A measure is valid if it truly measures the concept. Note that the validity of measures is different from the validity resulting from the study design, which is concerned with being able to say the results generally apply to the population (generalizability of findings).

Establishing the validity of measure through advanced statistical analyses is more typically a research activity, rather than an evaluation activity. However, validity can be more informally established as face validity. Face validity, in the simplest procedure, involves asking a panel of experts whether the questions appear or seem to be measuring the concept. If the panel agrees, then face validity has been established. Because face validity can be relatively straightforward, stakeholders and program staff can be involved and help establish this type of validity.

Time and resources used to establish face validity can be saved if existing instruments and questionnaires are selected. Several books are available that specifically review the validity and reliability of health-related instruments (Bowling, 1997), as well as websites (see the "Internet Resources" at the end of this chapter). Other sources for locating existing instruments include the published literature. Researchers who have developed instruments for specific constructs often publish information about those instruments in scientific journals. Another source is electronic databases of instruments, which are typically available through major universities. The Health and Psychological Instruments database, for example, contains published articles using health and psychological instruments, facilitating the search for an instrument applicable to a specific variable.

CONTEXTUAL CONSIDERATIONS IN PLANNING THE EVALUATION

Several broad considerations can influence the effect evaluation. Each of these considerations comes into play to varying degrees during the evaluation.

Budget

One major consideration is the budget—specifically, the cost involved in doing the outcome assessment and the feasibility of allocating such funds to the outcome assessment. This is akin to avoiding the Robin Hood syndrome of "robbing from the program implementation to pay for the evaluation." This problem may occur if the program effect evaluation was not included in the total program budget developed during the planning or implementation stage. A rule of thumb is that funds allocated for effect evaluation ought to amount to 10% to 20% of the program implementation budget. This translates into reducing the dollars for the program by 10% to 20% up front, before the program begins.

A budget for the effect evaluation ought to delineate costs for evaluation expenses, such as personnel wages or salaries, participant incentives, costs of copying and duplicating data instruments, fees for purchasing data, additional office expenses, statistical software licenses, data entry costs, and consultant fees. While it is difficult to set a minimum amount for an evaluation, these expenses can easily exceed $5,000 for straightforward outcome documentation and can reach $50,000 or more for an outcome evaluation that requires evaluation research. Once the evaluation budget has been negotiated and established, then the logistics focus on staying within that budget.

Evaluation Standards

Criteria for a good evaluation were established by the American Evaluation Association. Patton (1997) discussed these criteria in terms of four issues. The first criterion is the process by which decision making occurs regarding the evaluation. That is, a good evaluation is generated from a decision process that is inclusive and thoughtful. The second criterion is that stakeholders need to be able to believe the evaluation results and the evaluator. The third criterion is that stakeholders need to be able to trust the evaluation as being scientifically and ethically conducted and trust the evaluator as a person to do what is ethical and scientifically sound. The fourth criterion is that the most feasible and reasonable design is used, given the constraints and resources of the health program. Each evaluator has the responsibility of designing outcome evaluations that meet these criteria to the greatest extent possible.

Ethics

Another consideration when conducting an effect evaluation is the ethics inherent in conducting outcome assessments. Ethical considerations can affect not only the criteria for eligibility as program participant, but also eligibility for evaluation participants and procedures in the evaluation. From the perspective of some health agencies, program eligibility—not just program evaluation participation—of those in need may be both a moral and an ethical issue. In other words, the ethics of program eligibility needs to be addressed during the program development stage, and those decisions will affect the subsequent ethics of who is included in the evaluation.

The federal Office for Human Research Protections' (OHRP) spotlight on health programs receiving federal funds has highlighted the need for evaluators to participate in efforts to comply with federal regulations. One area of great concern is obtaining informed consent, as discussed in Chapter 17. Consultants from a local university can be helpful in navigating this process. In larger healthcare systems, the internal research review panel can be consulted for assistance in this area.

These caveats and considerations can create circumstances in which an ideal outcome assessment is not possible, despite efforts to make the outcome assessment scientifically rigorous. Recognizing this constraint early in the process and working with it as a limitation is a strength. The solution then becomes to focus on creating not a "perfect" assessment, but rather a "good enough" assessment; "good enough" outcome assessments use the best methodological design given the realities at hand.

One reason why a "good enough" outcome assessment is acceptable is that intervention effect evaluations differ from research in important ways (Table 11.2). The differences between research and evaluation can get blurry for some health program outcome assessments, but recognizing that they exist can help health program evaluators develop a strong "good enough" intervention evaluation. These differences may not be well understood by stakeholders, so education about how the evaluation will be different from research can help stakeholders have greater trust and confidence in the evaluation. A "good enough" evaluation needs to have the same characteristics as the criteria discussed earlier for all evaluations—namely, it must use a feasible design that produces credible, believable, and potentially useful findings.

Stakeholders

One consideration is the stakeholders of the program, and the need to take into account who wants to know what from the outcome assessment. Once the key outcome evaluation questions have been posed, it is important to ask stakeholders what they want to know about the program. Involvement of the stakeholders in the development of the effect evaluation can produce some real payoffs. Not only will they become invested in the findings, but they will be more likely to believe the findings. Because neither programs nor stakeholders are static, some outcome objectives might have been developed by people who are no longer involved with the program and hence may not be valued as highly by current stakeholders or still be relevant given the current circumstances. If the ultimate goal of the outcome evaluation is its use in future program or policy decisions, then stakeholder involvement is imperative. Also, involvement of stakeholders can result in an improved outcome assessment. Another benefit of stakeholder involvement is that expectations can be addressed; that is, if stakeholders' expectations are unrealistic given resource limits or methodological reasons, those expectations need to be acknowledged, discussed, and made more realistic.

At the end of the evaluation, the intended users of the evaluation need to be able to judge the utility of the design and recognize both the strengths and the weaknesses of the evaluation. The intended users may have different criteria for judging the quality of the evaluation, so they may need to learn about the methods used to carry out the evaluation. A debate about the possible findings before the evaluation is complete can help to uncover what would and would not be acceptable findings from the perspective of the stakeholders.

The creation of a long list of variables to be measured may be met with resistance and skepticism by stakeholders, particularly those who advocate for the protection of the participants. This reality reinforces the need for stakeholder involvement in the development of the effect theory and its evaluation. Nevertheless, in some circumstances it will be important to go beyond the objectives in data collection. For example, the evaluation can offer an opportunity to collect information deemed necessary for future program refinement or to update aspects of the community health assessment. The data collected for these purposes are best kept separate, with separate analyses and reporting of them.

For each element of an evaluation, both scientific and programmatic considerations apply (Table 11.6). These considerations have the potential to influence the ultimate design and implementation of the effect evaluations. Reviewing these differences and considerations with stakeholders can help establish realistic expectations and identify points on which consensus is needed. Whatever choices are being faced, ultimately the planners will need to be flexible so that the evaluation can adapt to the realities that are encountered (Resnicow et al., 2001).

ACROSS THE PYRAMID

At the direct services level of the public health pyramid, the evaluation of the outcome of direct services is the most straightforward, albeit not necessarily the easiest type of evaluation. It is straightforward in terms of the effect on individuals who receive the service. At this level, it is always individuals who complete questionnaires and about whom data are collected via secondary sources. For this reason, the means used to construct the questionnaire and collect secondary data are major considerations.

At the enabling services level, the same issues arise as at the direct services level of the public health pyramid—namely, the need to construct sensitive and valid measures and the reliability of the means used to gather secondary data. In addition, evaluators face the issue of how to identify program participants, given that enabling services are likely to be embedded within other services and programs. At the enabling services level, the unit of observation is more likely to become a point of consideration.

At the population services level of the public health pyramid, the major issue deals with aggregation of data and selection of the unit of observation.

Table 11.6   Summary of Evaluation Elements

Elements of Effect Evaluation	Science Considerations	Program Considerations
What to evaluate	Outcome and impact variables most likely to demonstrate the strength of the evidence for the effect theory	Highest-priority outcome and impact objectives, variables that meet funding agency requirements
Who to evaluate	Representativeness of sample and comparability to non-participants, ethics of assignment to the program or not	Accessibility of program participants, availability of easily accessed target audience members
When to evaluate	Onset and duration of effect	Convenience and accessibility of program participants
Why evaluate	Scientific contributions and generation of knowledge	Program promotion, refinement of program, funding agency requirements
How to evaluate	Maximize rigor through choice of measures and design and analysis	Minimize intrusion of evaluation into program through seamlessness of evaluation with program implementation

The inclination is to say that the population is the unit, but in actuality, the unit is most often an aggregation of individual-level data. True population measures would include the gross national product (GNP), population density, biodiversity, and community social capital. Data collection cannot be collected from an entire population, except by census. It is possible to use data from existing national surveys to develop a rate, which is then assumed to apply throughout the population. However, this assumption may be false at more local levels.

Often health programs at the population services level address public knowledge, public opinion, or community outcomes. Stead, Hastings, and Eadie (2002) suggest that for these outcomes, methods such as surveys, focus groups, document reviews, and audits could be appropriate tools, depending on the specific evaluation question.

At the infrastructure level, the evaluation itself is an infrastructure process. But if the program is intended to affect the infrastructure, outcomes are measured as related to the infrastructure. If the skills of public health employees (capacity building) are the program intervention focus, then individual-level data are needed to measure changes in their skills. If the intervention outcome of an infrastructure change is at another level of the pyramid—say, physical education to change a specific direct services practice—then the impact is measured as it relates to the other pyramid level. If, however, the program is intended to have an effect at the infrastructure level, then a major challenge is to construct measures that are at the infrastructure level. Although Halverson and associates (Corso, Wiesner, Halverson, & Brown, 2000; Halverson, 2000), along with others from the Centers for Disease Control and Prevention (CDC), have been working to develop infrastructure measures, these global assessments of the public health infrastructure may not be useful unless the programmatic intervention has sweeping policy impacts that would be measurable throughout the infrastructure.

DISCUSSION QUESTIONS AND ACTIVITIES

1. Develop a working plan for how you would involve stakeholders in the development of the intervention evaluation plan. How does your plan address timing and budget constraints? In what ways does your plan include attention to interactions and group processes? Which strategies will be used to address the four criteria for having a good evaluation question?

2. Select one of the five health programs implemented in Bowe County and Layetteville. Construct a levels of measurement table, similar to Table 11.5, for at least one outcome (dependent) variable in three different health or well-being domains.

3. What are the major problems in using secondary data sources, such as birth or death certificate data? What, if anything, can the evaluator do about these problems?

4. How do the steps in instrument development apply to making surveys cross-culturally appropriate? What effect might you expect in the data, and subsequently in the interpretation of those data, if surveys are not culturally appropriate?

INTERNET RESOURCES

Centers for Disease Control and Prevention

The CDC has a useful site called "Measurement Properties: Validity, Reliability, and Responsiveness" (http://www.cdc.gov/hrqol/measurement_properties/index.htm) that lists studies and research related to the validity and reliability of health status and quality-of-life measures.

Agency for Healthcare Research and Quality

AHRQ offers an online workshop titled "Collecting, Using, and Disseminating Health Data on Minority Populations" (http://www.ahrq.gov/news/ulp/minorpop/ulpmpop.htm) with information on data collection, dissemination, and secondary data sources specific to minority populations.

REFERENCES

Bauman, A. E., Sallis, J. F., Dzewaltowski, D. A., & Owen, N. (2002). Toward a better understanding of the influences on physical activity: The role of determinants, correlates, causal variables, mediators, moderators, and confounders. *American Journal of Preventive Medicine, 23*(2 Suppl.), 5–14.

Best, J. A., Brown, K. S., Cameron, R., Smith, E. A., & MacDonald, M. (1989). Conceptualizing outcomes for health promotion programs. In M. T. Braverman (Ed.), *Evaluating health promotion programs* (pp. 19–32). San Francisco: Jossey-Bass.

Black, T. R. (1999). *Doing quantitative research in the social sciences: An integrated approach to research design, measurement and statistics.* London: Sage Publications.

Bowling, A. (1997). *Measuring health: A review of quality of life measurement scales* (2nd ed.). Philadelphia: Open University Press.

Burke, V., Beilin, L. J., Cutt, H. E., Mansour, J., & Mori, T. A. (2007). Moderators and mediators of behaviour change in a lifestyle program for treated hypertensives: A randomized controlled trial (ADAPT). *Health Education Research, 23*, 202–217.

Cohen, J. (1960). A coefficient of agreement for nominal scales. *Educational and Psychological Measurement, 20*, 37–46.

Cohen, S., Underwood, L. G., & Gottlieb, B. H. (2000). *Social support measurement and intervention: A guide for health social scientists.* Oxford, UK: Oxford University Press.

Corso, L. C., Wiesner, P. J., Halverson, P. K., & Brown, C. K. (2000). Using the essential services as a foundation for performance measurement an assessment of local public health systems. *Journal of Public Health Management and Practice, 6*(5), 88–92.

Donaldson, S. I. (2001). Mediator and moderator analysis in program development. In S. Sussman (Ed.), *Handbook of program development for health behavior and practice* (pp. 470–496). Newbury Park, CA: Sage Publications.

Foshee, V. A., Bauman, K. E., Ennett, S. T., Suchindran, C., Benefield, T., & Linder, G. F. (2005). Assessing the effects of the dating violence prevention program "Safe Dates" using random coefficient regression modeling. *Prevention Science, 6*, 245–258.

Green, L. W., & Lewis, F. M. (1986). *Measurement and evaluation in health education and health promotion.* Palo Alto, CA: Mayfield.

Halverson, P. K. (2000). Performance measurement and performance standards: Old wine in new bottles. *Journal of Public Health Management and Practice, 6*(5), vi–x.

Hennessy, E. (1999). Children as service evaluators. *Child Psychology and Psychiatric Review*, *4*, 153–161.

Maticka-Tyndale, E., Wildish, J., & Gichuru, M. (2007). Quasi-experimental evaluation of a national primary school HIV intervention in Kenya. *Evaluation and Program Planning*, *30*, 172–186.

Patton, M. (1978). *Utilization evaluation*. Beverly Hills, CA: Sage Publications.

Patton, M. (1997). *Utilization focused evaluation*. Newbury Park, CA: Sage Publications.

Pedhazur, E. J., & Schmelkin, L. P. (1991). *Measurement, design, and analysis: An integrated approach*. Hillsdale, NJ: Lawrence Erlbaum Associates.

Resnicow, K., Braithwaite, R., Dilorio, C., Vaughan, R., Cohen, M. I., & Uhl, G. (2001). Preventing substance abuse in high risk youth: Evaluation challenges and solutions. *Journal of Primary Prevention*, *21*, 399–415.

Stead, M., Hastings, G., & Eadie, D. (2002). The challenge of evaluating complex interventions: A framework for evaluating media advocacy. *Health Education Research*, *17*, 351–364.

CHAPTER 12

Choosing Designs for Effect Evaluation

L. Michele Issel, PhD, RN, and Arden Handler, DrPH

Of the many factors contributing to the scientific rigor of an effect evaluation, design is key. In a health program evaluation, evaluators, as compared to researchers, may not have the same degree of control over timing, quality and amount of data collection, or amount of exposure to the intervention. Such constraints and realities contribute to the differences between evaluation and pure research. Much of the evaluation literature discusses design from a research perspective and is geared toward maximizing the scientific rigor of the evaluation. While this approach is needed and appropriate if sufficient funding is available, most small health programs will not have such resources. Most agencies are more focused on and have expertise related to providing or delivering health programs. Personnel in such programs understandably can become lost, confused, or overwhelmed when faced with the task of designing an effect evaluation. This chapter discusses designs from the perspective of evaluators and program managers who must address issues posed by program realities.

Several assumptions underlie the discussion in this chapter. The first assumption is that regardless of the program or agency, at least one design exists that is both scientifically the best option and realistically feasible for the program. A second assumption is that program personnel would choose the best scientific option if it was clear and easy to identify. Thus designs are described here with respect to their feasibility for both small, local, direct services programs for individuals and large-scale, full-coverage programs for populations. Most designs can be adapted for either individual-level or population-level interventions, if the same decision criteria are met. For simplicity, the explanation about a design is framed around the usual and customary use of that design.

377

A third key assumption is that there is a programmatic need to demonstrate that the participants or recipients have changed more than might happen by chance. This assumption means that only collecting data on whether the outcome objectives were met is not sufficient to meet the needs of stakeholders, including funders. Choosing the right design becomes critical in showing that changes to participants did not occur by chance or that one intervention is more effective than another. The last assumption is that the process evaluation has shown that the intervention was delivered as planned to the target audience. This assumption is critical in terms of then assuming that changes ought to be related to the intervention.

EVALUATION DESIGN CAVEATS

The *design* of the evaluation is the grand scheme that delineates when and from whom data are collected. Many types of designs are drawn from health and social sciences. The *methods* indicate the way in which the data are collected as part of the evaluation and typically consist of strategies such as surveys, interviews, or observations. Qualitative designs, another type of design, are reviewed in Chapter 15.

Evaluation designs can be very simple or extraordinarily complex. Most research textbooks cover designs and methods in considerable depth from a research perspective in which the researcher has a great deal of control over factors affecting the choice of a design. However, the choice of a design for an effect evaluation is complicated by the realities and limitations that are inherent in health programs.

Effect evaluation can be done from the perspective of a number of different disciplines, each of which has its own terminology for describing designs (Table 12.1). The social science of psychology typically focuses on individuals and uses experimental and quasi-experimental as the terminology to describe the major classification of designs. Health education mostly uses social sciences terminology for designs. Epidemiology and sociology are other disciplines from which to draw upon when developing the evaluation plan, particularly for full-coverage or population-based programs with target audiences that are populations. Another discipline that is relevant to the evaluation of health programs is health services research, which uses terminology drawn heavily from economics and social sciences. Designs from across these disciplines are available for use in program evaluation.

The terminology used throughout this chapter represents a blend of terms used in social sciences and epidemiology. Application of epidemiological designs to the evaluation of health programs is a fairly new phenomenon (Handler, 2002; Rosenberg & Handler, 1998). Given this more recent use,

Table 12.1   Contribution of Disciplines to Health Program Evaluation

Discipline	Typical Outcome or Impact Question	Typical Design Terminology
Psychology	Are outcomes for individuals in the program (recipients) different from those in the comparison or control group (nonrecipients)?	Experimental, quasi-experimental
Sociology	Are there changes over time that might be related to the implementation of the program?	
Epidemiology	Are cases (individuals who have the outcome characteristic) less likely to have had exposure to the program than controls (individuals without the outcome characteristic)?	Observational
Health services research	Does differential utilization of services (participation or not) by enrollees (target audience) and non-enrollees (non-target audience) lead to differential outcomes?	Experimental, quasi-experimental, clinical trial

Source: Modified from Handler (2002) with personal permission.

specific attention is given to understanding and applying epidemiology designs. In addition, this chapter introduces the terms *pre-test* and *post-test*, which have been adopted from social sciences. When we apply these terms to health programs, two points are worth stressing.

First, *pre* and *post* refer to the sequence of when data are collected; *pre* is any time before receiving the program intervention, and *post* is any time after receiving the program intervention. The precise timing of data collection depends, of course, on logistical issues. More importantly, however, it depends on the expected timing of the first program effects and the duration of those effects as articulated in the program effect theory. The timing of the pre-test and post-test data collection also ought to have been specified in the "by when" element of the outcome objectives.

Second, "test" is a convenient, shorthand term that refers to the measures being used to quantify the program effect. In other words, it is the measurement of the specific outcomes and impacts. When data are collected at the population or aggregate level rather than at the individual level, the pre-test equivalent is *baseline* data; the latter term is more commonly used in epi-demiology, public policy, and health services studies of populations.

CONSIDERATIONS IN CHOOSING A DESIGN

The aim in choosing a design is to come as close as possible to a design that is free of bias. An ideal design has three salient characteristics: (1) a comparison control or unexposed group that is typically as similar as possible to the experimental or exposed group, (2) measurement of the outcome variables before and after the intervention for unbounded health outcomes, and (3) minimal threats to internal and external validity. Designs that meet these three criteria allow the evaluator to make statements that attribute differences found between the two groups to the intervention—and only to the intervention. The following seven considerations become factors in the choice of a design.

Causality

The first decision in choosing a design is to decide whether it is important to determine if a cause-and-effect relationship (also known as a causal relationship) exists between receiving the health program interventions and the health outcomes. There is a direct relationship between the ability to show causality and the costs and complexity of the design (Bamberger, Rugh, & Mabry, 2006). Specifically, as the ability to show causality increases, so do the costs and complexity of the design (Figure 12.1). Thus these two factors become the first considerations in choosing a design.

While choosing to identify a causal relationship leads to a more costly design, such a design may be appropriate if the intervention is new or being adapted to a new target audience. Some designs are better suited than others to establishing a causal connection. This first decision is tempered by considering the need to balance the design with the skill and resources available to the health program personnel. A creative evaluator or evaluation team may devise a complex, scientifically rigorous design that may provide sound evidence for the effectiveness of the program. Nevertheless, unless resources for personnel, data collection expenses, consultants, and incentives for participants are available, the design will probably not be implemented as planned. As such, there will always be an element of needing to adapt the ideal to reality when conducting effect evaluations.

Bias

The choice of an evaluation design is also influenced by the need to have a design that is as free of bias as possible given the realities of the evaluation.

Figure 12.1   Relationship Between the Ability to Show Causality and the Costs and Complexity of the Design

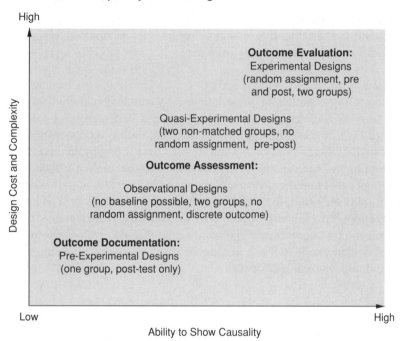

Bias in design refers to the extent to which the design is flawed and, therefore, more likely to lead to an inaccurate conclusion about the effectiveness of the health program. The flaws are categorized based on whether they affect the ability to generalize the findings to other populations (*external validity*) or whether they affect the ability to say that the intervention made a difference (*internal validity*) (Campbell & Stanley, 1963). Understanding the design flaws that constitute threats to the internal and external validity of each design helps in choosing a design that is as free of bias as possible, given the evaluation question and the circumstances. In general, designs with fewer flaws are more complex and costly and are usually more likely to demonstrate a causal relationship between the health program and outcomes.

Retrospective Versus Prospective Orientation

Another major consideration in the choice of a design is whether data are collected retrospectively or prospectively. *Retrospective designs* entail gathering data from the point of intervention backward in time. In other words, participants will have received the program before any baseline data are gathered or accessed. *Prospective designs* entail gathering data forward in time, beginning from a point prior to the initiation of the intervention. If the evaluation is planned during the development of the health program, a prospective design is possible and is generally the preferred approach. Retrospective designs limit the options for measurement and for the selection of comparison groups, whereas prospective designs require that evaluation resources be obtained prior to the start of the program.

Time Span

The length of time that is encompassed by the design—whether looking back or looking forward—needs to be considered. A design can be described as *longitudinal* if it includes multiple pre-tests, multiple post-tests, or both, with these tests spaced out over a duration of time. Longitudinal has the connotation of longer time spans, such as weeks, months, years, or decades, over which the pre-test and the post-test data are collected, although in reality data might be collected multiple times during one day, a few days, or a week. As the designs are described, it will be easy to imagine which are amenable to modification to become longitudinal. The two factors that determine whether a longitudinal design is appropriate in a particular situation are the intervention theory and the evaluation budget.

Groups

Yet another consideration in choosing an evaluation design is whether it is possible to identify and distinguish between participants and nonparticipants. There is inevitably an interplay between the design choice and the ability to know who did and did not receive the intervention. Choosing an evaluation design is linked to defining who is a participant and who is a nonparticipant for individual-level programs or who is a recipient and who is a nonrecipient for population-level programs. The process of defining participants versus nonparticipants can take place prospectively or retrospectively, but relies on information developed in the service utilization plan for program eligibility, screening, and recruitment. Careful screening and participation record keeping as the program proceeds become useful in distinguishing program recipients from nonrecipients. The group whose members received or participated in the program is called the *experimental, intervention,* or *exposed group,* whereas the group whose members did not receive or participate in the program is called the *control, comparison,* or *unexposed group.* The choice of terms is based on the evaluation design, the scope of the effect evaluation (individuals or a population), and the discipline of the evaluator. Related to the ability to identify the two groups is knowing whether it is possible and feasible to collect data from those who did not receive the program interventions. This, too, will influence the design choice.

Bounded Outcome

The last consideration in choosing an evaluation design is the type of outcome being evaluated. In the context of choosing a design, two broad classifications of health outcomes are distinguished: unbounded and bounded.

One class of outcomes has the possibility of existing before and after the program; these outcomes are, therefore, *unbounded* by time or an event. Most health conditions and behaviors fall into this group. Examples of unbounded outcomes include knowledge, attitudes, behavioral intentions, behaviors, and health or physical conditions that can exist before (and after) the program, such as blood pressure, immune status, weight, or depression. Because the health outcome or behavior is unbounded by an event, it is possible to collect data on the health outcome before the program begins.

The other classification of outcomes is *bounded*, meaning that that they occur only once and, therefore, are bound to an event and time. In epidemiology, these results are called discrete health outcomes. Birth and death are the prime examples of bounded health outcomes, as are low birth weight, adolescent pregnancy, or amputation of toes for diabetics. Some health behaviors also occur only once—for example, initiating breastfeeding after the delivery of a first child, self-efficacy of self-administered insulin after being started on insulin, or first experience of sexual abuse. For bounded outcomes, the program participants or recipients cannot provide pre-test information on these outcome variables because the outcomes occur only after the program has been implemented. For these types of outcomes, there is no naturally occurring pre-test or baseline value for the individual program participants. In addition, the variable used to measure bounded outcomes may sometimes be measurable only as a dichotomous variable. This, too, affects the design choice.

Individual-Versus Population-Level Interventions

Health programs designed for different levels of the public health pyramid will require different designs. Some designs are used when the intervention is delivered to individuals, whereas other designs are applicable only when the intervention is delivered to the population and the outcome is also measurable only at the population level. For population-level interventions, a design is required that captures the changes in the population rather than in individuals. Often the population-focused intervention takes time to manifest and show an effect, which then requires considering the time span aspect of the design. Some programs designed to change the infrastructure, such as the development of a regional referral network or a change in licensure requirements, may require the use of designs for populations because the recipients are populations rather than individuals.

Intervention and Observational Designs

Recall that the history of program evaluation has roots in educational evaluation. From that lineage came the classic book on evaluation designs, *Experimental and Quasi-Experimental Designs for Research*. Campbell and Stanley (1963), in this classic work, identified and described 16 different intervention designs: 3 pre-experimental, 10 quasi-experimental, and only 3 truly experimental. Designs that use random assignment of potential participants to either receive or not receive the program are called *experimental*, whereas designs that do not use random assignment are called *quasi-experimental* designs.

The assumption in the traditional literature (Cook & Campbell, 1979) is that exposure to the programmatic intervention is manipulated by the health professional, as typically occurs with health programs delivered to individuals and groups. *Manipulation* implies that those providing the program have some degree of control over the choice of who among those eligible receives the program. Designs that rely on such manipulation of the intervention, broadly called *intervention designs*, have different names depending on the discipline. For example, in epidemiology and clinical medicine, intervention designs are called clinical trials; in the social sciences, they are called experimental designs or quasi-experimental designs.

In program evaluation, experimental and quasi-experimental designs at the individual level are typically used when four conditions exist. First, information or data on the outcome variable usually exists before the program is delivered. Second, outcome information is usually collected from or on members of at least two groups. Third, an intervention takes place and is received by members of one of the groups. Fourth, after delivery of the intervention, data are collected from or on the same members of the groups as were collected pre-program. Evaluation questions that ask whether the intervention changed the unbounded outcome at the individual level are best answered through experimental and quasi-experimental designs (Handler, 2002; Rosenberg & Handler, 1998). This classification of designs is widely used and understood, but does not include all possible designs. What is lacking in this classification scheme are the observational designs that are primarily from epidemiology.

Observational designs, which come from the field of analytic epidemiology (Fos & Fine, 2000), were initially developed for situations in which exposures are not manipulated but are simply observed as they naturally occur. These designs are typically used to study what constitutes environmental or lifestyle risks. Historically, observational designs such as case-control and cohort designs were reserved exclusively for examining health risk factors and outcomes. However, as epidemiologists have become more thoroughly integrated into health services research and become actively involved in conducting program evaluations, use of observational designs to examine the relationship between receiving health program interventions and health outcomes has grown. When these designs are used for effect evaluation, they are no longer purely "observational." The fact that a program was created and delivered, and that an exposure to the program occurred, similar to an exposure to a toxin, amounts to a de facto manipulation of the exposure. Based on this logic, manipulation of the exposure to the program is no longer a useful way to distinguish between observational designs and intervention experimental and quasi-experimental designs when conducting program evaluations (Handler, 2002; Rosenberg & Handler, 1998). This trend toward a more interdisciplinary and integrated approach is consistent with the continuing evolution of designs and the science behind designs for program evaluation (Barnett & Wallis, 2005; Zuckerman, Lee, Wutoh, Xue, & Stuart, 2006).

An observational design is best used for program evaluation when the health outcome is bounded—that is, discrete (e.g., birth or death)—at the individual level because there are essentially no pre-test data on the outcome (Handler, 2002; Rosenberg & Handler, 1998). Although individual-level pre-test data are not available, baseline data on the population-level intervention may be available for health outcomes that occur only once. When this is true, designs for the population level become possible, such as time series designs, which typically fall into the quasi-experimental rather than epidemiologic typology.

Integrated Use of Designs: An Example

The following example demonstrates how both interventional and observational evaluation designs might be used to measure different components of a health program. Using the Bowe County birth defects prevention program, high-risk women planning a pregnancy receive education about nutrition and environmental hazards that contribute to neural tube defects. The program consists of preconceptional screening, nutrition counseling, the use of multivitamins prior to and during pregnancy, and cooking classes. Each component is evaluated for its effect on the use of vitamins, food choices, and presence of a neural tube defect in the infant.

For the preconceptional screening and nutrition education component, the outcome is increased dietary folic acid intake. At the beginning of the first nutrition education session, women provide information on their current food purchasing and dietary practices. The same women also provide data on their food purchasing behaviors at the end of cooking classes. The possibility that the same women provide both pre- and post-program data on their behaviors permits the program evaluator to choose from among a set of experimental or quasi-experimental designs.

The situation is different for the evaluation of effect of the program on the occurrence of a neural tube defect. Whether or not the women have had prior children, it is not possible to collect pre-test program data about the prevalence of neural tube defect because women in the program have not yet given birth. Consequently, the only evaluation design choices to evaluate this program effect are observational designs. For this intervention, an observational design such as a two-group prospective cohort study is ideal, because neural tube defect data can be collected after delivery from the birth records of women in the program (exposed) and from the birth records of a group of women not in the program (unexposed). At first pass, the collection of data from two groups after the intervention may seem like a post-test only nonrandomized design, which is considered a weak, nonexperimental design. However, when examining neural tube defects, a post-test-only design in the form of a cohort study, for example, is a robust design because it is not possible to have pre-test data at the individual level on the health outcome of interest (i.e., neural tube defects). Observational designs are used in evaluation for outcomes, such as birth weight, for which baseline data cannot be collected at the individual level, which contributes to their being used more widely in evaluations of public health programs.

CHOOSING THE EVALUATION DESIGN

Identifying Design Options

From the point of view of health program evaluation, designs can be more easily understood if we think of them as having three levels of ability to attribute effects to the program, yielding three groups of designs: outcome documentation, outcome assessment, and outcome evaluation. These three levels more readily correspond to the trade-offs and choices that program administrators and evaluators must make in choosing a design. It is more important for the effects of the intervention theory to be assessed than the outcome theory because, unless the casual factors are changed by the intervention and the health outcomes achieved, the longer-range health impacts will not occur. This chapter reviews only the most common designs, noting the types of bias that are likely to occur with each.

Ideally, feasible and possible design options can be identified before the program begins, to ensure that the strongest, most rigorous design possible can be implemented for the effect evaluation. Most of the stronger program evaluation designs must be implemented *before* recipients receive the program, necessitating that the evaluation be ready for implementation well before program implementation. Thus the placement of this chapter after the chapters on program implementation and monitoring is somewhat misleading and should **not** be interpreted as indicating when planning for the evaluation should occur.

An underlying assumption is that program managers and evaluators have some means of knowing that an individual or individuals received the program intervention. For population-level programs, such as a seat belt law or a mass media campaign, exposure to the program can be assumed for all members of the population, although it is sometimes possible to obtain precise measures of coverage. For programs at the direct services or enabling services level of the public health pyramid, indicators of having received the program can be obtained more directly.

Overview of the Decision Tree

To assist with the choice of an evaluation design, Figure 12.2 presents a flow diagram of the key questions that need to be asked. Each of the designs discussed in this chapter is shown in the decision tree. At each branch, a yes or no response to the key question leads either to a design or to a subsequent choice. At each choice branch, the program evaluator and the program staff need to confer and agree on which branch to follow.

The designs shown in the decision tree in Figure 12.2 are the ones most likely to be used in the majority of program evaluations. More complex designs do exist, such as the Solomon four-group design. Such complex designs are more likely to be used in research rather than in an applied setting, so they are not discussed or covered in this text. Also, the use of more than one comparison or control group or the collection of post-program data more than once (except for time series) is not reflected in the list of designs; these procedures are considered modifications to the basic designs that do not intrinsically alter their structure or rigor.

As can be seen in the decision tree in Figure 12.2, the questions of whether a comparison group is possible and whether the group members can be identified before the program begins are critical to determining the design. If the answer to both questions is yes, the resulting possible designs tend to be stronger. One question is rarely asked explicitly, however: whether the program is repeated. A yes response to this question allows for the possibility of the patched-up cycle design.

It is important to note that the first decision question is whether it is possible, either theoretically or practically, to collect any post-test or outcome data from program participants. These data might be obtainable either directly from

Figure 12.2   Decision Tree for Choosing an Evaluation Design, Based on the Design's Typical Use

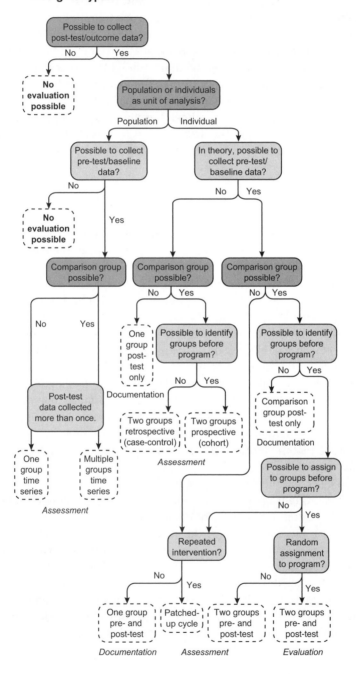

individual participants or indirectly from secondary sources, such as medical records or vital records. If the answer is no, then it is not possible to determine whether the program had any effect, and an evaluation is not possible.

The second branch of the decision tree focuses on whether the program, and hence the evaluation, is delivered to a population or to individuals. For population-based evaluations, it is highly desirable to have baseline data on members of the population to determine if an intervention effect occurred. If it is not possible to have such data, a strong evaluation design cannot be constructed. The discussion of population-level designs is interwoven into the discussion of designs for effect evaluations. In Figure 12.2, many of the designs can be used for either individual-level or population-level programs, as long as all other prior decision points are the same. In other words, designs primarily used for a population-level program could be adapted for use with individual-level programs.

In the following overview of designs, several of the designs can be used at either individual or population levels (Table 12.2). Using the design at the individual or population level does not change the assumptions that must be met, the timing of data collection, or the comparability of the groups. A few designs can be used at only one level—a restriction that is a result of the nature of the design.

In the following discussion, if a design is known by more than one name, all of the alternative names are given. This is the case for designs that are structurally the same but have roots in both epidemiology and social sciences.

Designs for Outcome Documentation

At a minimum, an evaluation ought to document the effect of the program in terms of reaching the stated outcome and impact objectives. Focusing on documenting an outcome from the point of view of the objectives often results in using designs that are called pre-experimental in social sciences terminology. These designs involve collecting data after program implementation (i.e., post-intervention). This procedure theoretically allows post-test data to be compared either to the stated outcome and impact objective targets or to pre-test data. These designs are frequently used by health program evaluators because they are not complicated and are comparatively inexpensive. Their simplicity also contributes to their wide intuitive appeal, and sometimes to their unintentional use.

It is important to understand that these designs are quite weak in terms of being able to attribute changes or differences to the program. Because of their weaknesses, these designs are appropriately used to document the level or degree of reaching the target stated in the outcome objective. Evaluators must remember, however, that these designs do not allow for the attribution of any

Table 12.2   Summary of Main Designs and Their Use for Individual- or Population-Level Effect Evaluations

Design	Level at Which Design Can Be Used	
	Individual	Aggregate, Population
One group, post-test only*		
One group, pre-test/post-test	X	X
Comparison groups, post-test only	X	X
Ecological study		X
One group, repeated measures or time series	X	X
Multiple group, repeated measures or time series	X	X
Two group, retrospective; case-control	X	
Two group, prospective; cohort	X	
Patched-up cycle	X	
Two group, pre-test/post-test	X	X
Two group, pre-test/post-test, with random assignment; randomized trial	X	X (Cluster trial if the groups are separate populations)

* Not recommended at either level.

causality to the program. Put simply, these designs can answer the evaluation question of whether any noticeable change or difference occurred, but they cannot identify the source of the change as the intervention.

In the social sciences, post-test-only designs, and particularly those without random assignment, are considered some of the weaker designs. They are considered weaker because these designs do not control the bias or threats to internal validity that occur due to differences that might exist in the outcome variables prior to the intervention. However, when using two-group designs for bounded outcomes at the individual level (e.g., cohort and case-control studies), concern about the weakness of the post-test only is unwarranted.

One Group, Post-Test Only

An evaluation that collects data on the outcome variable only from program participants and only after the program takes place is using a one-group, post-test-only design. A post-test-only design involves providing the intervention and then collecting data only on or from those who received the intervention, which makes it useful primarily for individual-level evaluations. This design is inexpensive and simple to understand, so it is often the decision of choice for smaller programs with limited budgets and for staff with minimal training in program evaluation. It may be the only option if the program was initiated before the evaluation could be started. It would also be the only design option if evaluators do not have access to members of the target audience who did not receive the program.

Findings based on the data from this design can be misleading because the design has two major biases, or threats to the internal validity of the evaluation: history and maturation. *History threats* are specific events that happen to participants between the beginning and the end of the program—these events might also explain the findings. *Maturation threats* arise when participants mature physically or emotionally between the beginning and the end of the program, independent of the program. In the post-test-only design, there is no information about participants except at one point in time; thus evaluators have no way of knowing whether external historical events or internal maturational processes affected the outcomes. As a consequence, this design has minimal usefulness in determining the effect of the program.

One Group, Pre-Test/Post-Test

An evaluation that collects outcome data only on or from participants before receiving the program and again after receiving the program is using a one-group, pre-test/post-test design. This design involves collecting data from program participants once at any time before and once at any time after they have received the program. It can be implemented readily by many direct services programs that collect data on a set of indicators before starting the program and again at exit from the program.

A major advantage of the one-group, pre-test/post-test design is that data can be analyzed for indications of the amount of change in program participants. Often the data are collected in a manner that allows for connecting the pre- and post-test data from a single individual. For this reason, the design is used mostly with individual-level programs, although a simple pre- and post-test one-group comparison can be made with population data as well. The difference between the before- and after-program scores or levels for the outcome variable is usually easy to calculate and to understand. In addition, because there is no expense involved in finding and gathering data from non-participants, this design has a relatively low cost.

The disadvantage of this design, as with the post-test-only designs, is that both history and maturation can affect the data. In addition, two other threats or problems may arise with this design. A *testing effect* occurs when the process of being involved in providing the pre-test data in some way affects the post-test data. For example, a questionnaire about exercise given at baseline may motivate program participants to exercise more, such that on the post-test data they may report more exercise because of the questionnaire, rather than because of the program. Another possible threat is *instrumentation*, in which the concern focuses on possible changes or alterations to how or which data are collected for the post-test as compared to the pre-test. Unless exactly the same information is collected in exactly the same way, the findings can be influenced by the data collection method, rather than by the program.

Comparison Group, Post-Test Only

An evaluation that collects data on or from participants as they complete the program, as well as from a group of nonparticipants from the target audience, is said to use a post-test-only design with a comparison group. In this third pre-experimental type of design, data are collected once from both program participants and another group that did not receive the program. Liller, Craig, Crane, and McDermott (1998) used such a design to evaluate the effect of a poison prevention program on children ages 5 to 9 in three schools. After providing the educational program, they interviewed children who had received the program at the intervention schools and a comparable group of children from three schools that had not received the program. They were able to show that the children in the intervention schools had "better" scores on poison knowledge than the comparison group.

The simplicity of this design keeps evaluation costs low, especially if the nonparticipants are recruited from a readily available source, such as a companion program or clinic. Like the one-group, post-test-only design, a post-test-only design with a comparison group may be the only option available if the evaluation was started late. Usually, the difference between the scores or levels for the outcome variable for the two groups is easy to calculate. Unfortunately, the difference may be incorrectly interpreted as an actual program effect, whereas in a stricter sense it may only suggest a program effect.

Although this evaluation design reduces the likelihood of instrumentation and testing threats, it is vulnerable to other threats—namely, program attrition and selection bias. *Attrition* is the loss of participants over time due to their dropping out of the evaluation, moving away, being lost to follow-up, or dying. Attrition increases for these reasons as the time span for data collection increases. *Selection bias* refers to the fact that program participants may differ significantly from those not in the program. Unless more extensive data are collected from everyone in the evaluation, the extent to which they differ in fundamental ways will never be known. A difference in outcome between the groups, if seen, may be attributable to factors other than the intervention.

To see how selection bias might affect evaluation results, suppose that the Special Supplemental Nutrition Program for Women, Infants, and Children (WIC) has initiated a breastfeeding education campaign. The program evaluator plans to compare breastfeeding knowledge and attitudes of postpartum women in WIC to those of postpartum women not in WIC. However, the group of women in WIC might differ in fundamental ways from the group of women not in WIC, including factors that influenced their decision to be WIC recipients. Perhaps any difference in the postpartum breastfeeding knowledge and attitudes of the two groups of women reflects those factors that influenced their decision to participate in WIC, rather than the prenatal breastfeeding program.

Another example of a comparison-group, post-test-only evaluation from the literature is informative. Klassen and associates (2002) matched women who attended a mammography program with friends and neighbors. They called the friends and neighbors "controls," connoting that they were not program participants. Data collection was done only once, after the program was complete and from both groups, making it a comparison-group, post-test-only design. However, the researchers incorrectly called this another type of design, a case-control design. This example highlights the potential confusion over correctly describing and labeling designs, and hence the potential challenges that program evaluators face when discussing designs with relevant stakeholders. Klassen and colleagues (2002) also claimed to have "matched" the program participants with their friends. True matching is done infrequently because of the cost involved in identifying and recruiting individuals who are completely like the program participants. Nonetheless, these authors' use of a convenient and accessible comparison group highlights the potential for thinking creatively about how to arrive at the best possible design and sample.

Ecological Design

In some instances, the evaluation seeks to understand if a relationship exists between an intervention and an outcome, but only at the population level. Evaluation of interventions designed and implemented to have effects on aggregates or populations could use several of the designs discussed in this chapter. One of the designs that can be used only with population-level data is the ecological study design drawn from epidemiology. The ecological study design considers the differences between groups rather than individuals (Morgenstern, 1995). This design is most often used to determine whether there is an association between an exposure and a health consequence at the population level. For example, Cech, Burau, and Walston (2007) used geographic data to assess whether the incidence of cleft palate was higher in locations with higher radium and radon concentrations. Others have proposed the use of ecological studies for evaluating the effects of policy, such as policies to reduce injuries (Stevenson & McClure, 2005). In the simplest form of ecological design, the exposed and unexposed aggregates are compared to aggregates with and without the outcome of interest. What distinguishes the ecological design is that there is no possibility of identifying individuals, so the comparison occurs only across aggregates.

A key advantage of the ecological design is its use of existing population data, often drawn from various sources. At the same time, this design can be subject to the *ecologic fallacy* (discussed in Chapter 14)—that is the evaluators may wrongly assume that group characteristics apply to all individuals in the group. Nonetheless, ecological studies can be helpful in assessing whether there is a relationship between a public health program intervention and a health outcome at the population level. For example, an ecological design would answer the question of whether there is a relationship between the percentage of counties in a state with smoking cessation programs and the percentage of counties that meet the *Healthy People 2010* objective for low birth weight.

Designs for Outcome Assessment

If more resources are available for understanding the degree of effect from the program, then more complex and costly designs can be used. In general, the quasi-experimental designs fall into this category, along with some observational designs.

The designs for outcome assessment answer the evaluation question of whether any noticeable change or difference seems related to having received the program. All of these designs are considered "stronger" than the outcome documentation designs because to varying degrees they attempt to minimize possible differences between groups that may be related to some effect from the program.

These designs involve at least post-program or intervention data collection, plus the use of a comparison group. The comparison groups in these designs are *nonequivalent*, meaning that the groups being compared are not necessarily statistically similar or matched. Nonequivalence occurs because membership in the comparison group is influenced by the factors that influence the choice of being in the program or not. Individuals who choose to receive the program may be different from those individuals who choose not to receive the program, and without extensive data on both groups it may not be possible to know how the two groups differ. Therefore, claiming that the program was the cause of differences in the outcome variable between the groups remains problematic.

Two observational designs can also be used for outcome assessment. Generally, the observational designs—cohort and case-control—are appropriate for bounded outcomes at the individual level. In the following subsections, designs for outcome assessment are described in terms of their use in program evaluation and their commonly used names. For each design, the biases inherent in that design are discussed. Again, the trade-offs involved in choosing one design over another need to be weighed in view of the specific program characteristics and the evaluation needs of the program staff, stakeholders, and funders.

One Group, Time Series

As shown in the decision tree in Figure 12.2, the one-group, time series design is one of two designs that can be used if an entire population is the unit of analysis for the program evaluation. Such a design makes sense if data have been collected for the same group at several time points before the program and the same data have been collected at several time points after the program. This design is also known as a single time series design because only one group is used; it is also referred to as an interrupted time series design because the program interrupts the baseline value of the outcome variable.

The one-group, time series design might be one of the few options available if the program is delivered to or received by an entire population—as is the case with interventions such as seat belt laws, water fluoridation, or health insurance for underinsured children provided through state health insurance programs. Because the unit of analysis can be the population rather than individuals, there is no assumption that exactly the same individuals contributed to the data at each time point. A time series, because it does not require following specific individuals, is often used in public health for evaluating policy effects on a population. It is also useful in evaluating programs that are delivered to only one distinct aggregate, such as a school that will be included in the program and evaluation, and for which the same data have consistently been collected over time.

The one-group, time series design can also be used with one group of individuals from whom data are collected multiple times over a long-term follow-up.

For example, all patients with diabetes at one clinic might be followed for several years, with data being collected, say, on their HgbA1c values and weight. During that time, if a major program intervention was introduced throughout the clinic, this design would enable evaluators to identify whether a change occurred among those patients from before and after the introduction of the program. Generally, if one group of individuals is followed over time and outcome data are repeatedly collected on them, the study design is called a *repeated measures design*. Whether data are collected from a group of individuals or the population as a whole, the caveats in choosing a one-group time series are the same.

The key consideration in choosing this design is the number of time points before and after the program at which data were collected and are available. For a variety of statistical reasons, the optimal number of time points to have is five before and five after the intervention (Tukey, 1977). For a program targeting a large population, such as a seat belt law, obtaining five years of highway fatality data before and after the law took effect may not be a problem. In other programs, such as a school-based program, where the data collection tools used with students, such as standardized tests, may be revised, having the same metric for five years before and after a program may be problematic. A reasonable rule of thumb, when the ideal is not possible, is to have a minimum of three years of data before the program was initiated and three years after the program was completed. Fewer than three years' worth of data makes it extremely difficult to statistically assess for the presence of a trend before and after the program.

The one-group, time series design has intuitive appeal, is easy to plan, and has a relatively low cost if the data already exist. An additional attractive feature of this design is that data other than physical health outcomes can be used. For example, Conrey, Grongillo, Dollahite, and Griffin (2003) used the rate of redemption of WIC coupons for produce at farmers' markets in New York as the outcome variable for a program designed to increase the use of farmers' markets by women in WIC. Their study is an example of how existing data from social services might also be appropriate for population-focused health programs.

Campbell and Russo (1999) have pointed out that, with the one-group, time series design, usually only effects from sudden and dramatically effective interventions can be identified and distinguished from the background, normal variations that occur over time. This shortcoming occurs because the design has several biases, of which history is the major problem. The other threats—maturation, instrumentation, selection, and regression to the mean—tend to be less problematic and have less effect on the conclusions. *Regression to the mean* refers to the tendency for the scores of different groups to become more alike over time. Thus, the longer the time period between the intervention and the collection of the post-test data, the more likely the two groups are to have no differences on the outcome variable. One major disadvantage of this design is the challenge in interpreting the amount of change in relationship to when the intervention occurred. It is possible that the change did not occur immediately and only after the program was introduced. The different patterns of the intervention–change relationship become evident only during the data analysis.

Multiple Group, Time Series

If data have been collected from a potentially affected population and a comparison population at several time points before the program, and the same data have been collected at several time points after the program on the same groups, a multiple-group, time series design is possible. The addition of at least one comparison population that did not receive the intervention is the most obvious way to improve on the one-group, time series design, so long as the data are from the same time frames for all groups. The classic example of this design is the comparison of two states, one with a seat belt law and the other without such a law. The annual mortality rates for motor vehicle accidents in both states are plotted across several years before and after enactment of the law. The rates in the two states are compared to determine whether the mortality rate in the state with the law declined more after the enactment compared to the mortality rate in the state without the law.

Because the multiple-group, time series design requires collecting data on or from at least two groups many times before and after the program, it is generally used with large aggregates, such as schools, or with populations. Nevertheless, the same logic applies when this design is used to evaluate programs for individuals. Using the earlier example of patients with diabetes who visit a certain clinic, it is easy to imagine a health system that includes several clinics, but where only one or two implement the intervention. In this case, there are naturally occurring multiple groups and repeated measures on the patients, which creates the time series.

The major advantage of this design is that few biases are likely to seriously affect the ability to draw conclusions regarding the program effect. In other words, the multiple-group time series is a very strong design to use with population-focused health programs. A major disadvantage of the design is that the same outcome variable data must have been collected on all populations being compared. If an outcome variable such as injury mortality is the outcome of interest, then the data are likely to be similar across groups. In contrast, if fetal death rates are the outcome variable of interest, because states use different metrics for collecting fetal death information, comparing changes in fetal death rates over time across several states may be problematic. Another disadvantage of time series designs (both single group and multiple group) is the need for more complex statistical analysis that takes into account the repeated measurement; conducting this analysis may require the services of a statistical expert.

Two Group, Retrospective (Case-Control)

If it is possible to identify individuals with and without the program outcome and to review their historical, existing data to determine which individuals received the program and which did not, a retrospectively constructed, two-group design is possible. This observational design, which is also called a case-control design, is used at the individual level. It is appropriate when, for whatever reason, the program evaluation is conducted after the program has started or has concluded, access to the individuals for data collection purposes is limited, and the outcome variable is bounded and discrete. In this design, those with the outcome are compared to those without the outcome, with regard to whether they were exposed to or received the program.

The retrospective two-group design is useful because the degree to which the program improved the likelihood of the desired outcome can be statistically calculated by comparing those with the outcome to those without the outcome based on whether they were exposed to the program. The exposed/not exposed and the outcome/not outcome relationships are often represented with a two-row by two-column table, called a 2×2 table. In the retrospective two-group design, knowing who falls into which of the four cells in the table becomes possible only after the program and the outcome have occurred; relevant data may be collected through a review of existing records that contain both program participation data and outcome variable data. Thus this design is feasible only if evaluators have access to those records and the information in those records includes data on both exposure to the program and the outcome variable.

A retrospective case-control design is generally used when the outcome is bounded. In other words, this design can be used when it theoretically is not possible to collect baseline or pre-test data on the outcome for the same individuals, as discussed earlier. For outcome variables that occur only once, the retrospective two-group (case-control) design is quite robust, meaning that it is a strong design (Handler, 2002; Rosenberg & Handler, 1998). The uniqueness of this design derives from the fact that individuals who have and do not have the outcome of concern are identified post hoc and then compared with regard to whether they received the program. In this sense, this design retrospectively assigns individuals to exposure groups.

The major advantage of the retrospective two-group design is that it can be used any time after the program has been implemented because it is not necessary to know before the beginning of the program who will be in the evaluation.

However, use of this design is not possible unless either the evaluator or program itself has collected data on program exposure, even if the information was not initially intended for evaluation purposes. Like other evaluation designs that are implemented after the program, the retrospective two-group design may be one of the few choices available if the evaluators were not involved in creating or choosing an evaluation design earlier in the planning cycle.

This design does have certain disadvantages. A major limitation relates to the ability to obtain high-quality data on exposure to the program, including whether the individual received the program and what intervention dosage was received. Although healthcare organizations have been increasing their use of data warehousing, there is no guarantee that the variables needed for the evaluation will be available or that they will have been collected in a consistent and reliable manner. The cost associated with the retrieval of existing data—a task that is necessary in all retrospective designs—will be lower if a comprehensive and stable management information system has been used for recording the data that need to be abstracted for the program evaluation. However, if budget constraints and data retrieval difficulties impose severe limitations on the number of individuals for whom adequate retrospective data are available, then the size of the sample can be a concern. A small sample size will affect the statistical conclusions that can be drawn about the effectiveness of the program.

Another potential problem is that, although the retrospective case-control design is robust, selection bias can be present. Data about why individuals were in the program will likely not be available, making it difficult to know whether any apparent program effect might have been due to a selective preference on the part of participants for receiving the program. Another major issue with the case-control design is recall bias—that is, inaccurate memory, particularly if the participants are asked about their having received the program. Recall bias can be circumvented if evaluators have access to records documenting participation in the program.

Two Group, Prospective (Cohort)

If the target audience is distinct, clearly defined, and can be followed forward in time as a group, it is called a *cohort*. If a cohort exists, then a prospective design becomes possible. Like the retrospective two-group design, the prospective design is used if there is no theoretical possibility of collecting pre-test outcome data on the same individuals because the outcome is bounded. Prospective cohort designs are widely used in the evaluation of health services when the outcomes of interest are health outcomes that occur only once for an individual. These characteristics render this design most suitable for individual-level evaluations.

Two versions of the prospective cohort design are distinguished; they differ based on whether it is possible to know at the outset of the evaluation who will receive the program. In Version I, it is not possible to know beforehand who will participate in or receive the program. The members of the target population are followed forward in time (prospectively) as a group (a cohort) for a given time period, and some individuals are exposed to the program and some are not. The evaluators determine who received exposure to the program at the end of the evaluation. In Version II, it is known before the program begins who will and will not participate in or receive the program. Both groups are followed forward as a cohort throughout the duration of the evaluation. In both versions of the prospective cohort design, at the end of the time period, the outcome variable is measured to determine whether the outcome is present among those exposed to the program intervention.

When evaluating the effect of a home visitation program for pregnant women on the prevention of child abuse, for example, it is possible to use a two-group, prospective cohort design. One group might consist of women in the program who are followed for a year; at the end of the year, the evaluators assess whether child abuse had occurred. The other group would include pregnant women, perhaps from a waiting list or from a list of women who had refused to receive the program, who are also followed forward in time, with child abuse measured at one year. At one year, the rate of child abuse for each group of new mothers would be compared. This example represents the Version II of a prospective cohort study design.

The prospective cohort design is appealing because data can be collected on key variables, such as relevant antecedent and moderating factors, from members of the target audience before exposure to the program. In this regard, this design does not rely on existing data, as the retrospective two-group design does. Also, if Version I is used, this design does not require knowing who will receive the program. The exposed and unexposed groups are identified at the end of the time period, based on data collected over the duration of the evaluation. If data collection occurs over a long time period, more individuals might potentially develop the outcome expected to result from the program intervention. This extended follow-up period is an important feature for programs with a potentially long time lag between intervention and evidence of outcome, such as those aimed at changing substance abuse behavior, long-term weight-loss programs, or long-term medical treatments.

The major disadvantages of a prospective design are the need to track individuals for a substantial time frame and the need to collect follow-up data on the outcome variable. Maintaining contact with the individuals in the evaluation for a period of time can be costly, as well as frustrating, particularly if those persons do not have stable lives or their whereabouts are not reliable.

Loss of participants due to attrition does have consequences for the validity of the design and the statistical conclusions that can be drawn. Although attrition of those in the evaluation can be addressed—and lowered—through a variety of strategies (Resnicow et al., 2001), these strategies are both costly and labor intensive.

Often it is not possible to actually determine who will be exposed to the program before the program begins. When program records are used to establish exposure, but the analysis proceeds from the exposure forward in time (the prospective element) to the outcome, then the design is best called a retrospective cohort design. An example of this design is an evaluation of five types of providers of prenatal care services: public hospital clinics, health department clinics, community clinics, private physicians' offices, and private hospital clinics (Simpson, Korenbrot, & Greene, 1997). In this study, all women on Medicaid from specific geographic regions were included in the evaluation, which sought to determine the association between prenatal care provider type and pregnancy outcome. The medical records of all women in the study regions who gave birth during the evaluation time period were reviewed. The evaluators noted where the women had received prenatal care, and then they compared the outcomes of the pregnancies across the types of providers. Despite the fact that the groups were retrospectively constructed, the design used in this study was prospective in that it followed the women forward through their pregnancy and reassessed the bounded outcome variables of birth weight and preterm delivery.

Patched-up Cycle

If only post-test data are available from a first group of program participants (a one-group, post-test-only design), but the program is being repeated, then a patched-up cycle design becomes possible. This design utilizes a technique for patching up the one-group, post-test-only design by adding a new group. Each time the program is offered, evaluators have the chance to collect data from participants before and after the program. The patched-up cycle design, also called the recurrent institutional design, allows the post-program data from participants in the first cycle to become the comparison group for the pre-program data for the next cycle of program participants. The design is termed "patched up" because the first cycle is a one-group, post-test-only design, the second cycle is a one-group, pre-test/post-test design, and the third cycle is a comparison-group, post-test design. The cycle can be repeated as many times as the program is offered, so there can be more than three cycles. The patched-up cycle design is also feasible if the first program was offered before the evaluation was started, but it is not too late to collect post-test data on the first set of program participants. The reliance on enrolling individuals in the program and collecting data from them makes this design most useful at the individual level.

The patched-up cycle design can be useful for health programs, such as health education programs, in which waiting for the program does not have serious health consequences. It allows for the collection of the pre-test data from potential participants who don't receive the intervention in the first cycle. The advantage of the patched-up cycle design is that statistical comparisons can be carried out in the interlude between each cycle of the program. Specifically, the cycle 1 post-test data may be compared to the cycle 2 pre-test data, the cycle 2 pre-test data may then be compared to the cycle 2 post-test data, and finally the cycle 2 post-test data may be compared to the cycle 3 post-test data. This set of comparisons allows the patched-up cycle design to compensate, to some extent, for the weaknesses of the design.

Another way to think of the patched-up cycle design is to note that it comprises three designs: (1) the one-group, post-test-only design of cycle 1; (2) the one-group, pre-test/post-test design of cycle 2; and (3) the post-test only with a comparison group. As a consequence, the biases and weaknesses of each of these three designs are present in the patched-up cycle design—specifically, maturation, regression, and history risks.

Two Group, Pre-Test/Post-Test

An evaluation that collects outcome variable data on or from program participants and nonparticipants, both before the program begins and after the program is complete, uses a two-group, pre-test/post-test design. This design is more formally called a nonequivalent, two-group, control-group design. It is theoretically similar to the population-level time series, but includes only two groups and fewer data points. It extends the post-test-only design discussed earlier by adding the collection of data from both program participants and nonparticipants before the program begins. In other words, pre-test and post-test data are collected from both program participants and nonparticipants on similar dates. This design has intuitive and practical appeal because data are collected only twice and because the statistical comparison of the two groups is relatively simple and straightforward.

In using this design, evaluators must attempt to ensure that the groups are as alike as possible, by carefully selecting the nonparticipants (i.e., the control group). However, without random assignment, evaluators do not have any assurance that the groups will be alike—hence the "nonequivalence" label. Selection bias is a major threat in the two-group, pre-test/post-test design. If sufficient information about members of both groups has been collected, such as demographic variables and relevant antecedent variables, the statistical analysis can be adjusted to account for the differences between the groups.

Another threat to this design is regression to the mean. This risk suggests that the design is best used with outcomes that are expected to occur relatively soon after the intervention, and the post-test data should be collected at that time point.

Designs for Outcome Evaluation Research

The last set of designs is the most costly and complex, but they enable evaluators to show that the program was truly the cause of the effect. Designs for outcome evaluation research answer the evaluation question of whether the change or difference can be attributed to having received the program. Experimental designs involve a program, an outcome measure, and a comparison from which change due to the program or intervention can be inferred. Only one of the several experimental designs is discussed here—the two-group, pretest/post-test design with random assignment. The other experimental designs are essentially variations on this design but because they are more complex, they are used only in evaluation research.

Experimental designs are expensive in terms of the number of evaluation participants needed to reach statistically sound conclusions and in terms of the amount of time required to track those in the evaluation sample. Methods for determining the number of evaluation participants needed are discussed in Chapter 13; specifically, the necessary sample size and power are explored. The distinguishing feature of all experimental designs is the use of random assignment.

Random Assignment

Random assignment is the process of determining on a random basis who receives the health program intervention and who does not. This concept is not to be confused with *random selection*, which refers to the random identification from the target population of who will be in the evaluation. Random assignment is essentially done using either a table of random numbers or the flip of a coin, so to speak, although more sophisticated methods of arriving at random assignment also exist. Random assignment is the basis for designs used in clinical trials (to use epidemiological or related terminology) and in experimental designs (to use social sciences language).

The advantage of using random assignment of participants to either the experimental/participant group or the control/nonparticipant group is that it creates comparison groups that are theoretically equivalent. In other words, by assigning evaluation participants to either the experimental or control group on a random basis, the possibility of the two groups being different is no greater than one might expect by chance alone. This consideration is critical, because it eliminates design biases that stem from groups not being equivalent. With random assignment, the two groups are as alike as is theoretically possible, so subsequent differences found in outcome variables can logically be attributed to the effect of the intervention.

Practical Issues

A reality for many health programs is that ethical concerns often preclude the use of random assignment to receive or not receive the program. For each program, the staff and stakeholders ought to discuss their comfort with random assignment. In the birth defects prevention program of Bowe County, it might be ethically acceptable to randomly assign women to the cooking program component, but it would be ethically unacceptable to randomly assign women to the prenatal vitamins component. In highly vulnerable populations or communities, experimental designs may not be ethically realistic or even acceptable to stakeholders. Stakeholders may object to studies using these designs because not all who need the program are able to receive it due to the random assignment. For example, a community agency may have a moral objection to not offering a health promotion program to all who are at high risk. However, if a new program is compared to the standard program, then health program evaluators might choose an experimental design that allows the unexposed group members either to receive the standard program or to receive the new program after the exposed group receives it. Similarly, if the program has limited slots, instead of establishing a waiting list, participants can be randomly assigned to participate. These approaches to random assignment help minimize ethical concerns yet maintain rigor in the evaluation.

Other practical issues exist with experimental designs. First, the target population needs to be sufficiently large to have both an experimental group and a control group. Second, the program interventions must be robust, meaning that the interventions must have a statistical probability of having an effect. Experimental designs are *not* appropriate if any element of the effect theory is poorly substantiated or if the intervention theory predicts only a small change in the outcome variable.

An evaluation of an educational intervention with older African Americans (Walker, 2000) may have failed to find any program effect as a result of both of these challenges to an experimental design. In this case, the intervention for the experimental group consisted of spiritual and hypertension-related messages delivered by programmed telephone calls. The control group received only the spiritual messages via the programmed telephone calls. Both groups also received pamphlets and home visits by a health educator. Thus the only difference between the experimental and control group interventions was the hypertension-related messages were provided to the experimental group. It is likely that receiving such messages would produce only a small change in hypertension management behaviors. In addition, there were only 43 people in the experimental group and 40 people in the control group. This would be considered a small sample size, especially for attempting to find the small effect from the hypertension-related messages provided to the experimental group. The strong experimental study design might have been undermined by having a weak intervention and a small sample size. In other words, the choice of design must be considered in light of the whole program and the evaluation plan.

A third issue that arises with the use of experimental designs is that logistically the evaluation team and budget must be able to accommodate the large number of evaluation participants needed for random assignment to work as intended. When random assignment is undertaken with too few participants, the two assigned groups may not be theoretically equivalent. For these reasons, random assignment, as an approach to the construction of control groups, is rarely, if ever, used in health programs that are not research projects.

Two Group, Pre-Test/Post-Test, with Random Assignment (Randomized Trial)

If individuals from the target audience are randomly assigned to receive the health program or not, and data are collected from those who receive the program (experimental or intervention group) and those who do not (controls or comparison group) both before and after receiving the program, then a two-group, pre-test/post-test, with random assignment design was used. This design is very similar to the two-group, pre-test/post-test design described earlier, except that random assignment is used. Although technically incorrect to some extent, the term "experimental group" is used in the health and evaluation literature instead of "cases" as a way to denote that random assignment to receive the program was used.

This design, which is also called a randomized clinical trial, is often considered the "gold standard" in medical treatment research. Because it is the most rigorous of all possible designs, innumerable examples of this design exist, especially in the evaluation of medical treatments and pharmaceuticals. Nevertheless, the same design can also be used with behavioral interventions. For example, Morone, Greco, and Weiner (2008) randomly assigned individuals to a mindfulness meditation program or to a wait list. Data collected at baseline and 8-week and 3-month follow-ups showed that those who had received the program had reduced chronic pain and increased physical function.

The two-group, pre-test/post-test, with random assignment design is generally perceived as being used only with individuals and medical treatment. In reality, the same design can be used with aggregates, such as schools, or with populations, such as geographically distinct communities. When applied to groups rather than individuals, the design might be called a *cluster trial;* when entire communities are randomly assigned, it is termed a *community trial.* Both the evaluation question and the unit of analysis are different when groups or populations are randomly assigned to receive the intervention; the issue to be determined becomes which program or program component works better (St. Pierre & Rossi, 2006).

Biases associated with this design are minimal because of the use of equivalent groups. The major bias is the differential attrition that results if underlying but unknown causes prompt members of either the experimental group or the control group to drop out of the evaluation. This factor then results in a systematic difference between the groups, which affects the ability to attribute causality to the programmatic intervention. To avoid problems associated with differential attrition, evaluators need to carefully follow both groups and determine who is and who is not still in the groups at the end of the intervention. As mentioned earlier, the major disadvantage of this design is the complex logistics involved in using random assignment.

DESIGNS AND FAILURES

As mentioned in Chapter 6, there are two types of failure that program evaluators attempt to identify or avoid, to which a third type of failure can now be added (Figure 12.3). Table 12.3 summarizes the strategies for avoiding each type of failure.

The first type of failure is process failure, in which the service utilization plan is not sufficiently implemented, thereby resulting in no or inadequate implementation of the intervention. Avoiding process theory failure involves careful program oversight and implementation. The process or monitoring evaluation, rather than the effect evaluation, provides insights as to whether a process theory failure occurred.

The second type of failure concerns the effect theory. If the program interventions did not or could not lead to the desired program impacts and outcomes, then the rationale for choosing those interventions may have been flawed. If a high-quality evaluation found no effect and the process evaluation verified that the intervention was provided as planned, then an effect theory failure may have occurred. However, both the process evaluation and the outcome evaluation must have been conducted and must have provided sufficient scientific data to reach the conclusion that effect theory failure occurred. In particular, the outcome evaluation must have been designed to assess for causality; this would have involved the use of experimental designs. Unless these approaches were used, it is impossible to conclude that only an effect theory failure took place.

Figure 12.3   Three Sources of Program Failure

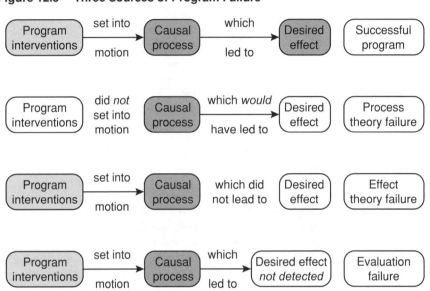

Source: Adapted from Weiss (1972).

The third type of failure is directly related to the evaluation—namely, that it failed to correctly identify an effect that resulted from the interventions. If the evaluation was flawed with regard to the sample, the measures used, the design, or the statistical tests, then the findings regarding the success of the program are questionable. To prevent an evaluation failure, it is necessary to adhere to the highest level of rigor possible given the programmatic realities (Table 12.3). If adequate resources are available and it is critical to greatly minimize the risk of evaluation failure, then certain steps can be taken to avoid this outcome. However, these steps are costly and involve more stringent research methodologies. For example, if measurement is seen as a possible source of an evaluation failure, then additional, complementary, or redundant measures may be used to validate the measures used in the evaluation. To avoid evaluation failure due to inappropriate design choice, evaluators can use a decision flowchart, like that shown in Figure 12.2.

ACROSS THE PYRAMID

At the direct services level of the public health pyramid, health programs focus on individuals. Many of the designs discussed in this chapter can be used

Table 12.3   Approaches to Minimizing Each of the Three Types of Program Failure

	Process Theory Failure	Effect Theory Failure	Evaluation Failure
Definition	The interventions were not sufficiently implemented to (potentially) affect the health problem being targeted	The interventions did not or could not affect the health problem being targeted	The evaluation methods, design, or sample was inappropriate, such that the true effects of the program were not detected
Design and methods considerations	Ability to link process data with effect data at an individual level	Ideally use random assignment; consider timing with regard to finding maximum effect from program	Tailor instruments to participants and specific impact expected; maximize internal and eternal validity
Sample considerations	Ideally include all program participants	Ideally use random assignment and random selection	Select equivalent intervention and control groups; have adequate sample size to achieve high power

with programs at this level. It is a fairly straightforward matter to randomly assign individuals to the program group or to the nonprogram group. As one might imagine, this approach may present ethical difficulties. Rather than randomly assigning individuals to either the program or control group, participants can become their own controls, as in a pre-test and post-test design, or future participants may serve as controls while they remain on a waiting list. Overall, the effect evaluations of health programs at the direct services level can resemble or be straightforward research in terms of the sampling technique and design used. In terms of cost, depending on the type of data collected and the frequency of data collection, evaluation designs at the individual level can range from relatively inexpensive to expensive.

At the enabling services level, health programs focus on groups of individuals and are provided in a wider range of contexts. Programs at this level will be the most challenging to evaluate in terms of their outcomes, for several reasons. One challenge is to identify and recruit a comparison group that has the same characteristics as the program participants. Another challenge relates to the fact that health services programs at this level are probably not suited to experimental designs, though they may be appropriate for quasi-experimental designs. At a minimum, pre-test and post-test designs can be used for evaluation purposes. In addition, depending on the program, random assignment might be possible, particularly at the group or community level.

At the population-based level, health programs are provided to entire populations. Although this broad scope of delivery does not preclude the use of experimental designs, it does limit the evaluation options to designs that can reasonably be implemented with populations. Time series designs are especially useful for evaluating population-level programs. Evaluations that use existing data on populations will be the least costly to conduct, whereas community intervention trials with random assignment will be the most expensive of all designs.

At the infrastructure level, programs focus on changing the working of the healthcare organization or the public health system. At this level, the outcome evaluation question will determine whether the evaluation deals with the changes in the infrastructure or the changes to the health status of clients. This distinction, in turn, influences the type of design that is needed to answer the intervention effect question. A time series would be appropriate if the focus is on a long-term change for which data are available at the individual or population level across many time points, as might be the case for a policy analysis of funding for health departments. In contrast, if the program focuses on the knowledge of individual workers, many of the designs that use pre-test and post-test data and comparison groups at the individual level might be appropriate.

DISCUSSION QUESTIONS

1. Chapter 8 introduced the concepts of full- and partial-coverage programs. Which evaluation designs are more appropriate for full-coverage programs and which are more appropriate for partial-coverage programs? Justify your response.

2. Suppose the county board of supervisors has asked you, as an evaluation consultant, to evaluate the immunization program for older persons and the community-based adolescent violence prevention program, both of which are offered throughout Bowe County. You have been asked to suggest at least three design options for how to evaluate each program, based on complexity and cost. Use the table you created in response to Discussion Question and Activity 2 in Chapter 11. Which three designs would you propose and why?

3. Which evaluation designs are susceptible to biases due to history and maturation? Explain.

4. Under what conditions would it be accurate to state that a program caused the improvements in a specific health outcome?

INTERNET RESOURCES

Numerous resources for study designs are available; only a few are listed here to show the variety. As you explore websites with content on research designs, you will notice differences in nomenclature, based on the discipline of the authors.

Garson

A nice list of designs is available from Garson at http://www2.chass.ncsu.edu/garson/pa765/design.htm, along with definitions.

Introduction to Research Design and Statistics

This website, from a course developed by Philip Ender at the University of California at Los Angeles, lists the designs using the classic X O R descriptions: http://www.gseis.ucla.edu/courses/ed230a2/designs.html.

Center for Evidence-Based Medicine

The Center for Evidence-Based Medicine summarizes the advantages and disadvantages of the major design types: http://www.cebm.net/study_designs.asp#sectional.

REFERENCES

Bamberger, M., Rugh, J., & Mabry, L. (2006). *Real world evaluation: Working under budget, time, data and political constraints.* Thousand Oaks, CA: Sage Publications.

Barnett, J. J., & Wallis, A. B. (2005). The missing treatment design element: Continuity of treatment when multiple post observations are used in time-series and repeated measures study designs. *American Journal of Evaluation, 26,* 106–123.

Campbell, D. T., & Russo, M. J. (Eds.). (1999). *Social experimentation.* Thousand Oaks, CA: Sage Publications.

Campbell, D. T., & Stanley, J. C. (1963). *Experimental and quasi-experimental designs for research.* Boston: Houghton Mifflin.

Cech, I., Burau, K. D., & Walston, J. (2007). Spatial distribution of orofacial cleft defect births in Harris County, Texas, 1990 to 1994, and historical evidence for the presence of low level radioactivity in tap water. *Southern Medical Journal, 100*, 560–569.

Conrey, E. J., Grongillo, E. A., Dollahite, J. S., & Griffin, M. R. (2003). Integrated program enhancements increased utilization of Farmers' Market Nutrition Program. *Journal of Nutrition, 133*, 1841–1844.

Cook, T. D., & Campbell, D. T. (1979). *Quasi-experimentation: Design and analysis issues for field settings.* Chicago: Rand McNally.

Fos, P. J., & Fine, D. J. (2000). *Designing health care for populations: Applied epidemiology in health care administration.* San Francisco: Jossey-Bass.

Handler, A. (2002). Lecture notes. Retrieved July 14, 2003, from http://www.uic.edu/sph/mch/evaluation/index.htm

Klassen, A. C., Smith, A. L., Meissner, H. I., Zobora, J., Curbow, B., & Mandelbatt, J. (2002). If we gave away mammograms, who would get them? A neighborhood evaluation of a no-cost breast cancer screening program. *Preventive Medicine, 34*(1), 13–21.

Liller, K. D., Craig, J., Crane, N., & McDermott, R. J. (1998). Evaluation of a poison prevention lesson for kindergarten and third grade students. *Injury Prevention, 4*, 218–221.

Morgenstern, H. (1995). Ecologic studies in epidemiology: Concepts, principles and methods. *Annual Review of Public Health, 16*, 61–81.

Morone, N. E., Greco, C. M., & Weiner, D. K. (2008). Mindfulness meditation for the treatment of chronic back pain in older adults: A randomized controlled pilot study. *Pain, 134*, 310–319.

Resnicow, K., Braithwaite, R., Dilorio, C., Vaughan, R., Cohen, M. I., & Uhl, G. (2001). Preventing substance abuse in high risk youth: Evaluation challenges and solutions. *Journal of Primary Prevention, 21*, 399–415.

Rosenberg, D., & Handler, A. (1998). Analytic epidemiology and multivariate methods. In A. Handler, D. Rosenberg, C. Monahan, & J. Kennelly (Eds.), *Analytic methods* (pp. 77–136). Washington, DC: Maternal and Child Health Bureau, Health Resources and Services Administration, Department of Health and Human Services.

Simpson, L., Korenbrot, C., & Greene, J. (1997). Outcomes of enhanced prenatal services for Medicaid-eligible women in public and private settings. *Public Health Reports, 112*, 122–132.

St. Pierre, R. G., & Rossi, P. H. (2006). Randomize groups, not individuals: A strategy for improving early childhood programs. *Evaluation Review, 30*, 656–685.

Stevenson, M., & McClure, R. (2005). Use of ecological study designs for injury prevention. *Injury Prevention, 11*, 2–4.

Tukey, J. W. (1977). *Exploratory data analysis.* Reading, MA: Addison-Wesley.

Walker, C. C. (2000). An educational intervention for hypertension management in older African Americans. *Ethnicity and Disease, 10*, 165–174.

Weiss, C. (1972). *Evaluation.* San Francisco: Jossey-Bass.

Zuckerman, I. H., Lee, E., Wutoh, A. K., Xue, Z., & Stuart, B. (2006). Application of regression–discontinuity analysis in pharmaceutical health services research. *Health Services Research, 41*, 550–561.

CHAPTER 13

Sampling Designs and Data Sources for Effect Evaluations

In planning and developing the evaluation of the effects of a program both sampling and data collection methods will arise as critical decisions. The third critical choice for an effect evaluation is the design. Designs for evaluation are covered in depth in Chapter 12.

Both sampling and data collection decisions ought to be addressed from the point of view of having the most rigorous, scientific approach possible, given the various realities of the health program. This chapter reviews both sampling and data collection methods with the intent of presenting the issues and possible solutions that can be used across a variety of programs. For program evaluation purposes, the term *sample* refers to the groups whose members were chosen to be part of the evaluation and who were selected from among those who received the program and from the target audience who did not receive the program. Although *sampling* is more generally associated with research, the way in which the sample is selected for the effect evaluation can have a major influence on the results of the evaluation. As a consequence, important considerations for developing a sampling plan are covered and a brief review of calculating response rates is provided here. The content covered will help program managers, evaluators, and stakeholders make the best possible choice of a sampling design, given the type of program, the resource limitations, and any time constraints. Likewise, the method for collecting the evaluation data is another key choice in planning an effect evaluation, and the major types of data collection methods are reviewed in this chapter.

SAMPLING REALITIES

Devising a plan for selecting who will actually be included in the evaluation of program effects is often a creative—albeit technical—endeavor that consists of two basic steps (Rossi, Freeman, & Lipsey, 1999). The first step is to identify program participants and the target population. This step applies regardless of the design chosen. For outcome evaluation designs, the second step is to develop a plan to select an unbiased sample from the target population and from among program participants. When discussing sampling, statisticians use the term "population" to refer to the group from which a sample is selected. This group may or may not be the same as the larger target population of the program.

Unlike sampling for research projects that are under the control of investigators, sampling for evaluations places several constraints on evaluators. The foremost limitation is the number of people who can or did participate in the program. If the health program was a small health education class, then including all program participants in the evaluation sample may be feasible. In contrast, if the health program was delivered to the population at large, such as a public awareness campaign or passive protection through policy implementation, then it becomes necessary to select individuals from within the population for the evaluation. A corollary constraint to the number of program participants is the size of the target population, which can vary from a country, if a national health policy is being evaluated, to a small, discrete group, such as adults between the ages of 75 and 80 with glaucoma who live within a small geographic location. Because nonparticipants in the target audience become controls, the number of potential controls also needs to be taken into consideration.

The second sampling constraint is that it is not always clear who was a member of the target audience and, more importantly, who was a participant. Such blurring of lines occurs when there is either unclear program eligibility or inadequate service utilization documentation. Unless the program has clearly delineated criteria for membership in the target population and for designating a participant, it may not be possible to know who ought to have received the program and who actually received it. This fuzziness can make it difficult or impossible to know who is appropriately classified as a member of the exposed/experimental group versus the unexposed/control group. Hence, there is a need to have developed clear eligibility guidelines and procedures as part of the process theory. Ambiguous group membership may also result if the evaluator has limited access to or ability to identify program participants. This situation could arise if the program has poorly maintained records or if it is provided anonymously on a drop-in basis. A lack of such information makes it difficult to classify who was or is in the exposed/experimental group and unexposed/control group, which in turn has implications for both design choice and sampling strategy. Just as being able to delineate program participants begins with the process theory, the issue of obtaining information about who the program participants are can also be addressed during the development of the process theory.

A third constraint involves how participants are classified by the program, meaning which criteria are used to assign evaluation participants to either the program/experimental group or the control group (i.e., those individuals not receiving the program). In some programs, participation in the program is not a clear-cut, dichotomous variable. This fuzziness is particularly likely with programs that have multiple components that may be provided by multiple providers, or programs that are implemented over an extended time. For example, Manalo and Meezan (2000) were interested in evaluating family support programs that varied with regard to actual content. The typology used to classify the family support programs (the unit of analysis) proved problematic when these authors attempted to evaluate outcomes across programs, which limited their ability to draw conclusions about the effectiveness of different types of programs. Thus a key part of the sampling strategy is the development of a definition of "participation" in the program. This definition may be the same as the definitions developed for the process evaluation and may be based on a wide variety of criteria, ranging from hours of intervention received to membership in a health policy target population.

The approach chosen for constructing the evaluation sample, along with the design choice, has implications for the ability to draw statistical conclusions. The more carefully the evaluation needs to compare program participants (exposed/experimental) to nonparticipants (unexposed/control), the more carefully sample selection needs to proceed in terms of making the groups as alike as possible. In such cases, random assignment is an important element of the evaluation plan. For example, if the program being evaluated delivers a novel intervention and the evaluation is akin to evaluation research, then attention to random assignment becomes relevant. In contrast, for most local, ongoing, or smaller health programs, the efforts and resources required to accomplish random assignment are beyond the scope of what is needed or expected by stakeholders.

SAMPLE CONSTRUCTION

Two broad classifications of sampling approaches are distinguished: probability sampling and nonprobability sampling. Within each of these two approaches are sample types based on increasingly complex methods used to derive the sample. Table 13.1 summarizes the differences between the probability and nonprobability sampling techniques.

If each member of a population has a known chance, or probability, of being chosen to participate in the program, then the sample is said to be a *probability* or *random sample*, depending on the discipline. To have a random sample requires having a list of all possible evaluation participants and then randomly

Table 13.1   Probability and Nonprobability Samples and Their Usage

Type of Sample	Key Characteristics	Situations When Preferred
Probability	Each population element has a chance of being selected; known probabilities of selection	When evaluation must demonstrate causation (i.e., experimental or quasi-experimental designs); effect evaluation of a novel program
Nonprobability	Unknown probabilities of selection	Outcome documentation and assessment designs; no sampling frame; very small population size; hard-to-reach population

selecting who is included in the effect evaluation. A probability sample, in theory, allows the evaluator to create groups that ought to be the same when statistically compared. This type of sample is recommended if the evaluation is seeking to demonstrate that the program, and only the program, was responsible for the outcome—in other words, causation. Ideally, probability samples are used with outcome evaluation designs—specifically, experimental or some quasi-experimental designs. A probability sample would be used in an effect evaluation only if the program delivered a novel intervention and, therefore, was being studied for its effectiveness. Most evaluations of ongoing or smaller programs will encounter one of two barriers to using a probability sample: the ethical issues inherent in randomly selecting evaluation participants, and unavailability of a sufficiently large sampling frame for random selection.

The other approach to sampling does not rely on chance to select members of the population for participation in the evaluation, so it is called a *nonprobability* or *nonrandom sample*, depending on the discipline of the evaluator. With this sampling technique, there is no attempt to randomly select individuals for participation in the effect evaluation. Nonprobability samples are used with outcome documentation and outcome assessment designs. None of the nonprobability. sample types enables evaluators to say that the samples in the evaluation are representative of the population at large, the population in need, or participants.

Hard-to-Reach Populations

Hard-to-reach populations refers to individuals who are not easily identifiable or readily accessible for participation in intervention programs or program evaluations (Faugier & Sargeant, 1997). Typically, hard-to-reach individuals are members of rare subgroups within a population and are not readily identifiable in commonly available lists such as telephone directories. Health programs, for example, often address sensitive issues or health behaviors that are not legal. Recruiting evaluation participants from hard-to-reach groups, such as intravenous drug users or individuals with AIDS (Faugier & Sargeant, 1997) will be even more difficult than recruiting participants for the actual program. Yet, to have rigor and a defensible evaluation, it may be imperative to include such individuals in the evaluation.

A variety of strategies have been developed as means to include individuals from hard-to-reach populations in a sample. One strategy is random-digit dialing (Blair & Czaja, 1982), which involves calling phone numbers based on randomly generating the last four digits of the telephone number. This approach overcomes the problem of accessing individuals with unlisted phone numbers. Another technique is capture–recapture (Larson, Stevens, & Wardlaw, 1994), which involves using two or more lists or observational periods to identify unique individuals who might be eligible for participation.

Another set of techniques goes by a variety of names: multiplicity, referral, or snowball sampling (Rothbart, Fine, & Sudman, 1982). With this approach, a key informant provides a referral to other potential participants, each of whom then provides additional referrals, and so on. Over time, the list of potential participants snowballs, growing through a multiplicity of referrals. This approach has been successfully used to access very specific subgroups.

Another technique for reaching the hard-to-reach is venue-based sampling (Muhib, Lin, & Stueve, 2001). This strategy entails going to specific types of locations to find potential participants. It was first developed as a means to reach very high risk individuals whose high-risk behaviors were associated with specific locations, such as bath houses, gay bars, or tattoo parlors. Based on this logic, going to alternative high schools to recruit high-risk adolescents into an evaluation of the pregnancy prevention program could be considered using venue-based sampling. A similar technique is time–space sampling (Muhib, Lin & Stueve, 2001).

This brief overview of techniques to obtain a sample from hard-to-reach populations ought to bring to mind that these same approaches could have been used to recruit the actual program participants. If this is the case, then at the time of the program recruitment, a process ought to have been in place for simultaneously recruiting hard-to-reach individuals into the evaluation of the program.

Sample Size

The question of how many evaluation participants—whether individuals, families, or communities—are needed in the evaluation can be a complex issue. Evaluators face a raft of practical considerations, such as fiscal limitations, logistics of data collection and management, and accessibility challenges. Statistical considerations also complicate matters. In a pure research study, the investigator first chooses a level of probability that a significant result might be found by the study if the program, in fact, was successful. This level is called the *power*, and it is usually chosen to be between 80% and 90%. The number of study participants needed to achieve that level of power is then calculated. When the power is set higher, meaning a higher probability that a significant result will be found if the result truly exists, more subjects are needed. Also, if a large number of moderating, mediating, intervention, or antecedent variables will be included in the evaluation and analyses, then more evaluation participants are needed. The other key element in calculating the sample size is the degree of difference that is expected, called the *effect size*. This difference can be based on the degree of difference between pre-test and post-test data or between program participants and nonparticipants.

The statistical process of analyzing the relationships among the power of a study, the type of statistical tests to be done, the number of variables, the effect size, and the sample size is called a *power analysis*. Black (1999) summarizes the issues involved in such an analysis by showing that four factors affect the power of a statistical test: the sample representativeness and size, the quality of the measurement in terms of reliability and design, the choice of the statistical test, and the effectiveness of the intervention (Figure 13.1). Several software programs can be used to perform the calculations necessary for a power analysis (see the "Internet Resources" list), many of which are available via the Internet. Whether freeware or copyright programs are used, the power analysis requires a clear understanding of the sample, the size of the anticipated effect of the program, and the statistical tests that will be used.

The power analysis might lead the program evaluator to refine, modify, and solidify aspects of the evaluation design that are under the control of the evaluator in an effort to enhance the study's power. However, for most program evaluations, the number of evaluation participants may already be determined, perhaps because funding is limited or because the program has already been provided. In such circumstances, the power analysis works backward from the given sample size to provide the evaluator and the stakeholders with a sense of how realistic the chances are that the evaluation will find a meaningful difference if one exists. With a predetermined sample size, the design of the evaluation takes on greater importance in determining whether the possibility exists of finding a significant difference that might be related to the program. In addition, the power analysis may reveal that the possibility of finding a program effect is so unlikely as to make an outcome evaluation questionable, such that an outcome

Figure 13.1   Factors Influencing Sample Size

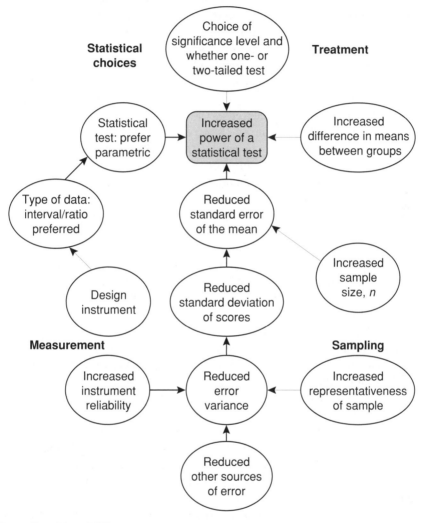

Source: From Black (1999).

documentation or assessment approach might be a better approach for evaluating the program's effectiveness. The evaluator must then make the difficult choice of whether to proceed with the evaluation, search for alternative approaches to the evaluation or data analysis as assessed by the power analysis, or determine whether it is feasible to modify the evaluation in ways that will increase the power.

Calculating Response Rates

During and at the conclusion of the evaluation, the response rate is a key factor that influences the interpretation of the results. *Response rate* is the percentage of individuals who were invited to participate in the evaluation and who actually participated in the evaluation. Response rate is mentioned in conjunction with sampling because of the need to keep in mind that the best possible response rate depends on having a sampling strategy that not only is rigorous but also yields the most possible participants in the evaluation. A basic response rate—say, for a survey—is calculated as the number of usable surveys divided by the number distributed, times 100%; this calculation yields a percent response. The same formula can be used with slightly different numerators and denominators if the goal is to provide more detailed information about response rates for different groups in the evaluation or for different portions of the evaluation. Response rates typically range from a high of 80%, which is achieved with considerable effort and expense, to a low of less than 30%, which is typical for a mail survey for which minimal incentives for participation are provided.

A plethora of minor variations on that basic formula exist, which then lead to minor differences in the response rate, depending on three key factors. The first key factor is whether those invited to participate are ultimately eligible to participate in the evaluation. It is easy to imagine situations in which many people are invited to become part of the evaluation but, after going through a brief set of screening questions, are found not to fit the criteria for participating in the evaluation. Subtracting the number found ineligible from the number invited leads to a more realistic denominator of "invited persons who are eligible." A second key factor that affects the response rate is whether, once invited and found to be eligible, people agree to participate. The third key factor that affects response rates is whether evaluation participants complete their participation in the evaluation. Partially completed participation, such as a half-completed self-administered questionnaire, also affects the calculations of the response rate.

It is amazing how many reasons individuals cite for refusing to participate in an evaluation. Tracking both the number and reasons for refusing or declining to participate is required for evaluation research, in which the evaluation has approval from the human subjects protection board. To the extent that any of the three key factors might affect the final interpretation of the evaluation findings, it will be important to set up a mechanism to track invitations, eligibility, refusals, and completions.

Nonresponse Bias

Regardless of whether evaluators have a detailed and well-constructed sample design, some evaluation participants will inevitably fail to provide data for any number of reasons. Efforts must be made to minimize these nonresponses so as to increase the response rate. A low response rate, less than 50%, is important for two reasons. First, those who reply may not be like those who do not reply, biasing the sample and having subsequent consequences on the data and findings. The extent to which any differences between nonparticipants and participants alter the findings is called *nonresponse bias*. Second, it is costly to try to achieve the desired sample size by continually attempting to identify and obtain data from "replacements."

Nonresponse may be due to *attrition*, meaning that program participants or control subjects are no longer part of the evaluation or the program. Attrition occurs for various reasons: no longer fitting the criteria for being in the program or the evaluation, loss to follow-up, death, or declining or refusing to continue. Attrition is a normal part of the evaluation process, and the sample size must be based on the expected loss of 10% to 40% of participants. Attrition rates are particularly crucial for outcome assessment and outcome evaluation designs, because they affect the final sample size and can affect the balance of participants and nonparticipants sought through a carefully constructed sampling method.

Some individuals selected for the evaluation will be difficult to reach or to convince to participate in the evaluation. Aggressive recruitment efforts may be needed in such situations. For example, evaluators may need to make multiple attempts to contact these individuals, using different media (telephone, email, and letter) at different times by different voices. The number of attempts made to reach an individual needs to be carefully weighed against the possible appearance of harassing the individual, and the extent to which repeated attempts and refusals will affect the quality of the data eventually obtained. In many situations, evaluators—and particularly external evaluation consultants—have little or no control over who is in the program and little or no control over who is selected for the evaluation. In such instances, additional efforts are needed to address the program staff as key stakeholders in the evaluation and to train or educate them about recruitment and retention techniques. Actions of program staff with regard to how the evaluation is presented and supported can dramatically influence the participation and response rates.

Incentives

Incentives, such as money, gift certificates, or small tokens of appreciation, are effective in increasing participation in research. Many individuals participate in research for humanitarian reasons, such as their desire to contribute to making life better for others and to advance science (Agarwal et al., 2007). Alternatively, some program participants may have a culture characterized by the attitude "pay me to participate," which is particularly likely for high-risk individuals who view monetary incentives as additional income (Slomka, McCurdy, Ratliff, Timpson, & Williams, 2007). Thus it is likely that at least some participants in evaluations of health programs will expect a monetary incentive. An extensive body of literature exists on the use of incentives in research (Huby & Hughes, 2001) and the monetary amounts that are most effective in increasing the response rate. This knowledge needs to be used in developing the data collection procedure, along with common sense and a working understanding of the community standard for incentives for a comparable request of participants' time and effort.

Designing the monetary incentive must take into account both the total amount and the payment schedule. The amount must not be so great that it would be perceived as coercive, nor should it be so small as to not be an incentive. The payment schedule for providing evaluation data needs to be congruent with the frequency with which participants are asked to provide data. The rule of thumb is that incentives ought to be provided at each data collection point.

Consider an evaluation of a six-week diabetes self-management class for Layetteville residents. If class participants are asked to complete a survey before the first class and at the end of the last class, then the incentive could be for the same amount and payments could be delivered at the time the surveys are returned. However, if the participants are asked to undergo physical testing before the class, then the incentive may need to be larger to reflect that greater burden on the participant. If the evaluation is longitudinal with data collection at six months and one year after the classes have ended, then a slightly larger incentive may be needed for those time periods as a way to keep participants' interest in the evaluation study.

SAMPLING FOR EFFECT EVALUATIONS

Sampling for Outcome Assessment

Using a nonprobability sample, as is done in outcome assessments, tends to be simple and not costly (Table 13.2). For many smaller, locally based, or agency-specific health programs, a nonprobability sample will be adequate for the evaluation. This type of sample allows for a statistical comparison of differences between program participants and nonparticipants.

A nonprobability sample can be constructed in several ways (Table 13.2). These types of samples come from the social sciences. A *convenience sample* is constructed by inviting whoever is accessible or available to participate; it is an inexpensive means of obtaining a sufficient number of evaluation participants. In a *purposive sample*, the evaluation participants are typically chosen based on a specific characteristic, thereby ensuring that the program

Table 13.2   Comparison of Main Types of Samples with Regard to Implementation Ease, Degree of Representativeness, and Complexity of Sampling Frame

Type of Sample	Implementation Ease	Representative-ness to General Population	Sampling Frame
Nonprobability			
Convenience	Easiest	None ensured, but may occur by chance	Willingness to participate in the evaluation
Purposive	Easy	None	Specific character-istics of interest
Quota	Moderately easy, but must track number in each quota category	None ensured, but possibly represen-tative of those with characteristics by chance	Specific character-istics of interest
Snowball	Somewhat difficult	None; likely to be biased	Network of initial participants
Probability			
Simple random	Easy-to-use random-number chart	High	Entire population
Stratified random	Moderate, because must first choose stratification vari-able and then stra-tum categories	High	Entire population, but must have information to assign individuals to strata
Systematic	Easy to select each nth from a list	Moderately high; lower if the listing sequence is not random	List of possible evaluation participants

Table 13.2   Comparison of Types of Samples with Regard to Implementation Ease, Degree of Representativeness, and Complexity of Sampling Frame *(continued)*

Type of Sample	Implementation Ease	Representative-ness to General Population	Sampling Frame
Probability			
Random route	Difficult, because must define area, construct a random route, and then choose nth house for inclusion	Moderate to poor, depending on the diversity or homogeneity of the residents in area chosen and the availability of residents	Geographically accessible area
Cluster or nested sampling	Moderate once the cluster has been identified	Moderately high if using random selection of clusters and individuals within clusters	Population with naturally occurring nested clusters

participant and nonparticipant samples are balanced with regard to that characteristic. A *quota sample* also involves selecting participants based on a specific characteristic, but the proportion of evaluation participants having that characteristic is proportional to their representation in the population at large. For example, if age is important in the evaluation and 10% of the population of participants at large is more than 80 years old, then the evaluation sample must meet a 10% quota of 80-year-old participants. A *snowball sample* is achieved by asking current evaluation participants who have a specific characteristic to identify or nominate other individuals they know who also have the characteristic of interest. As mentioned earlier, this type of sampling is useful for accessing hard-to-reach populations and when a list of names of potential evaluation participants does not exist. As more evaluation participants name others, the snowball of evaluation participants grows.

Overall, these sampling strategies are easy to implement and explain to stakeholders and, therefore, are likely to be used in program evaluations. Each sampling design varies with regard to the ease of implementation, the degree of representativeness of the larger population, and the sampling frame used—in other words, the basis for inclusion in the evaluation sample.

Sampling for Outcome Evaluation

If it is crucial to demonstrate that the health problem was changed (and presumably improved) in program participants, then a probability sample is recommended as part of the program evaluation. Such a sample is also necessary in a needs assessment if the assessment is intended to accurately estimate the rate of a health problem in a population. A *probability sample* is one in which all potential members of the evaluation have a known probability of being selected to participate in the evaluation. The major barrier to obtaining a probability sample is that evaluators may not have control over who receives the program, especially if the outcome evaluation is not designed during program development. Probability samples are used to increase the external validity of the evaluation; however, for the vast majority of program evaluations external validity is less of an issue than the biases and threats inherent in the design.

Achieving known probability of selection involves randomly selecting potential participants. Several types of probability samples can be constructed, depending on the specific method used to identify and then select members of the evaluation sample. Random selection of evaluation participants, whether individuals, classrooms, or neighborhoods, from the entire population of possible participants can be done in one of several ways, with each technique resulting in a different type of probability sample. A simple probability sample, for example, is constructed by using a table of random numbers to select individuals from a known list of possible participants. The other types of probability samples involve increasingly more complex selection procedures from increasingly more specific groups within the population.

The various probability sample types are explained in greater detail in various textbooks (e.g., Bamberger, Rugh, & Mabry, 2006). Most local or agency-based program planning efforts and evaluations are not likely to have the resources required to construct and obtain these more complicated samples. The costs associated with the sampling effort increase in proportion to the complexity of the probability sample because of increases in the number and qualifications of personnel needed to "find" the individual selected, and because of increases in the amount of time required first to establish the sampling procedures and then to carry out those procedures. The sample type chosen may be influenced by the ease of implementing that technique, the degree of representativeness of the target population, and the complexity of the sampling frame.

DATA COLLECTION METHODS

Methods refers to techniques used to collect data, whereas *design* is the overall plan or strategy for when and from whom data are collected. Design is discussed in Chapter 12. Methods generally fall into one of two categories: those for collecting primary data (i.e., the generation of new data) and those for collecting secondary data (i.e., the use of existing data). The evaluation method needs to be consistent with the purpose of the evaluation and the specific evaluation question. The following discussion of methods and data sources focuses on collection of both primary and secondary quantitative data. Methods to collect qualitative data are sufficiently different to warrant a separate discussion (see Chapter 15). The most common form of primary data collected is through the use of surveys and questionnaires. For each health and well-being domain, various sources of data can be used to generate information (Table 13.3).

Surveys and Questionnaires

A *survey* is a method that specifies how and from whom data are collected, whereas a *questionnaire* is a tool for data collection. Typically surveys use questionnaires to collect data; for example, the U.S. Census is a survey that uses a questionnaire to collect data on all persons who reside in the United States. In most cases, residents complete a pen-and-paper questionnaire. However, in some instances, a census taker completes the questionnaire while talking with the individual. Although the distinction between a survey and a questionnaire is important for the sake of clear thinking, generally the word "survey" implies the use of a questionnaire.

Questionnaire Construction Considerations

Much has been written about ways to construct health questionnaires (e.g., Aday & Cornelius, 2006), ways to write individual questions on the questionnaire (Aday & Cornelius, 2006; Krosnick, 1999), and techniques to have sets of questions form a valid and reliable scale (DeVellis, 2003; Fowler, 1995; Pedhazur & Schmelkin, 1991). Several key points can be drawn from these resources that are paramount to developing a good health program evaluation questionnaire.

To the extent possible, evaluators should use existing questionnaire items and valid and reliable scales so that they can avoid spending precious resources "reinventing the wheel." An example of existing items is the U.S. Census Bureau race/ethnicity categories. These race/ethnicity items can be used rather than creating new race/ethnicity categories for a particular evaluation (see Table 2.2). An advantage of using existing items is that it provides some assurance that the items are understandable. Existing scales also can be

Table 13.3 Example of Data Sources for Each Health and Well-Being Domain

Health Domain	Examples of Data Sources
Physical health	Survey data: self-report Secondary data: medical records for medical diagnoses Physical data: scale for weight, laboratory tests Observation: response to physical activity
Knowledge	Survey data: self-report, standardized tests Secondary data: school records Physical data: not applicable Observation: performance of task
Lifestyle behavior	Survey data: self-report Secondary data: police records Physical data: laboratory tests related to behaviors, such as nicotine or cocaine blood levels Observation: behaviors in natural settings
Cognitive processes	Survey data: self-report, standardized tests of cognitive development and problem solving Secondary data: school records Physical data: imaging of brain activity Observation: problem-solving tasks, narrative
Mental health	Survey data: self-reported motivation, values, attitudes Secondary data: medical records diagnostic category Physical data: self-inflicted wounds, lab values Observation: emotional bonding
Social health	Survey data: self-report, social network questionnaires, report of others Secondary data: attendance records of recreational activities Physical data: not applicable Observation: interpersonal interactions
Resources	Survey data: self-report Secondary data: employer records, county marriage records, school records Physical data: address Observation: possessions

used, which makes it possible to compare evaluation participants with those with whom the scale was previously used. However, if the target audience has a unique characteristic—for example, a specific medical diagnosis—that is relevant to understanding the effect of the program, then comparison to existing scales may not be the optimal choice.

Instruments also need to be appropriate for diverse ethnicities and possibly multiple languages. In terms of instruments, cultural sensitivity has two dimensions: the surface structure, which consists of the superficial characteristics, and the deep structure, which consists of core values or meanings. This second dimension is sometimes called cultural relevance. Attention to both careful translation and cultural relevance is especially needed for questionnaires that are being used for the first time with a different cultural group, such as was done by Yu, Wu, and Mood (2005). Willis and Zahnd (2007) found that, in addition to issues of translation and cultural adaptation of the content, problems arose from the basic questionnaire item construction and from erroneous assumptions about the background and lives of the cultural group.

One type of scale that is likely to be discussed with regard to evaluating health programs is the use of client goals. MacKay, Somerville, and Lundie (1996) report that this evaluation technique has been used since 1968. Program staff may be inclined to count the number of client goals attained as an indicator of program success; indeed, the temptation is to consider this quantity as outcome data that are very readily available. Unfortunately, this crude measure of client outcome is highly problematic from an evaluation perspective. The main problem is that unless the goals are highly standardized for specific health problems, there can be great variability in the goals set. Similarly, unless strict criteria have been established for determining whether a client goal was reached, biases among program staff may influence client assessments. The use of goal attainment scaling, in which a Likert-type scale specific to each goal is used, still poses serious problems (MacKay, Somerville & Lundie, 1996) and, therefore, its use ought to be severely curtailed.

To assess the readability, ease of completing, and overall appeal of the questionnaire, a pre-test or pilot test is advised. Involving stakeholders in this activity is encouraged for two reasons: it helps the evaluators have a better questionnaire given the target audience, and it helps stakeholders anticipate what the evaluation data will include. Key considerations are to keep the language simple, use an easy-to-follow format and layout, and break down complex concepts into more easily understood ideas. Even if evaluation participants are expected to be well educated, people are more likely to complete questionnaires that are easily and quickly read.

Verify that what is in the questionnaire corresponds to the program outcome objectives. Evaluators are often tempted to add "just a few more questions" because the opportunity exists or because the information might be interesting to know. A shorter questionnaire is both better and more likely to be completed. A good rationale for going beyond the program objectives in what is collected is if those data will be used for subsequent program planning or to refine the current program.

Regardless of the care taken to construct a questionnaire, whatever can be misinterpreted or be done wrong will inevitably happen. For example, questionnaires that are copied double-sided on single pages that are stapled together are guaranteed to have skipped pages. Unless the questionnaire is administered by an interviewer who is well trained, do not use "skip patterns" that direct respondents to skip questions based on a previous response. These complicated patterns quickly become confusing, and the well-intending respondent may answer all questions, including those items that ought to have been skipped. Using skip patterns is really appropriate only for questionnaires used with interviewing.

Survey Considerations

Any survey, whether done in person or via mail or email, needs careful planning. The process by which the questionnaire is distributed and returned to the evaluator must be thoroughly planned to minimize nonresponse and nonparticipation rates. That process is as critical as the quality of the questionnaire to the success of the evaluation. One technique for developing a well-crafted survey plan is to imagine and role-play each step in the process, and to follow the paper from hand to hand.

Increasingly, questionnaire data are collected electronically, whether via agency computers, hand-held devices used in the field, Internet-based surveys, or client-accessed computers. The same advice about the need to have a carefully crafted data collection plan applies to the use of electronic data collection: follow the answers from the asker to the responder through data entry to computer output. Each of these steps is needed to be able to accurately and feasibly collect the data and constitutes the survey design.

Response Biases

A threat to the quality of questionnaire data, and especially to self-report data from individuals, comes from the various types of *response bias*, the intentional or unconscious, systematic way in which individuals select responses. One of the most common types of response bias, known as *social desirability*, is answering questions in a manner intended to make a favorable impression (Tan & Grace, 2008). Social desirability is a powerful motivator and has been widely measured in program evaluations in which there is the potential for the participant to want to please the evaluators or when the participants believe there is a socially correct answer they are supposed to give. Response bias can also occur as a result of the respondent falling into a pattern of just giving the same response, regardless of the question or his or her true opinion or feeling. Response bias can be difficult to anticipate. Nonetheless, evaluators would be wise to consider that both response bias and random errors inherent in the way the variables are measured can interactively produce questionable or even totally undesirable data (Table 13.4).

Secondary Data

Secondary data are data that have already been collected and are now being used for a purpose that is secondary to their original purpose. Some sources of existing data are appropriately used to assess the effect of health programs; others are not. Each source of secondary data must be carefully considered with regard to its quality. Evaluators must decide whether the data are actually needed to answer the evaluation question.

Vital records—namely, birth certificates, death certificates, and disease registries—are a major source of secondary data for health program evaluators. Birth records contain a wealth of information on prenatal variables, delivery complications, and infant characteristics. These records are usually not available for up to a year past the date of the birth of the infant, so evaluations of prenatal programs that are designed to affect birth outcomes will not be able to include data from birth records immediately following the program. If

Table 13.4 Interaction of Response Bias and Variable Error

		Variable Error	
		Low	**High**
Bias	**Low**	Ideal: high range of honest responses on good measure	Questionable but acceptable data from high range of honest responses on poor measure
	High	Questionable but acceptable data from skewed responses (i.e., toward socially desirable responses) on good measure	Unusable data due to skewed responses on poor measure

the evaluation is longitudinal and focuses on trends, then birth record data may be useful. However, pinpointing the time of the programmatic intervention may be challenging. In addition, for community-based interventions, sampling comparable communities for comparison of birth data will need to take into account how to select the two communities using the address information on the birth certificates. These same caveats to using birth data apply to data from death certificates or disease registries.

Medical records, case files, or insurance claims may also contain information desired for the evaluation. However, data abstraction from these sources entails using a form to record the variables of interest. Several issues must be considered before embarking on data abstraction. First is the quality of the data as recorded and available for abstraction. Because the data in such records are collected for clinical purposes rather than evaluation purposes, the information can be inconsistent and vary by the practitioner recording the data. If the evaluator has reason to believe that data in the records are reliably recorded, the evaluator must then devise a reliable way to abstract the data. This effort will involve training individual data abstractors. If any interpretation of the record information is required, guidelines for what will be recorded and decision rules for interpretation must be understood and applied consistently by all of the data abstractors. Typically, the goal is at least 80% agreement between any two abstractors on the coding of data from a single data source.

Another source of secondary data is national surveys, such as the National Health and Nutrition Examination Survey (NHANES) or the National Family Planning Survey (NFPS). These and several other surveys are conducted periodically by various federal agencies with a health focus, including the Occupational Safety and Health Administration. These data sets have often been used for community assessment. Data from these surveys are publicly accessible through the Internet; they can be used for evaluation of population-level programs. Some data sets have restrictions or stipulations on their use that must be addressed before they can be used. A drawback to using these broad surveys is that the most recent data can be as much as two years old. As secondary data sets, they may be of limited value in determining the effect of small-scale programs. By contrast, they may be highly useful if the effect evaluation focuses on a population-level health program, such as a state program, and the timing is such that immediate information is not critical.

The use of large secondary data sets for the evaluation of programs faces the challenge of overcoming conceptual issues, such as associating the variables available in the data set to the program theory and determining the reliability and validity of the data. Other pragmatic considerations arise as well, such as selection of subsamples and the need to recode data. In addition, data

from some national surveys may not generate results applicable to rural populations (Borders, Rohrer, & Vaughn, 2000). Overall, the evaluator needs to be
cautious and have a specific rationale for using large secondary data sets for
an effect evaluation.

Physical Data

Biological samples, anthropometric measures, and environmental samples
are examples of physical data that may be needed to evaluate a health program.
Biological samples include things such as blood, urine, or hair; anthropometric
measures are typically height, weight, and body mass index; and environmental
samples range from ozone to bacteria counts in water supplies to lead levels in
fish. The decision regarding inclusion of physical data in the evaluation ought
be based on the health program goal and objectives, as well as the determination of whether the intervention and causal theories underlying the health program are sufficiently well substantiated to justify the cost and effort needed to
collect physical data, especially if laboratory tests are necessary.

As with the collection of other types of data, physical data need to be collected in a consistent manner. Evaluators may not have control over laboratory
processing, so they need some assurance that any laboratory results are reliable.
Evaluators need to be familiar with the laboratory standards for processing the
samples and take steps to minimize factors that would lead to erroneous variation in results. Another consideration with regard to physical data, and specifically biological data, is the cost involved in collecting, storing, and processing the
data. Generally, use of biological data in an evaluation can be quite an expensive
proposition, and evaluators need to be proactive in budgeting for these expenses.

ACROSS THE PYRAMID

At the direct services level of the public health pyramid, health programs
focus on individuals. As a consequence, the sample frame is more likely to be
accessible and knowable to the evaluators. If this is the case and the program
is sufficiently large, a simple probability sample of the program participants is
possible. However, getting a probability sample of nonparticipants may be
more difficult.

At the enabling services level, health programs focus on groups of individuals and are provided in a wider range of contexts. Programs at this level of the
pyramid will be most challenging to evaluate in terms of their effect, for several reasons. First, the sampling frame is less likely to be knowable and accessible to the evaluators, which will necessitate that the evaluation sampling
plan be creative and carefully tailored to the program realities. Second, some
of the options may require the use of statistically constructed control groups.

Third, response biases are more likely because of the challenge in accessing or collecting data from participants in enabling services programs.

At the population-based level of the public health pyramid, health programs are provided to entire populations. Although this does not preclude the use of probability sampling designs, it does limit the evaluation options to those sampling methods that can reasonably be implemented with populations.

At the infrastructure level, programs focus on changing the workings of the healthcare organization or the public health system. The effect evaluation question will determine whether the evaluation concentrates on the changes in the infrastructure or the changes to the health status of clients. This distinction, in turn, influences the sample that is needed to answer the intervention effect question.

DISCUSSION QUESTIONS AND ACTIVITIES

1. Identify at least one sampling issue that would be particularly relevant at each level of the public health pyramid. Which strategy could be used to minimize these problems?

2. Conduct an Internet search for power analysis software. From among the programs you find, select two (that are freeware) and experiment with them. What information is required to conduct the analysis? In what ways does the need for that information affect how you would proceed with planning the outcome evaluation?

3. Participation rates for three programs in Layetteville and Bowe County are given in Exhibits 9.2 and 9.3. Review the information for the violence prevention program delivered in schools to individual students and the adult immunization program. Given that information, which type of effect evaluation samples would you suggest for each of those programs, and why?

4. Issues related to obtaining good response rates were discussed in this chapter. Make a list of those issues. Which ones could be anticipated? Which are preventable? For the problems you listed, give at least one possible means of minimizing or preventing the response problem.

5. Use the following information to determine the sample size needed. You plan on conducting a paired t test with program participants, using their pre-test and post-test data. Alpha significance is set at .05, and the standard deviation on the outcome measure was reported in the literature to be 3.5, with a mean of 12.0. You would like 80% power.

INTERNET RESOURCES

Research Methods Knowledge Base

William Trochim's website for research includes a discussion of sample types with both graphics and formulas: http://www.socialresearchmethods.net/kb/sampling.php.

Statistics Canada

This Canadian website has useful explanations about sampling: http://www.statcan.ca/english/edu/power/ch13/probability/probability.htm.

American Association for Public Opinion Research

For some program evaluations, the response rate will be very important. The website found at http://www.aapor.org/responserates has an Excel spreadsheet already set up to calculate response rates. However, it does require having counts for ineligibles and refusals.

Power Analysis

Power analysis and determination of sample size can feel intimidating. However, using programs can provide some reasonable estimates and allow you to better understand the trade-offs between sample size and power. A Google search will yield many power analysis resources. The two listed here are examples of what can be found. A free power analysis program, GPower (http://www.psycho.uni-duesseldorf.de/aap/projects/gpower/index.html) is accessible over the Internet and is based on the work of Cohen (the father of power analysis). A slightly more primitive but very functional calculator comes from a website from a Harvard course (http://hedwig.mgh.harvard.edu/sample_size/size.html); this calculator is intended more for clinical experimental designs that would be applicable for evaluation of small, pilot programs.

REFERENCES

Aday, L. A., & Cornelius, L. J. (2006). *Designing and conducting health surveys: A comprehensive guide* (3rd ed.). San Francisco: Jossey-Bass.

Agarwal, S. K., Estrada, S., Foster, W. G., Wall, L. L., Brown, D., Revis, E. S., et al. (2007). What motivates women to take part in clinical and basic science endometriosis research? *Bioethics, 21*(5), 263–269.

Bamberger, M., Rugh, J., & Mabry, L. (2006). *Real world evaluation: Working under budget, time, data and political constraints.* Thousand Oaks, CA: Sage Publications.

Black, T. R. (1999). *Doing quantitative research in the social sciences: An integrated approach to research design, measurement and statistics.* London: Sage Publications.

Blair, J., & Czaja, R. (1982). Locating a special population using random digit dialing. *Public Opinion Quarterly, 46*(4), 585–591.

Borders, T. F., Rohrer, J. E., & Vaughn, T. E. (2000). Limitations of secondary data for strategic marketing in rural areas. *Health Services Management Research, 13*(4), 216–222.

DeVellis, R. (2003). *Scale development: Theory and application* (2nd ed.). Thousand Oaks, CA: Sage Publications.

Faugier, J., & Sargeant, M. (1997). Sampling hard-to-reach populations. *Journal of Advanced Nursing, 26*(4), 790–797.

Fowler, F. J., Jr. (1995). *Improving survey questions: Design and evaluation. Applied social research methods series: Volume 38.* Thousand Oaks, CA: Sage Publications.

Huby, M., & Hughes, R. (2001). The effects of data on using material incentives in social research. *Social Work and Social Sciences Review, 9,* 5–16.

Krosnick, J. A. (1999). Maximizing measurement quality: Principles of good questionnaire design. In J. P. Robinson, P. R. Shaver, & L. S. Wrightsman (Eds.), *Measures of political attitudes* (pp. 37–57). New York: Academic Press..

Larson, A., Stevens, A., & Wardlaw, G. (1994). Indirect estimates of "hidden" populations: Capture–recapture methods to estimate the numbers of heroin users in the Australian Capital Territory. *Social Science & Medicine, 39*(6), 823–831.

MacKay, G., Somerville, W., & Lundie, J. (1996). Reflections on goal attainment scaling (GAS): Cautionary notes and proposals for development. *Educational Research, 38*(2), 161–172.

Manalo, V., & Meezan, W. (2000). Toward building a typology for the evaluation of services in family support programs. *Child Welfare, 79*(4), 405–429.

Muhib, F. B., Lin, L. S., & Stueve, A. (2001). A venue-based method for sampling hard to reach populations. *Public Health Reports, 116*(suppl 1), 216–222.

Pedhazur, E. J., & Schmelkin, L. P. (1991). *Measurement, design, and analysis: An integrated approach.* Hillsdale, NJ: Lawrence Erlbaum Associates.

Rossi, P. H., Freeman, H. E., & Lipsey, M. W. (1999). *Evaluation: A systematic approach* (6th ed.). Thousand Oaks, CA: Sage Publications.

Rothbart, G. S., Fine, M., & Sudman, S. (1982). On finding and interviewing the needles in the haystack: The use of multiplicity sampling. *Public Opinion Quarterly, 46*(3), 408–421.

Slomka, J., McCurdy, S., Ratliff, E. A., Timpson, S., & Williams, M. L. (2007). Perceptions of financial payment for research participation among African-American drug users in HIV studies. *Journal of General Internal Medicine, 22*(10), 1403–1409.

Tan, L., & Grace, R. C. (2008). Social desirability and sexual offenders: A review. *Sexual Abuse, 20*(1), 61–87.

Willis, G., & Zahnd, E. (2007). Questionnaire design from a cross-cultural perspective: An empirical investigation of Koreans and non-Koreans. *Journal of Health Care for the Poor and Underserved, 18*(4 suppl), 197–217.

Yu, M. Y., Wu, T. Y., & Mood, D. W. (2005). Cultural affiliation and mammography screening of Chinese women in an urban county of Michigan. *Journal of Transcultural Nursing, 16*(2), 107–116.

CHAPTER 14

Quantitative Data Analysis and Interpretation

Patton (1997) suggested that, during the development of the evaluation plan, evaluators develop a hypothetical data template—that is, a set of hypothetical data that might result from the evaluation data collection. Based on these hypothetical data, the evaluators could then ask the stakeholders what they would want to know from that data and which actions or decisions they would make based on the findings. This mind exercise serves two functions: it allows the evaluator to educate the stakeholders with regard to the evaluation design, and it helps establish realistic expectations regarding the findings of the evaluation. Then, when data analysis is in progress and the stakeholders are involved in interpretation of the data, they will be better prepared to understand both the data and its limitations. Patton's advice extends the involvement of the stakeholders from the program planning into its evaluation.

Needless to say, both stakeholders and evaluators will be focused on whether the program makes a difference. Program effect evaluations are essentially efforts to identify whether a significant degree of change occurred among program participants, compared to the rest of the target audience. Attention to the design of the effect evaluation, sample selection, and methods used to collect data lays the foundation for the subsequent statistical tests and affects the overall trustworthiness of the statistical findings. This chapter provides a rudimentary review of statistical tests, but is not intended to duplicate material available in statistics textbooks. The focus here is on the relationship of the statistical test to the design and sample, with an emphasis on understanding the implications of the statistical results in terms of program effect.

DATA ENTRY AND MANAGEMENT

Data collected for the effect evaluation will need to be computerized, if they were not collected in a computerized format. Data collected on paper, as is often the case with surveys, need to be entered into a computer database or spreadsheet so that evaluators can conduct statistical analyses. The software to be used for data analysis must be chosen before beginning data entry. Be assured that given the powerful computing capacity of today's computers and the ever-growing size of computer memory, desktop computers can readily accommodate evaluation data sets and the software used to analyze them.

A key consideration in the choice of statistical software is the sustainability of the evaluation. Put simply, if program staff and stakeholders are expected to be involved in the data entry and analysis, then their computer skills and interests need to be considered in choosing software. For the majority of program evaluations done by agencies, today's widely used spreadsheet and database programs are both adequate and convenient. In fact, such software is typically included in software packages such as Microsoft Office.

The convention for entering data into a spreadsheet is that each row represents a person (a participant in the evaluation) and each column represents one variable. A variable in this situation is one survey question—that is, one item of data/information. Each column must contain no more than one, discrete, distinct question. If a question contains several items with "yes or no" responses, then each item is actually a question. In this way, the number of yes and no responses for each item can be counted. Setting up the spreadsheet is a crucial component of data management.

If the evaluation plan calls for outsourcing the data analysis, entering the data into a standard spreadsheet is recommended. The data files can then be read by more sophisticated statistical software. The commercially available statistical software programs, such as SPSS, Stata, or SAS, have become increasingly user-friendly and are marketed widely to larger organizations interested in ongoing evaluations and data management. These statistical software packages include components that facilitate doing highly complex statistical tests used in research that may not be available in software intended for business.

Another choice is to use free statistical shareware, such as EpiInfo. EpiInfo may be downloaded via the Internet from the Centers for Disease Control and Prevention. This software is particularly helpful for program evaluations in which relative risks and odds ratios need to be calculated. EpiInfo was designed to be used internationally and to be compatible with as many systems as possible. Its ease of use and inclusion of statistics needed for some health program evaluations can make it an appropriate statistical software choice.

Data management includes not only the choice of software, but also the management of the flow of paper and the oversight of the electronic files. The paper flow issues include tracking data entry, storage of original paper questionnaires and consent forms, and destruction of paper records. A rule of thumb is that paper ought to be kept for as long as the evaluation is active and until the final report has been distributed. This rule also applies to the electronic files. Of course, creating backup files and having a standard procedure for naming the files are mandatory.

A critical step that can take a noticeable amount of time and effort is *data cleaning*. This process involves checking the data for obvious data entry errors. Data cleaning is important because without good data, the statistical results are meaningless. The need for data cleaning can be minimized by planning during the development of the instrument or questionnaire and careful adherence to the data collection procedures. Data cleaning begins with reviewing the frequency distributions of all variables. First look for values that do not seem reasonable or plausible, such as a participant's age being 45 when the program is for adolescents and is based in a regular high school, or a negative value for the number of days in a program that was calculated based on subtracting dates. If an unrealistic value is found, the next step is to review the data for the individual and determine whether (1) the data were incorrectly entered, (2) the value is plausible, or (3) the value is so unlikely that the data ought to be considered as missing. Keeping an incorrect value in the data can drastically alter the mean, standard deviation, and subsequent statistical tests.

The data also need to be reviewed for *skip patterns*—that is, systematic nonresponses to items on a questionnaire. If specific items have low response rates, then their use in subsequent analyses should be called into question. As with unreasonable values, including an item with a low response rate has implications for the subsequent statistical analysis. Including items that have missing data decreases the total number of respondents included in any analyses that includes that item, which can result in distorted and unstable statistics.

Outliers

Outliers are those variables with reasonable, plausible, yet extraordinary values; they lay outside the normal or at the extreme ends of a distribution curve. Outlying values can occur as a result of errors in the measures or instruments, data entry errors, or unusual but accurate data. Common examples of outliers in health care include the rare patients who incur extremely high hospitalization costs, as would be the case for a very-low-birth-weight infant, and the long lengths of stay for individuals with a rare but serious illness or with complications from a procedure.

Authors of statistical textbooks warn of the effects on statistical results when outliers are included in the data analysis (e.g., Kleinbaum, Kupper, Muller, & Nizan, 1998; Pedhazur & Pedhazur-Schmelkin, 1991). Outliers dramatically influence the results of statistical tests by shifting the mean and increasing the variance. Although complex statistical methods can correct for the effects of outliers, these methods are more complicated than necessary for most program evaluations. Essentially, evaluators need to decide whether to keep the outlier in the analysis or to exclude the outlier based on some defensible rationale. The rationale for exclusion is often based on determining some cut-off point for the values to be excluded.

The decision to include or exclude an outlier is made on a case-by-case basis. One factor that can influence the decision is the sample size in the evaluation study. Statistics based on smaller samples will be more dramatically affected by outliers. For example, an evaluation of change in HbA1c levels might be studied in 20 people. If one person had a decrease of more than 50% in this level while everyone else had a decrease of between 0% and 10%, the average percent decrease will be larger than if that one individual were excluded from the analysis. In contrast, if data from 200 people are collected, with the same range in decrease, the one individual with a 50% decrease in HbA1c level will have less effect on the average decrease.

Linked Data

Linked data refers to a data set that results from merging data from more than one source so that a more comprehensive set of variables becomes available for the subjects in the data set. Recall that for health programs, individuals, neighborhoods, or states could be the subjects of an effect evaluation. The types of data that are linked for health program evaluation, therefore, can include survey data with survey data, vital records data with survey data, vital records data with population surveys, survey data with administrative data, or population survey data with population survey data. Use of linked data may be necessary if the evaluation question focuses on outcomes for which data exist from a variety of sources. Linked data can be helpful throughout the stages of program planning and evaluation, from community assessment to effect evaluation.

One reason to use linked data is to connect program participation to outcome data. The study by Reichman and Hade (2001) is an example of linking participation data with outcome data; these authors matched a list of participants in a prenatal program with birth data from vital records in order to evaluate the outcome of the program. Another reason to use linked data is to have program outcome data associated with services utilization (process) data. For example, Meuleners, Hendrie, and Lee (2008) linked mortality data, hospital data, and data from mental health information systems to study readmission rates for persons who had experienced interpersonal violence. A third reason to use linked data is to validate self-report responses. For example, Robinson, Young, Roos, and Gelskey (1997) linked health insurance administrative data about individual patients with the self-reports from those individuals regarding having chronic health conditions. This strategy does, however, leave the evaluator with the dilemma of which data to believe and use.

The basic steps involved in linking data are simple, although their implementation is often far from simple. First, the data sets to be merged need to be in compatible software files. As software has become more standardized, it has become easier to create data files that are compatible. Nonetheless, software compatibility must be checked before beginning the linking process. Second, at least some variables about the individuals must be the same in both data sets. In other words, there needs to be a set of variables—called matching variables—that are the same in both data sets, and those variables must relate to only one individual. Thus each file needs to be checked for having the matching variables. Third, matching variables are used as the criteria for linking the data from each file and merging the data into one file.

Two major issues arise when using linked data: confidentiality and accuracy. For the majority of health program evaluations, data about individuals will be linked. This effort requires that some unique identifiers of the individual exist in both data sets, such as date of birth, Social Security number, or medical record number. Having data that identifies individuals with their data can raise ethical concerns, however. As a consequence, there must be strict, comprehensive, and careful procedures to remove the unique person identifiers after completing the merge of data files. Accuracy can be an issue in terms of correctly linking the files so that all data for a specific person are really about that person. Achieving accurately linked files requires using a complex algorithm for matching variables. For example, if there are two "Mary Smith" entries in the files, birth date and marital status may be needed to distinguish between the two Mary Smiths so as to link the files correctly.

SAMPLE DESCRIPTION

Once the data are clean, then the statistical analyses can begin. Always begin the analysis with a careful examination of the sample or samples by reviewing frequency statistics on each group (participants only, control group only) for any obvious unexpected differences. If the frequencies appear to be as expected, the evaluator can proceed to statistical comparisons. If any frequencies are not as might be expected, the data should be more carefully reviewed. For example, if the mean age for the participants looks considerably higher than for the control group, use a comparison test to assess whether there is a statistical difference for the two groups.

As a general rule, if an experimental/exposed group and a control/unexposed group were used in the design, the evaluator should begin with a statistical comparison of the participant and the control groups on basic demographic variables. This step can be important as a means to convince stakeholders and others that the subsequent differences were not related to demographic differences. In other words, if no statistically significant differences are found, then it is safe to say that the participants were similar to the population from which they were selected. This speaks to generalizability of the results and the external validity of the evaluation. If statistically significant differences between the participant and control groups are present, acknowledge and discuss possible reasons for the differences. This action speaks to the trustworthiness of the evaluator. It may be important, then, to consider using the statistically different demographic factors in subsequent analyses, as moderating factors, to diminish their influence on the statistical findings about the effect of the program.

THINKING ABOUT CHANGE

In terms of program effect evaluation, *change* is measured as a difference. In many ways, change is a relative term because it is detectable only by comparison. The amount of change detected is influenced by what is being compared—a fundamental characteristic of change that must be understood by evaluators, program staff, and stakeholders alike. Also, connecting the measure of change back to the outcome objective target values is important.

Change as a Difference Score

Change generally is measured three ways. The first way to measure change is to subtract an initial baseline score before the intervention from a subsequent score after the program. The term *score* is used generically to refer to a measure of the health outcome, whether it is a lab value, a cognitive test score, or a health services utilization rate. The first difference score is calculated with the following basic formula:

$$\text{Amount of change} = \frac{\text{Sum (each post-test score} - \text{each pre-test score)}}{\text{Number of paired scores}}$$

To calculate change using this formula requires having data from only one group, making it the only option for evaluations that used a one sample pre-test/post-test design. For each individual, a difference score is calculated and then averaged across all the participants.

The second way to measure change is to subtract the mean score of the group who received the program from the mean score of the group who did not receive the program:

$$\text{Amount of change} = (\text{mean participants' post-test score}) - (\text{mean nonparticipants' post-test score})$$

To calculate change using this formula requires having data from both the experimental group and the control group after the intervention has been received. However, given that a nonequivalent-group, post-test-only design is weak, this formula is seldom used.

Designs that include two groups and both pre-test and post-test data are stronger and provide additional data for estimating the program effect. If data have been collected from both the experimental group and the control group before and after the intervention, as would be the case in some quasi-experimental designs and true experimental design, formulas 1 and 2 can be combined:

Amount of change = (mean participants' post-test score −
mean participants' pre-test score) −
(mean nonparticipants' post-test score −
mean nonparticipants' pre-test score)

This formula gives a more precise measure of change because it uses all of the relevant data. First calculating the amount of change in participants and in nonparticipants would be especially important for health programs that have a longer duration and for target audiences that would experience natural changes over that time period. The remaining difference is more likely due to the program. A between-group mean change is essentially this third formula and is often used to report the findings of clinical trials. For example, Eser, Yavuzer, Karakus, and Karaoglan (2008) used this method to report the effect of balance training in a randomized trial.

Issues with Quantifying Change from the Program

Before evaluators can determine the program effect, five conceptual challenges to understanding change must be addressed. In this section, each challenge is explained and possible approaches to resolving the challenge are presented. These challenges may potentially influence the interpretation of the statistical findings.

Direction of Desired Outcome: Increase or Decrease

The direction of the change becomes important for selecting appropriate calculation techniques, interpreting the statistical results, and finally presenting the findings. For example, in Layettevillle the adolescent pregnancy prevention program sought to decrease the birth rate for adolescents from a baseline of 37.6 births per 1000 adolescent girls, whereas the congenital anomalies prevention program sought to increase the use of prenatal vitamins from a baseline of 80% to 98% use by pregnant women. Thus, when a change score is calculated for each of the programs, the result of subtracting the pre-intervention value from the post-intervention value will have different signs for the two programs. The decrease in adolescent pregnancy takes the form of a positive number, whereas the increase in prenatal vitamin use appears as a negative number. If a multicomponent program has objectives with targets that go in both directions, confusion is likely to ensue. There may be no way to avoid this problem, so taking care in the reporting and presentation may be the only path. One solution to this dilemma is to report the change as an absolute number. Alternatively, all outcome objectives and values might be characterized as phrases (e.g., "improvement") in a way that gets around having a mix of positive and negative numbers, both of which reflect improvement.

High Level of Desired Outcome at Baseline or Pre-Test

One difficulty faced by population-focused programs is that behavioral change in the population follows the diffusion of innovation curve (Rogers, 1983). Innovations, as new and novel ideas or products, become adopted over time by a greater number of people. This process is referred to as *diffusion* of the innovation through the population. The difficulty created by diffusion is that, with a higher prevalence of the desired health behavior before the program, it becomes more challenging to increase the prevalence of the health behavior. This dilemma arises because those who are the last to adopt a change are known to be the most resistant to change.

One approach for addressing this issue is to take into account the initial prevalence of the health or behavior when estimating the effectiveness of the intervention [Hovland, Lumsdaine, and Scheffield (1949), cited in Green & Lewis (1986)]. To do so, the change in the percentage of a population with the behavior after the program is compared to the percentage of the population without the behavior before the program. Because it is more difficult to achieve an equal increase in a behavior when the baseline value is already high, this approach is weighted in favor of improvements in a population with a high baseline. The result is an increasingly higher number as the pervasiveness of the desired health outcome increases at baseline. In general, a higher number is better, though it can be misleading. A major shortcoming of this approach is that it does not take into account the desired outcome level, as reflected in the outcome objectives.

Relationship of Change to an Outcome Objective Target Value

Mohr (1992) argued that the simple difference scores as given between the participants and nonparticipants or between pre-program and post-program scores or rates do not provide information on how effective the program was in terms of whether it was weak or strong. To overcome this shortcoming, he proposed a ratio that captures the amount of change achieved in relationship to the amount of change planned as given in the objective target value:

$$\text{Effectiveness ratio} = \frac{\text{post-test score} - \text{pre-test score}}{\text{target score} - \text{pre-test score}}$$

The target score is the level that the program intended to achieve, as stated in the outcome objectives. Keep in mind that this formula is applied to one group at a time, so it does not compare experimental and control groups. The formula is useful, however, in contrasting the program effect at two sites.

Consider, for example, two clinics that are participating in Bowe County's program to increase folic acid intake among women of childbearing age, where the change in prenatal vitamin use is one outcome indicator. In Clinic A, after the counseling intervention, 70% of the women take the vitamins—an increase of 10%. The effectiveness ratio for this clinic is .26 (Table 14.1). Clinic B has a baseline rate of 85% and also had an increase of 10% of women taking the vitamins, but its ratio is .77. Thus, although both clinics had a 10% increase or improvement, Clinic B appears more successful because of the higher baseline rate. Although the two clinics had a 10% increase, Clinic A started much farther from the target value, so it has a much lower effectiveness ratio than Clinic B, whose baseline was closer to the target value. Of course, this ratio still does not help us understand the extent to which the program addressed the health problem.

For many health problems, public health programs are designed to address gaps or disparities in health status. Accordingly, the aim of the program is to reduce the existing gap. To estimate the extent to which the gap remains, a different formula is needed, known as the target adequacy index:

$$\text{Target adequacy index} = \frac{\text{target score} - \text{post-test score}}{\text{target score} - \text{pre-test score}}$$

One advantage of the target adequacy index is that it can be used with either the program outcome objective target values or a standard target rate, such as one taken from the *Healthy People 2010* objectives. This index essentially highlights the absolute gap between the target and current levels. As a consequence, it is helpful in revising target objectives for subsequent iterations of the program and in raising awareness among the stakeholders of the difficulty in achieving the target objectives.

Relationship of Change to Intervention Effort

The effectiveness of a program can also be thought of in terms of the ability of the intervention to generate change. Abelson (1995) proposed a formula that takes into account both the intervention effect size and the size of the factor that caused the effect—namely, the intervention effort or dosage. The

Table 14.1   Calculation of Effectiveness and Adequacy Indices: An Example

	Bowe County		Interpretation
	Clinic A	**Clinic B**	
Outcome objective target value	98%	98%	Value established for the outcome objective
% taking prenatal vitamins at baseline	60%	85%	Baseline or control values
% taking prenatal vitamins post-program	70%	95%	Outcome values
Pre-program to post-program change	70%–60% = 10%	95%–85% = 10%	Simple amount of change in outcome variable
Effectiveness ratio	$\dfrac{70\%-60\%}{98\%-60\%} = .26$	$\dfrac{95\%-85\%}{98\%-85\%} = .77$	Ratio of actual to planned effect; reveals that the selection of the target rate influences interpretation of effectiveness
Target adequacy index	$1 - \dfrac{98\%-70\%}{98\%-60\%} =$ $1 - .73 = 27\%$	$1 - \dfrac{98\%-95\%}{98\%-85\%} =$ $1 - .23 = 77\%$	Gives a relative closeness to reaching the outcome target value, given the baseline; indicates the gap remaining to the target value
Intervention efficiency	$\dfrac{70\%-60\%}{10 \text{ min}-5 \text{ min}} =$ 2% per minute	$\dfrac{95\%-85\%}{15 \text{ min}-5 \text{ min}} =$ 1% per minute	Gives a measure of improvement per unit of intervention effort (Using minutes of counseling intervention)

effect size is the mean value of the outcome variable for the experimental group minus the mean value of the outcome variable for the control groups. The intervention causal size is the amount of the intervention each group received, generally thought of as dosage. The intervention efficiency score, or what Abelson calls the causal efficacy, uses both the effect size and the cause size:

$$\text{Intervention efficiency} = \frac{\begin{array}{c}(\text{mean post score experimental group}) - \\ (\text{mean post score control group})\end{array}}{\begin{array}{c}(\text{amount of intervention experimental group}) - \\ (\text{amount of intervention control group})\end{array}}$$

The intervention efficiency score provides insight into the amount of effort required to produce the amount of change observed. In Table 14.1, Clinic A has a higher intervention efficiency score (percent increase per minute of counseling) compared to Clinic B because more intervention time was given in Clinic B for the same amount of increase in women taking prenatal vitamins. Ideally, an intervention theory that is evidence-based and carefully aligns interventions with desired outcomes ought to lead to a higher intervention efficiency index. But as the Clinic A versus Clinic B example shows, the intervention dosage (minutes)—and not the intervention type (counseling)—made Clinic B appear less efficacious. Only by examining the process evaluation data would the program evaluator or program manager be able to determine the source of the variation between the two clinics.

The intervention efficiency score is critical for linking the outcomes and the processes. Table 14.2 shows a 2×2 matrix demonstrating how the intervention efficiency score gives useful planning information. As shown in Table 14.2, the ideal outcome would be to have large effects from small causes, and the least desirable outcome would be to have small effects from large causes. The intervention efficiency score is calculated using the effect evaluation data. However, during the planning stage, hypothetical data could be used, thereby providing some parameters for setting expectations. In any event, the intervention efficiency score would be one source of information for making decisions regarding continuing, modifying, or ceasing a program.

Unmeasured Factors Adding to the Difference

Calculating change as the difference between pre-program and post-program data gives a net program effect, which is the amount of intervention effect on participants compared to any effect on the comparison group, given the amount of error due to the design and measures used. Under ideal conditions, there would be no design or measurement error, so the amount of difference between participants and members of the comparison group would be the true amount of change from the program. Of course, real conditions make it more difficult to know the true and complete amount of change attributable

Table 14.2   Intervention Efficiency as a Relation of Effect Size and Causal Size

Causal Size	Effect Size	
	Small Effect	Large Effect
Small Cause	Neutral intervention efficiency	High intervention efficiency
Large Cause	Low intervention efficiency	Neutral intervention efficiency

to the program (Figure 14.1). Any of a variety of knowable and measurable, but not controllable, factors may influence the amount of difference or change that is statistically found, such as growth, aging, or recent media reports. For example, media reports might influence study participants to change a behavior, such that the change cannot be attributed solely to the program. In addition, unknowable or unanticipated, and hence unmeasured, factors can influence the amount of difference or change that is statistically found, such as sudden disasters, epidemics, and policy changes. Clearly, statistical findings are only as accurate and trustworthy as the design and measurement allows.

Figure 14.1   Contributing Factors to the Total Amount of Change

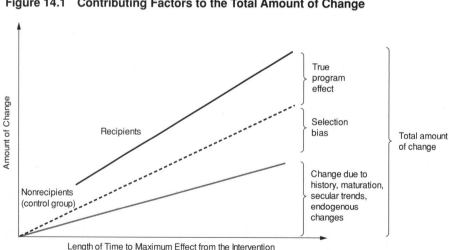

Clinical and Statistical Significance

The presence of statistical significance does not necessarily equate to practical or clinical significance. An excellent example of this phenomenon is the statistically significant increase in birth weight frequently found in a variety of prenatal programs. The amount of additional birth weight is often in the range 5 to 10 grams, which is a very minor—not clinically important—increase, except for very small newborns. *Statistical significance* indicates how likely one would be to get the result by pure chance, whereas *clinical significance* relates to how likely the intervention is to have a noticeable benefit to participants. Effect evaluations of health programs ideally seek to establish both the statistical and clinical significance of the program. Statistical significance may not directly translate into practical importance, as is the case in making programmatic or policy decisions. For these reasons, the discussion of statistical analysis presented here and the associated exhibits distinguish between significance tests and tests that indicate the degree of effect from the program.

ACROSS LEVELS OF ANALYSIS

Health programs can be designed to produce effects across the various levels of the public health pyramid. Effect evaluations of programs designed for and delivered to individuals will yield the most straightforward data for analysis. When programs are designed and delivered to a unit of individuals, such as a family, a school within a district, or a work unit within an agency, the effect evaluation will have data collected about that unit; items on a questionnaire will ask about things that happen "in our family," "in my school," or "in my department." Analysis of data collected from individuals about a unit must take the unit into account, which is accomplished by aggregating the data. *Aggregation* means summarizing data from across participants within one nested unit so as to create a variable at the unit level of analysis. The advantage of using aggregated data is that a different pattern exists for aggregates. Thus the evaluator is able to describe the characteristics of the aggregates, compare results across aggregates rather than across individuals, and identify associations between characteristics of aggregate and program or other variables. Epidemiological patterns can be more noticeable when comparisons are made across aggregates. For example, comparing data about different clinics, schools, or worksites may provide more useful information than focusing on individuals within those units.

Although aggregation of data makes sense for public and community health program evaluation, the notion of not maintaining an individual level of analysis may be uncomfortable or unfamiliar to clinicians who are trained to rely on data about each individual. Neither aggregated nor individual-level analysis is right or wrong. Instead, each results in different information about program effects.

If the evaluation is focused on an aggregate, such as a family, community, population, or work unit, the first step in aggregation is to analyze the data from the perspective of the within-unit variable. If those within the unit are more like one another than they are like the rest of the sample—in other words, if there is a low amount of variability among those within the unit—then it is acceptable to create a score per unit by aggregating the unit members' data to form a unit-level variable. The unit is then statistically considered as though it were a single participant. Various statistical tests, such as the intraclass correlation (ICC) or the eta-squared value, are used to determine the validity of aggregating the data (Blise, 2000). Alternatively, some statistical software may use data from individuals for analysis across units and analyses of units within units, such as students in classrooms in schools in districts. Use and interpretation of these complex statistical tests will require statistical consultation and guidance. The important point is that statistical procedures for dealing with and analyzing aggregated data exist and may be appropriate for effect evaluations that are conducted for an evaluation research purpose.

If the analysis focuses on a health outcome and a characteristic of a unit (such as a school, department, or community), then analysis might potentially find a higher correlation between the units than among the individuals. This outcome is known as an *ecological correlation*. Black (1999) stresses that these ecological correlations are important to consider in terms of the intent of the research. The correlation between units is acceptable as a finding if the intervention was aimed at the unit and the outcome being assessed occurred at the unit level. Conversely, if the evaluation was intended to identify changes in participants across units, then the analysis should remain at the individual level.

In summary, statistical analysis of effect evaluation data follows all the conventions of statistical analysis of research data. Evaluators need to be cognizant of the interplay between how the health program is delivered, how the evaluation data are collected, and which statistical tests are carried out. A word of caution is in order, however. If large amounts of data have been collected and the statistical tests first used to assess for a change revealed no program effect, there will be inclination to begin data dredging. *Data dredging* is the process of continuing to analyze the data in ways not originally planned—in other words, looking and looking and looking until some significant finding is found. Data dredging will eventually yield statistically significant findings, if only by chance. Therefore, unnecessary additional statistical tests ought to be avoided.

STATISTICAL ANSWERS TO THE QUESTIONS

Before beginning statistical analysis, program evaluators should review the program outcome objectives and the questions for the effect evaluation. The questions help keep the analysis focused, thereby minimizing evaluators' inclination to go searching for significant findings (i.e., data dredging). Staying close to the evaluation questions also ensures that the key concerns of stakeholders are addressed first. Unfortunately, the process of choosing the best statistical procedure and tests can quickly devolve into a guessing game. This review is not intended as a comprehensive review of basic statistical principles; rather, it emphasizes the practical relationship between the evaluation questions and the statistical tests performed. The purpose of this section is to provide guidelines for choosing statistical tests and decreasing the amount of guesswork involved. Given that spreadsheet and database software greatly facilitate doing the mathematical calculations, it is imperative to have a framework for choosing the best and most appropriate statistical test.

Table 14.3 lists a set of questions that need to be answered to arrive at an appropriate statistical analysis plan. Figure 14.2 graphically shows the factors that determine a statistical approach. For the purposes of this discussion, the focus of analysis refers to whether the effect evaluation is seeking to answer questions about comparison of groups, associations among two or more variables, or prediction of outcomes. This review of statistical data analysis is organized by those three dominant analytic approaches used in effect evaluations.

Table 14.3 Factors That Affect the Choice of a Statistical Test: Questions to Be Answered

1. How many groups did the design result in: one, two, or more? Were they paired/matched, independent, or a population?

2. What is the focus of the evaluation question: comparison, association among variables, or prediction of outcomes?

3. Which level of measurement was used for the dependent variable and for the independent variables: nominal, ordinal, interval/ratio? If interval/ratio measures were used, do the data have a parametric or nonparametric distribution?

4. What is the interest and capacity of the stakeholders for understanding statistical analyses?

Figure 14.2   Summary of the Three Decisions for Choosing an Analytic Approach

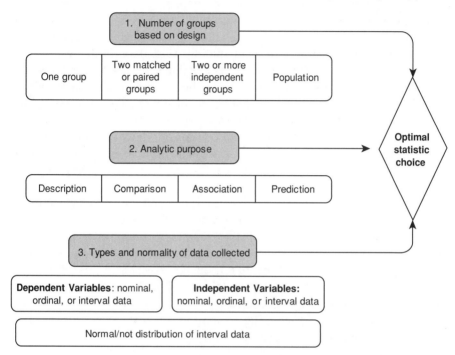

Using the level of intervention and level of analysis as two dimensions, the possible foci of analysis can be assigned. Table 14.4 is based on the assumption that the evaluation data were collected at the same level as that of the program intervention. A careful look at this table reveals that statistical tests of comparison and association can be used widely and that prediction tests are recommended only when the level of intervention and the level of analysis are the same, unless the help of a statistician is available. In addition, analyses cannot be done at levels where the data are more discrete (lower) than the level at which the programmatic intervention was delivered—hence the blank cells in Table 14.4.

When discussing the types of statistical analyses that are appropriate for comparison, association, and prediction, a useful distinction is the difference between analysis procedure, measure of magnitude, and test for significance. This distinction is rarely emphasized in statistical textbooks. The essential

Table 14.4   Analysis Procedures by Level of Intervention and Level of Analysis (Assuming Data Collected at Same Level as Analysis)

Level of Analysis	Level of Program Intervention			
	Individual	**Aggregate**	**Population**	**Infrastructure**
Individual	Comparison tests; Association tests; Prediction tests	If individuals can be identified, then: Comparison tests; Association tests	If individuals can be identified, then: Comparison tests; Association tests	If individuals can be identified, then: Comparison tests; Association tests
Aggregate	Not appropriate	Comparison tests; Association tests; Prediction tests	If subgroups can be identified, then: Comparison tests; Association tests	If subgroups can be identified, then: Comparison tests; Association tests
Population	Not appropriate	Not appropriate	Comparison tests; Association tests; Prediction tests	Comparison tests; Association tests; Prediction tests
Infrastructure	Not appropriate	Not appropriate	Comparison tests; Association tests; Prediction tests	Comparison tests; Association tests; Prediction tests

question for effect evaluations is either "How much difference did the program make?" or "How strongly was the program related to the effects?" Measures of magnitude answer this question. In contrast, the question of "Was the difference more than would happen by chance?" is answered with tests of statistical significance. For each measure of magnitude, there is a corresponding test of significance. Both Aday (1996) and Newcomer (1994) draw attention to the importance of knowing both the magnitude and the significance of results when evaluating programs.

Description

The first step in any statistical analysis focuses on description. *Descriptive statistics*, also called exploratory data analysis or univariate statistics, yield information of the most basic nature, such as frequency counts, mean, mode, percentages, and dispersion of values. Do not underestimate either the power and information contained in descriptive statistics (Tukey, 1977), or the ease with which most stakeholders can understand them. Descriptive statistics can be applied to all types of data, regardless of the design. These statistics are used to answer evaluation questions such as "What were the demographic characteristics of program participants and comparison groups?," "How were the scores on the pre-test and the post-test distributed?," and "What percentage of the program participants reached the target set in the objectives?" If the level of measure involves ordinal and interval variables, descriptive statistics can include measures of central tendency (mean, mode, and median) as well as measures of variation (range, variance, and standard deviation). These statistics were reviewed in Chapter 5, in the discussion of defining the health problem. Spreadsheet and database software programs can readily compute descriptive statistics, and the results can be displayed easily with the associated graphics package.

The central tendency, frequency distributions, and variation of variables form the foundation for further statistical analyses. The review of the variance needs to determine whether the amount of variance is similar in both the experimental and control groups. This information helps the evaluator select the appropriate statistical tests for comparisons and correlations. Evaluators should spend time reviewing these descriptive statistics, because the distribution of values often gives the first understanding about a program's participants and effects. Also, when the statistics for each variable are reviewed, evaluators may be able to obtain insights into unique characteristics of participants or unexpected distributions. Such observations may lead to additional, and sometimes unplanned, analyses.

Another reason to do descriptive analyses is to assess whether the data are normally distributed. Data collected at the nominal or ordinal levels of measurement can be used only in *nonparametric* statistical tests. Data collected at the interval level of measurement and whose distribution follows the normal distribution curve are called *parametric*. However, if the interval or ratio-level data are not normally distributed, nonparametric statistical tests must be used. Table 14.5 summarizes the major nonparametric and parametric statistical tests that are used for comparison, association, and prediction.

Table 14.5   Commonly Used Parametric and Nonparametric Statistical Tests for Comparison, Association, and Prediction

Type of Data	Complexity of Question about Effect		
	Comparison	Association	Prediction
Parametric	Difference scores, *t*-tests of difference of means, variance analyses (ANOVA, ANCOVA)	Correlations (Pearson's), hierarchical analyses	Time series, regression analyses, logistic regression analyses
Nonparametric	Chi-square tests based on contingency tables	Chi-square tests based on contingency tables, odds ratio, relative risk, other (i.e., Sign test, Wicoxon, Kruskal–Wallis)	Log-linear and probit regression analyses

Comparison

Comparison questions can ask for a within-group comparison—that is, determinations of whether baseline (pre-test) scores are different from the follow-up (post-test) scores. Comparison questions also are appropriate for between-groups comparisons—that is, determination of whether program participants are different from nonparticipants or from members of the control group. These comparison questions can be posed at the individual level of analysis as well as at the aggregate and population levels. Table 14.6 summarizes the major types of comparison analysis procedures that are appropriate for each level of analysis. Of course, which level of measurement is employed and whether the variables are parametric will influence the final choice of statistical procedure.

Comparisons between groups using only nominal data (for both the outcome variable and the independent variables) are performed by using one of the various versions of the chi-square test. Whether the groups are related/matched and how many groups are compared (Black, 1999, p. 436) can make a difference in which statistic is optimal. Between-groups questions addressed with such analyses focus on some version of "Are participants are statistically more likely to have characteristic *y* compared to nonparticipants?" Some

Table 14.6   Main Types of Comparison Analyses Used, by Level of Analysis, Assuming the Variables Are at the Same Level of Measurement

| Level of Measurement | Comparison-Focused Analyses | | |
	Analysis Procedures	Measures of Magnitude	Tests of Significance
Nominal by nominal data	Difference scores, chi-square tests based on contingency tables (i.e., McNemar, Fisher's exact)	Percent or mean difference, phi coefficient, Cramer's V, lambda	p value
Ordinal by ordinal data	Median test, Mann–Whitney U test, Kruskal–Wallis test for three or more groups, Sign test, Wilcoxon matched-pairs signed rank test, Friedman two-way analysis for three or more groups	Lambda, uncertainty coefficient, Goodman and Kruskal's gamma, Somer's d, eta coefficient	p value
Interval by interval data	t-test (independent samples), paired t-test (related samples)	Difference between means	p value, confidence interval

health program evaluation questions focus on comparing populations, such as those that seek to determine rates in different states of health behaviors derived from the BRFSS. These simple comparisons are made by using the same statistical tests used with individual-level data. However, because the population, rather than a sample, is used, slightly different equations are used.

Association

Most evaluations aspire to answer more than comparative questions. Questions about relationships or associations among variables are asked, such as whether receiving more interventions is related to a greater amount of change or whether the amount of change is associated with a specific characteristic of program participants. Correlational statistics or other statistics of association do not provide information on the temporal sequence of variables and, therefore, do not provide information about causation. Instead, *correlational* analyses indicate the strength of the relationship and whether the relationship is such that the variables vary directly or inversely. An inverse relationship between the variables, such as increasing age and decreasing tissue resilience, is indicated by a negative correlation.

Table 14.7 provides a summary of the main tests of association. To choose the appropriate statistical test, evaluators must consider the level of measurement needed, the parametric character, and the number of groups used in the analysis. Table 14.8 provides an example of the tests of the strength of association that could be used with data at different levels of measurement. Using the anti-violence program to prevent adolescent deaths due to gunshot wounds as an example, the dependent variables are the ICD-10 code for the injury, the

Table 14.7   Main Types of Association Analyses Used, by Level of Analysis, Assuming Variables Are at the Same Level of Measurement

Level of Measurement	Association-Focused Analyses		
	Analysis Procedures	Measures of Magnitude	Tests of Significance
Nominal by nominal data	Fisher's exact for 2 × 2 table, chi-square or independent samples, McNemar or Cochran Q for related samples	Relative risk, coefficient of contingency, phi coefficient, Cramer's V, lambda	p value, confidence intervals
Ordinal by ordinal data	Chi-square, Spearman rank order	Kendall's coefficient of concordance, Kendall's tau a, tau b, tau c, Somer's d, Spearman rank order coefficient	p value
Interval by interval data	Multiple regression analyses	Pearson correlation coefficient, intraclass coefficient	p value
Mixed	One-way analysis of variance (ANOVA) for nominal by interval data	Eta coefficient	p value for F statistic

Table 14.8   Example of Statistical Tests for Strength of Association by Level of Measurement, Using Laytonville Adolescent Anti-Violence Program

	Dependent Outcome Variables		
Independent Predictor Variables	**Nominal** (e.g., ICD-10 for injury)	**Ordinal** (e.g., rank among schools in terms of number of injuries)	**Interval** (e.g., number of students with emergency room admissions)
Nominal (e.g., race of student)	Cramer's C (two or more groups), phi (if two groups), chi-square	Chi-square, Mann–Whitney	Student's t-test, ANOVA, Kruskal–Wallis
Ordinal (e.g., rank among school in terms of test scores)	Probit regression	Spearman's rho, Kendall's tau, Spearman rank order, eta coefficient	Spearman's rank, linear regression
Interval (e.g., number of hours of anger management education)	Logistic regression	Pearson product moment r	Pearson's r, multiplecorrelation coefficient, linear regression

rank of the school in terms of number of injuries, and the number of school days missed due to gunshot wounds, and the independent variables are the race of students, the rank of the school in terms of standardized test scores, and the number of hours of anger management education. Table 14.9 continues with the anti-violence example by showing how the design of the evaluation further affects the statistical analysis plan.

At the individual level, in addition to contingency table analysis procedures for nonparametric data, correlation analyses are possible with parametric data. When the correlational analysis includes a copious number of variables, the likelihood increases that some pairs will be significantly related. Therefore, is it wise to lower the alpha value from $p < .05$ to either $p < .01$ or $p < .001$ to provide a more conservative statement about what was statistically significant. One approach to reducing the number of variables in the analysis is to exclude

Table 14.9   Examples of Statistical Tests by Evaluation Design and Level of Measurement, with Examples of Variables

Designs	Nominal by Nominal (e.g., ICD-10 for injury by race)	Interval by Interval (e.g., number students with emergency room admissions by hours of work anger management education)	Interval by Nominal (e.g., number students with emergency room admissions by student race)
One group (i.e., pre-test/ post-test)	Chi-square	Pearson correlation, logistic regression	Point biserial coefficient
Two groups, independent	Chi-square, $k \times 2$ tables	One-way analysis of variance (ANOVA)	Chi-square
Two groups, related or matched	McNemar change test	t-test for related or matched samples	McNemar

variables based on a logical basis, such as not possibly being related (i.e., hair color and height).

Moderating and Mediating Variables

The causal theory for the program may include either moderating or mediating variables. If data on these variables were collected as part of the effect evaluation, then those data can be used to assess whether their presence changes the strength of correlation between the intervention and the health outcome. Although inclusion of moderating and mediating variables can quickly complicate the statistical analysis, there is at least one simple way to use those data: A moderating or mediating variable can be used as a control variable in the correlation between the health outcome variable and the intervention variable. This approach yields a partial correlation that has been adjusted for the effects of the control variable.

Prediction

Questions about how much of an effect a programmatic intervention might have on individuals, aggregates, or populations are basically questions of causation. Causal questions are the most difficult to answer, despite the fact that most stakeholders want an answer to the most fundamental causal question of "Did our program cause the health improvement?" Table 14.10 summarizes key statistics that can help predict future outcomes.

To answer causal questions, it is absolutely necessary to have data from a rigorous quasi-experimental or true experimental design. In other words, answering causal questions is not only a matter of statistical analysis but one of design. Unless a design has been used that enables the evaluator to essentially eliminate alternative causes and that provides a time line for the effects, the cause-and-effect relationship between the program and the health outcome cannot be substantiated. The statistics used for causal evaluation questions are essentially the same as those used for assessing relationships and associations, except that the findings can be interpreted as causal rather than only as indicating relationship. If there was no randomization, then the statistical approaches yield association information only. However, because the statistical procedures for prediction forecast a trend, that trend is often interpreted as prediction.

One major variation on the basic correlational analysis is regression analysis, sometimes called trend analysis (Veany & Kaluzny, 1998). Regression analysis allows for prediction, in terms of extrapolation and interpolation, based on a best-fit line (Black, 1999; Pedhazur & Pedhazur-Schmelkin, 1991). As a tool, regression analysis answers evaluation questions such as "How

Table 14.10 **Main Types of Prediction Analyses Used, by Level of Analysis, Assuming Variables Are at the Same Level of Measurement**

Level of Measurement	Prediction-Focused Analysis		
	Analysis Procedures	**Measures of Magnitude**	**Tests of Significance**
Nominal by nominal data	Probit regression analyses	Correlation coefficient (r^2)	F-test
Ordinal by ordinal data	Trend analyses	Correlation coefficient (r^2)	F-test
Interval by interval data	Time series, regression-discontinuity	Beta coefficient	F-test, confidence intervals
Nominal by interval data	Logistic regression	Entropy concentration	F-test

much more improvement might occur with more intervention?" and "As participant characteristics $x1$ and $x2$ increase, how much change will occur in the health outcome?" Regression analyses are based on the correlation of independent variables with the dependent variable and on the strength of the association among independent variables.

Time series analysis requires collecting data on the same sample, using the same measure at multiple time points. Such analyses, based on the multiple regression model, can be used with data such as number of motor vehicle accidents per year, number of Medicare enrollees per month, number of infants diagnosed with ear infections per week, or, prototypically, closing value of the New York Stock Exchange on each day. If a health program was provided that was expected to affect, then the time series analysis would provide insights into whether a change was observed in the pattern across time.

Many health program evaluation questions focus on changes across time, rather than change at a single point in time among participants. This is often the case in evaluations of full-coverage programs, for which no control group may exist. Typical across-time evaluation questions are "To what extent is there a decline in the health problem from year to year?" and "To what extent was there a change in the health outcome from before the program or policy was implemented to after it was established?" To answer such questions, a longitudinal design for data collection is commonly used, such that data are collected from the same individuals, on the same variables, at multiple points in time. Analysis of the repeated measures collected from the same sample becomes complex because an underlying association inevitably exists between the individual and the data; each data set is not independent of the subsequent data set because the same people provided the data. If the level of measurement is at the interval level, then ANOVA tests are appropriate.

INTERPRETATION

Patton (1997, p. 314) suggests using nonstatistical comparisons in program evaluation as a means of assessing programs. Comparisons can be done with the statistical findings and any of the following: the program goals, the impact objectives, benchmarks from other programs, results of similar programs, professional standards regarding the health problem, and intuition or educated guesses. These less scientific but practical comparisons do provide insights into the relative success of the health program, and they may highlight general areas of success and inadequacies.

In any study, spurious findings and surprises can occur. A *spurious finding* is one that is incidental to the evaluation question or that is an artifact of poorly understood factors. Spurious findings are generally curiosities that can be discounted as the result of measurement error and random chance. In contrast, *surprise findings* are not related to the evaluation questions, but cause one to say, "Hmmm" (Abelson, 1995). Surprise findings can either support the health program interventions or not; in some cases, they may lead to new descriptive insights. For example, if the evaluation measured x, but the finding is that the average value of x is considerably higher or lower than in the literature or than common sense would dictate, then the evaluator may be surprised. Surprises can be used as a basis for further exploration or for making revisions to the program or the evaluation plan. Surprises, while not common, are important and need to be valued and acknowledged, as they may inspire further questions and lead to new knowledge.

Four Fallacies of Interpretation

Green and Lewis (1986) suggest that four types of errors can occur when interpreting evaluation data. One fallacy is equating effectiveness with efficiency. *Effectiveness* is the extent to which results are achieved, whereas *efficiency* is a ratio of amount of effort or resources to the amount of effect achieved. Another way to think of this fallacy is in terms of the cost per unit of health improvement. There may be a point of diminishing returns, at which application of additional resources and efforts may not result in large gains in effect. Here the use of intervention efficiency ratio becomes important: The issue is how much more is required in the organizational or service utilization plan to obtain each additional unit of effect from the program.

Another fallacy is assuming that a constant rate of progress or health improvement will or has occurred. The rate of change may be variable or sporadic for many reasons. For example, for population-focused services, such as mass media awareness campaigns, the diffusion of innovation curve (Rogers, 1983) will be evident if population adoption of a new behavior is part of the effect theory. The rate of change may also vary depending on the characteristics of the recipient audience.

The assumption that ongoing improvement—that is, the inexorable forward movement of change—can be achieved is another fallacy. Program effects can be affected by time, such as relapse, lack of reinforcement or follow-up, memory failure, and program dropouts. Any one of these or similar factors can cause the health problem or condition to return. The extent to which it is possible to identify ongoing improvement can be influenced by the timing of data collection relative to the expected beginning of the effect. There are at least five ways in which a lack of forward movement in the degree of change can occur; each can be visualized graphically (Figure 14.3). In Figure 14.3a, the change over

---

Figure 14.3   Five Ways That the Rate of Change Can Be Altered

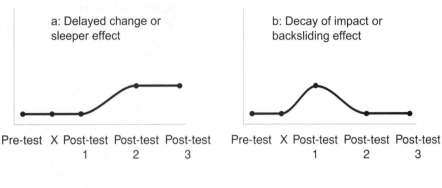

a: Delayed change or sleeper effect

b: Decay of impact or backsliding effect

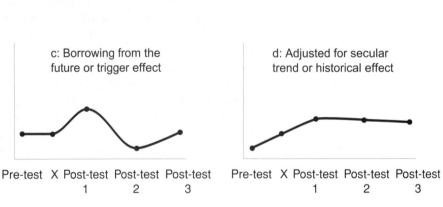

c: Borrowing from the future or trigger effect

d: Adjusted for secular trend or historical effect

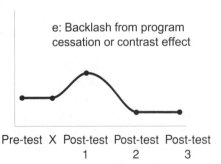

e: Backlash from program cessation or contrast effect

Note: X indicates the intervention. Y axis reflects amount of change from none to high.

time reflects a delayed change called a *sleeper effect*. In Figure 14.3b, the program effect is seen following the intervention, but then a gradual return to the baseline rate, known as *backsliding*, occurs. Sometimes, as shown in Figure 14.3c, anticipation of the intervention leads to adopting the behavior before the program has actually started (*trigger effect*). If factors influence the rate irrespective of the program, this is reflected in *historical effects* (Figure 14.3d). Finally, a *backlash* can occur if the program is discontinued, such that the long-term rates are worse than the rates before the program began (Figure 14.3e).

The fourth fallacy is underestimating the complexity of the change process. Behavioral change within individuals involves multiple stages (Prochaska, DiClemente, & Norcross, 1992) and is, in turn, influenced by multiple factors. Similarly, achieving physical changes through a health intervention can be complex, involving medications, procedures, and behaviors. Underestimating the complexity inherent in achieving change in the target audience—whether that audience consists of individuals, families, communities, or organizations—can lead to oversimplification of the interpretation of the findings. In addition, what is noticed in the findings will be affected by what was articulated in the program effect theory, especially the theory of intervention, partly because the effect theory guides the decisions regarding what is measured and when. Therefore, better causal and intervention theories that explain or predict the change and possible contributing factors to either maintaining the status quo or changing are more likely to lead to an evaluation that can minimize the risk of falling prey to this fallacy.

Ecological Fallacy

The ecological correlation mentioned previously should not be confused with the ecological fallacy. The latter fallacy has been an issue in program planning and evaluation for more than 20 years (Milcarek & Link, 1981). The *ecological fallacy* is the assumption that a group characteristic applies to all individuals within that group. For example, if a group of participants had an average of a high school education, the ecological fallacy would be to assume that any member of the group had a high school education. This fallacy involves interpretation of the findings in a way that is not being completely truthful to the data. Perhaps the group of participants actually includes many persons with college degrees and many persons with only an eighth-grade education; the presence of both subgroups would yield an average of 12 years of school.

Johnson and Caron (2006) found that the ecological fallacy was used by members of the public in estimating the risks for their community based on state data. Their findings hint at a natural human tendency to draw erroneous conclusions based on the flawed logic of an ecological inference. Various statistical approaches, such as multilevel modeling, can be helpful in understanding the extent to which a group characteristic truly applies to individuals within a group. Also, a move away from ecological or observational designs produces data that do not require making assumptions about individuals based on group characteristics.

ACROSS THE PYRAMID

At the direct services level of the public health pyramid, health programs focus on individual change. Therefore, most of the analysis will revolve around identifying changes within subjects, such as pre-test/post-test changes in program participants. Health programs at the direct services level are likely to be highly tailored and relatively small. The small number of participants should prompt concerns about having a sufficient sample size for statistical analysis. If the sample size is less than 30, the choice of statistical tests is affected. However, because it may be easier to identify nonparticipants in the program (controls), statistical tests may be available that can compare those groups.

At the enabling services level, health programs focus on groups and changes evident in those groups. Issues related to levels of analysis are of major importance at this level of the public health pyramid. If data from individuals within units (whether families, schools, social networks, or agencies) are to be aggregated, then statistical tests for within- and between-group variance need to be performed. Most of the data analysis needs to focus on identifying differences between groups in the amount of change for each group.

At the population services level of the public health pyramid, it becomes more difficult to have nonparticipants. Therefore, it is more likely that statistical tests will involve trend analysis of population data or time series analysis. In some cases, it may be possible to compare populations, such as counties or states. Because the population mean is known, as is the mean of the sample, a different set of statistical tests becomes possible.

At the infrastructure level, there are likely to be two major foci to the outcome evaluation: the change among participants who are part of the infrastructure, and the change in the population before and after the infrastructure change. In the first case, the statistical tests chosen will depend on the design of the program. For example, public health workers in several different counties may receive the same training program. The analysis could occur at the individual level of analysis and compare program participants with nonparticipants. Alternatively, data from the workers might be aggregated to have a higher level of analysis (i.e., county) and participating counties then compared with nonparticipating counties. If the evaluation was concerned with the health status of those served by the infrastructure, a trends analysis could be carried out to identify whether a change occurred in the health status of county residents after the training program was finished. These are just a few examples of the interaction between impact evaluation question, design, and statistical analysis.

DISCUSSION QUESTIONS AND ACTIVITIES

1. What are the pros and cons of aggregating data to have a higher level of analysis? Under which conditions would aggregation be the preferred approach to handling the impact evaluation data?

2. The adult immunization program of Bowe County has reached the effect evaluation stage. Data have been collected from individuals on their motivation to get immunized, use of the enabling service of transportation to the clinics has been tracked, and random telephone calls throughout the county have asked about recollection of the mass media campaigns. The evaluation team is now developing a plan for the statistical analysis. What would be your questions to the team about the data? Depending on the answers, which recommendations would you make?

3. It is common for stakeholders to essentially ask, "How can you prove that our program had an effect?" What would be your standard, simple, "sound bite" response to this question?

4. What is the importance of having both an effect size and significance? Which would be more important to subsequent decision making about continuing a program?

5. Evaluations of the five programs in Layetteville and Bowe County could potentially benefit from having linked data. For at least two of the health programs, identify at least two databases for linking the data and give a brief outline of how you would link the data.

INTERNET RESOURCES

Have fun with statistics—really! The websites identified here can help make statistics real, and statistics can sometimes be easier to understand when you see the numbers change.

Seeing Statistics

The Java applets at the *Seeing Statistics* webbook (http://www.seeingstatistics.com/) are awesome.

Statistical Education through Problem Solving (STEPS)

The STEPS webpage (http://www.stats.gla.ac.uk/steps/glossary/index.html) gives brief definitions of statistical tests.

Steve's Attempt to Teach Statistics (StATS)

If you prefer a more congenial approach to statistics, try Steven Simon's page (http://www.childrensmercy.org/stats/model.asp), which has examples and screen shots of SPSS and printouts. His statistics Koans are enlightening and entertaining.

Duke University

The Duke Statistics webpage (http://www.isds.duke.edu/sites/java.html) has links to applets that allow visualizing what happens.

Decision Tree for Statistics

The online decision tree for making statistical choices found at http://www.microsiris.com/Statistical%20Decision%20Tree/ takes you through a series of decision questions.

GraphPad.com: *Intuitive Biostatistics*

This website clearly links the number of groups to some of the possible statistical tests: http://www.graphpad.com/www/book/Choose.htm.

REFERENCES

Abelson, R. P. (1995). *Statistics as principled argument.* Hillsdale, NJ: Lawrence Erlbaum.

Aday, L. A. (1996). *Designing and conducting health surveys* (2nd ed.). San Francisco: Jossey-Bass.

Black, T. R. (1999). *Doing quantitative research in the social sciences: An integrated approach to research design, measurement, and statistics.* London: Sage Publications.

Blise, P. D. (2000). Within-group agreement, non-independence, and reliability. In K. Klein & S. Kozlowski (Eds.), *Multilevel theory, research and methods in organizations* (pp. 349–381). San Francisco: Jossey-Bass.

Eser, F., Yavuzer, G., Karakus, D., & Karaoglan, B. (2008). The effect of balance training on motor recovery and ambulation after stroke: A randomized controlled trial. *European Journal of Physical and Rehabilitation Medicine, 44,* 19–25.

Green, L. W., & Lewis, F. M. (1986). *Measurement and evaluation in health education and health promotion.* Palo Alto, CA: Mayfield.

Hovland, C. F., Lumsdaine, A., & Scheffield, F. D. (1949). Experiments on mass communication. New York: John Wiley. In Green, L. W. & Lewis, F. M. (1986). *Measurement and evaluation in health education and health promotion.* Palo Alto, CA: Mayfield Publishing.

Johnson, B. B., & Caron, C. (2006). Evaluating public responses to environmental trend indicators. *Science Communication, 28,* 64–92.

Kleinbaum, D., Kupper, L., Muller, K. E., & Nizan, A. (1998). *Applied regression analysis and other multivariable methods* (3rd ed.). Boston: Duxbury Press.

Meuleners, L. B., Hendrie, D., & Lee, A. H. (2008). Hospitalisations due to interpersonal violence: A population-based study in Western Australia. *Medical Journal of Australia, 188,* 572–575.

Milcarek, B. I., & Link, B. G. (1981). Handling problems of ecological fallacy in program planning and evaluation. *Evaluation & Program Planning, 4*(1), 23–28.

Mohr, L. B. (1992). *Impact analysis for program evaluation.* Newbury Park, CA: Sage Publications.

Newcomer, K. E. (1994). Using statistics appropriately. In J. Wholey, H. Hatry, & K. Newcomer (Eds.), *Handbook of practical program evaluation* (pp. 389–416). San Francisco: Jossey-Bass.

Patton, M. Q. (1997). *Utilization-focused evaluation* (3rd ed.). Thousand Oaks, CA: Sage Publications.

Pedhazur, E., & Pedhazur-Schmelkin, L. (1991). *Measurement, design, and analysis: An integrated approach.* Hillsdale, NJ: Lawrence Erlbaum Associates.

Prochaska, J., DiClemente, C., & Norcross, J. (1992). In search of how people change: Applications of addictive behaviors. *American Psychologist, 47,* 1102–1114.

Reichman, N. E., & Hade, E. M. (2001). Validation of birth certificate data: A study of women in New Jersey's Healthy Start program. *Annals of Epidemiology, 11,* 186–193.

Robinson, J. R., Young, T. K., Roos, L. L., & Gelskey, D. E. (1997). Estimating the burden of disease: Comparing administrative data and self-reports. *Medical Care, 35,* 932–937.

Rogers, E. M. (1983). *Diffusion of innovations* (3rd ed.). New York: Free Press.

Tukey, J. W. (1977). *Exploratory data analysis.* Reading, MA: Addison-Wesley.

Veany, J. E., & Kaluzny, A. D. (1998). *Evaluation and decision making for health services* (3rd ed.). Chicago: Health Administration Press.

CHAPTER 15

Qualitative Methods for Planning and Evaluation

Thus far the approach to health program planning and evaluation has been essentially quantitative in approach. Numbers are used in the needs assessment; numbers are used in budgeting and documenting the implementation of the services utilization plan; numbers are used to quantify the amount of effect on individuals receiving the program. However, stories are equally valid and important in health program planning and evaluation. Therefore, this chapter focuses on qualitative designs and methods. Much has been written on ways to conduct qualitative research and on strategies to ensure rigor in such research (Kirk & Miller, 1986; Lincoln & Guba, 1985; Strauss & Corbin, 1998), and there is no pretense of covering all that is currently known about qualitative research. As with the chapters reviewing quantitative methods, this chapter simply reviews qualitative methods, with particular emphasis on the use of these methods for health program planning and evaluation.

QUALITATIVE METHODS THROUGHOUT
THE PLANNING AND EVALUATION CYCLE

Throughout the planning and evaluation cycle, data are collected. The use of qualitative methods is an option for that data collection. During the assessment stage of the planning process, qualitative methods are suitable for gaining insights into the needs, problems, barriers, and issues faced by the target population. Also, during the assessment and planning stages, qualitative methods yield data essential to develop and delineate program elements before initiating a program. Similarly, qualitative methods can help generate the program theory, especially the effect theory, so that it incorporates the explanatory models of the target audience and the theory-in-use of program staff if a program is being revised. During the process monitoring phase, qualitative methods can take the place of quantitative methods, particularly for sensitive programs that function at the direct services level of the public health pyramid, and can broaden the observational field in terms of adding new types of information. During the effect evaluation phase, qualitative methods can enhance the explanatory power of the evaluation design and data. Also, by providing analyses of processes and individual cases, qualitative data can help explain why or how outcomes occurred. In other words, information from the qualitative data can be used to improve the effect theory upon which the program was based.

Qualitative approaches give a voice, both literally and metaphorically, to stakeholders. This effect is important because it makes stakeholders feel valued. The act of speaking to someone and telling a story generates feelings that are substantively different from the feeling generated by responding to a survey questionnaire.

QUALITATIVE METHODS

The first challenge faced by evaluators and program planners is to select the best qualitative method to answer the questions at hand. Qualitative methods have emerged from a variety of philosophical perspectives, each of which has influenced the development of the associated methodology. These underlying perspectives influence which evaluation questions might be answered from that perspective (Table 15.1). Thus the choice of a qualitative method is based on whether it is the best method given the question being asked and with the understanding that several methods might be applicable to more than one perspective (Table 15.2). The following sections review the major and most widely used qualitative methods, with particular attention being paid to how each method is useful in health program planning and evaluation.

Across the qualitative methods, a major concern is the amount of time it takes first to gather and then to analyze the data. The nature of the qualitative methods is such that the amount of time necessary to interview, observe, or interact to gather the data tends to be longer than the amount of time required to gather data via a survey or other quantitative methods typically used in program planning or evaluation. In addition, the iterative and intensive data analysis process is longer than for quantitative data analysis. These factors make qualitative methods more costly to use than a survey method. Table 15.3 summarizes the benefits and challenges for each of the qualitative methods discussed here.

In-Depth Individual Interview

The most widely known and used of the qualitative methods is the in-depth, open-ended questioning of an individual. Using questions that require more than a yes or no response, encouraging explanation, and allowing for story

Table 15.1   Comparison of Qualitative Perspectives with Regard to the Basic Question Addressed and the Relevance to Health Program Planning and Evaluation

Perspective	Basic Question Addressed	Planning and Evaluation Relevance
Content analysis	Which themes are in the text?	Thoughts and perspectives revealed in the text and dialogues
Critical analysis	How has power shaped it?	Participants' views of their ability to be in control of the health problem and the solutions; staff's view of their autonomy in improving the program
Ethnography	What are the norms and values (culture)?	Participants' cultural forces that contribute to the problem and acceptance of the program
Grounded theory	What are the relationships (theory)?	Explanations that participants and staff have for the health problem and possible solutions
Phenomenology	What does it mean to the person?	Participants' meaning of content and the problem being addressed

Table 15.2   Comparison of Major Qualitative Perspectives with Regard to the Method Used

Perspective	Typical Methods
Content analysis	Focus groups, surveys with open-ended questions, narrative designs
Critical analysis	Individual in-depth interviews
Ethnography	Case study, participant observation, observations
Grounded theory	Individual in-depth interviews
Phenomenology	Individual in-depth interviews

Table 15.3   Summary of Key Benefits and Challenges to Using Qualitative Methods in Planning and Evaluation

Method	Key Benefits	Key Challenges
Case study	Allows for understanding of context as an influence on the program or participant	Complex, overwhelming amount of data: definition of case
Observations	Can identify sequence of causes and effects, may identify new behaviors or events	Difficult to obtain reliable data unless recording devices are used, sampling frame difficult to establish
Individual in-depth interviews	Provides rich insights into personal thoughts, values, meanings, and attributions	Identifying individuals who are willing to be open
Focus groups	Inexpensive given the amount and type of data collected, get collective views rather than individual views	Need training in managing the group process, need good data-recording method
Survey with open-ended questions	Very inexpensive method of data collection	Poor handwriting and unclear statements can make data useless
Narrative designs	Very inexpensive methods of data collection; provide insights into social and cultural influences on thoughts and actions	Require special training in data analysis; may not have credibility with stakeholders; difficult to select the text most relevant to the health problem or program

telling lead to information that is detailed, personal, and often reflective. This type of data is preferred when meanings and attributions are the focus and when new or fresh insights into a poorly understood phenomenon are sought. Typically, individuals who are interviewed are purposively selected based on a narrow set of criteria. Interviewers may be program recipients, stakeholders in the program, or members of the target audience.

In-depth interviews can used be throughout the planning and evaluation cycle. For example, Kissman (1999) conducted in-depth interviews with homeless women, thereby identifying gaps in services to these women. This methodology, as compared with use of a survey method, was particularly appropriate given that one of the obstacles identified by the women was their inability to read. In-depth interviews can also be used to understand the effects of the program. For example, Issel (2000) interviewed women who had received prenatal comprehensive case management and learned from the women what they experienced as outcomes of having received that service.

Data Collection

Conducting in-depth interviews requires skill on the part of the interviewer. The interviewer needs to be sensitive to cues of the interviewee about when to stop the interview, as well as when and how to ask for clarification when the interviewee is either using slang or not providing an easily interpreted story. The ability and skill of the interviewer are critical to conducting a "good" interview that gathers sufficient details to make analysis less complicated, yet has not disrupted the flow of ideas from the interviewee.

In-depth interviews can be done almost anywhere that the interviewer and the interviewee mutually feel comfortable and secure in terms of maintaining confidentiality. Interviews conducted in the office of the program staff would not be a good idea, particularly if information is sought from individuals who feel vulnerable or who are in a lower power position. More neutral territory is better, whether that is the interviewee's home or, for example, the local library.

Sometimes the interviewee is referred to as a *key informant*, denoting that the individual is unique in possessing information of a specific nature. Key informants are more likely to be useful during the community assessment and planning stages, as they would have knowledge of system processes and barriers to services and can draw upon a range of experiences to comment on any generic issues. Data collected from in-depth interviews with key informants are analyzed in the same manner as data collected from any other interviewee.

Written Open-Ended Questions

Sometimes surveys include an open-ended question or two to which respondents can provide qualitative information. Typically, questions such as "Anything else?," "What was the best/worst?," and "What suggestions do you have?" are used. Such questions can be added to community assessment, process monitoring, or impact survey questionnaires. Because responses to such questions are generated by the individual, rather than by the researcher, the responses are of a qualitative nature.

The major limitations associated with collecting qualitative data with written open-ended questions are that people often do not write legibly, are not articulate, or provide extremely brief responses. These factors can make it impossible to interpret their responses, rendering their data useless. Giving more explicit instructions and providing sufficient space to write detailed responses can help minimize these problems. However, if the information from the questions is considered crucial, then other methods for collecting the data ought to be considered. Nonetheless, open-ended questions on a survey can be beneficial. Such questions, as compared to a survey of close-ended questions, provide respondents with an opportunity to express themselves; as a consequence, they are likely to feel "heard." Also, the response may provide sufficient information to generate an initial set of categories for a close-ended question. Ultimately, it is the discretion of the evaluator to decide whether the data are analyzable and useful. The analysis steps described later in this chapter can be applied to this rather limited, but potentially fruitful, set of qualitative data.

Focus Group

The *focus group* method of collecting qualitative data involves conducting an interview with a group of individuals, thereby taking advantage of the group dynamic, which itself can lead to discussions and revelations of new information. For some individuals, a group setting for interviews is less intimidating. By participating in focus groups, individuals within the group can confirm or disconfirm the experiences and views of others. This "instant feedback" aspect contributes to the focus group method being somewhat more efficient than in-depth individual interviews, which require a separate interview for validation of interpretations.

Data analysis follows the general steps used for analyzing in-depth interviews. Thus those familiar with that data analysis procedure will be capable of analyzing focus group data. The difference is that the findings are not person specific, but are considered already validated during the group process.

The efficiency aspect of the focus group method has led to its use in health program planning and evaluation. For example, Affonso, Shibuya, and Frueh (2007) conducted focus groups with both elementary school-aged children and adults to inform their development of a school-based violence prevention program; these focus groups were conducted in a manner consistent with the local culture of Hawaii. Clapp and Early (1999) used focus groups to study the perceptions of outcomes from alcohol and substance abuse prevention programs. They were able to identify potential outcomes from such programs, as well as a program effect theory that was implicit in the understandings of the focus group participants.

Both of the preceding examples involve the use of focus groups during the planning stage so as to refine the program effect theory and more accurately select potentially sensitive indicators of program impact. Because of their exploratory nature, focus groups are better suited to use during the community assessment and program planning phases. This method of qualitative data collection may not be as useful for outcome assessments because it may be inappropriate to ask individuals to reveal in a group setting what difference the program made to them. In some situations, focus groups can be appropriate as one method to collect process monitoring from staff.

Data Collection

The steps involved in selecting focus group members, conducting the focus groups, managing the group process, and analyzing the data have been explicated by various authors (Krueger, 2000; Morgan, 1998; Stewart, Shamdasani, & Rook, 2007). The types of questions posed to a focus group are constructed as open-ended questions. To maximize the data provided by the group members, the focus group leader actively directs the discussion by seeking clarification and by eliciting views and opinions from members more inclined to be quiet. Data are collected as either audio recordings or extensive written notes, and sometimes both; audiovisual recordings are rarely used. The process of recording can be somewhat intrusive, especially if the group members are not comfortable with a tape recorder or are distracted by the note taker. Thus the physical location of the recorder and the note taker with regard to the focus group members becomes a conscious choice of how *not* to influence the interactions of the group members.

The most immediately noticeable challenge is the logistics of scheduling a meeting with the 8 to 12 members of a focus group. Along these lines, it can be difficult to predict which combination of individuals will be optimal for producing insightful data. A balance between homogeneity and heterogeneity of group members is needed, but can be difficult to anticipate. The selection of focus group members, otherwise called the sampling strategy, ought to be guided by the notion that people who are alike are more likely to communicate with one another. At the same time, some degree of differences among the members stimulates discussion and promotes clarification.

Another challenge relates to capturing the data produced by a focus group. People frequently talk when others talk, and they often have voices that are difficult to identify on audiotapes. Similarly, taking handwritten notes inevitably misses some comments. For this reason, more than one data-recording technique is often used.

Observation

Using one's own eyes to collect data is another qualitative method. While one could look and count things, when a person is looking at the behavior of others and making interpretations about that behavior, the nature of the data becomes more subjective—that is, more qualitative. Observational methods vary widely and range from nonparticipatory techniques, such as using rooms with one-way mirrors to observe parent–child interactions, to very participatory techniques, such as assuming the identity of a program participant to experience what participants experience. Observations also occur across a wide variety of settings—from natural, such as a home or street corner in the neighborhood of the target audience, to less naturalistic, such as a clinic or lab.

Data Collection

Depending on the purpose of using an observational method, the specific procedures used to conduct the observation and record the data will vary. Nonetheless, there are some commonalities. First, training is needed with regard to what will be observed. For example, if the purpose is to assess the quality of interaction between program staff and participants, then dyadic or triadic actions and reactions will be the focus. If the purpose is to assess whether program participants have acquired a skill taught in the program, then the sequence of actions taken by the participant when in the situation requiring the skill will be the focus. In both process monitoring and the effect evaluation examples, many other events, interactions, and factors occur simultaneously that are not immediately relevant to the purpose and, therefore, are not recorded or noted during the observation.

Data collection can be accomplished in several different ways. One technique relies on audiovisual recordings. Although this data collection method is likely to capture all events or interactions of interest, it is also the most intrusive from the point of view of the person being observed. The advantage of using recording is that data can be analyzed by several different analysts. Repeated viewings of the recordings can also help ensure that an important event or interaction of interest is not missed.

Another approach to collecting data involves coding events or interactions as they occur, preferably with a standardized data collection tool. For example, Farley and colleagues (2007) observed the physical activity of children using a reliable tool that had categories for levels of activity. Such coding can be done on paper or using electronic aids. This approach has the advantage that the observer uses recording equipment that may be less intimidating to those being observed. Given that electronic equipment and recording devices are increasingly thought of as normal, and that equipment continues to decrease in size, a well-trained data collector can often use these devices discreetly. The disadvantage is that the quality of the data depends on the accuracy of the observer's coding; verifying the accuracy of the coding can also be complicated and expensive.

The most qualitative approach to collecting observational data entails making detailed notes and keeping a log of occurrences and observations after one is no longer doing the observation. This method relies heavily on the recall accuracy and memory of the person who made the observations as well as his or her ability to record what was observed with minimal interpretations in the description. While this approach to data collection is most susceptible to biases and inaccuracies, it is also the least intrusive.

Observational data can be analyzed as sequential data (Bakeman & Gottman, 1997), which means that the sequence in which interactions, behaviors, or reactions occurs is viewed as a pattern that is subject to specific statistical analytical procedures. Using the process monitoring example given earlier, suppose a program staff member initiates a question (call it Q1) and the participant looks away (call it LA1), followed by the question being repeated (Q1). The Q1→ LA1→ Q1 sequence is what is analyzed. This approach to analysis of observational data is a bit closer to a quantitative approach than if the observation data were collected as general categories of behaviors, events, and interactions. Using the outcome evaluation example, suppose a participant is observed in a real-life situation and context and is unaware of being observed. In this case, the data collected will be more like field notes, so analysis is more likely to follow the approach used with other types of qualitative data (described later in this chapter).

Depending on the method used to record the observations, the data may be susceptible to recall or observational bias. This is particularly the case if the observer is a participant-observer who is not at liberty to record the observations as they actually occur. Observation has other potential disadvantages. For example, deciding on a sampling frame can be difficult. In other words, the number of observations needed to be confident that the behavior could have occurred at a usual rate and in a usual manner may not be readily knowable. As with most qualitative methods, another disadvantage of the observation method is that the amount of time and resources required for data collection can be problematic. These disadvantages are offset by the advantage of potentially identifying behaviors and events that might become known only through observation. The flexibility and variety of techniques that can be used to collect the data can be viewed as another advantage.

Case Study

A *case study* is an empirical inquiry into existing phenomena in their real-life contexts when the boundary between what is being studied and its context is not clearly evident. Typically, case studies use multiple sources of data (Yin, 2004). The case is determined based on the question being asked; thus it could consists of an individual, a classroom, an organization, a program, or an event. The case study methodology is particularly useful for gaining insights into an entire program (Veney & Kaluzny, 1998) because the program is the unit of analysis (i.e., case). Typically, case studies address questions of how or why something occurred, and there is no attempt to experimentally control what happens. If the case study method is used during the assessment phase, then there is not yet a program, and thus what constitutes the case is unclear. If the case study method is used for the effect evaluation, then either the program implementation is an event that is the focus of the case study or the program itself is the case.

The methodology for conducting a case study is given by Yin (2004) and Stake (1995). Both authors argue that, as with any design, attention needs to be paid to the generation of the research question and rival hypotheses, and to the use of methods and techniques that enhance scientific rigor of the study. Stake (2000) summarizes the responsibilities of those doing case study research as being similar to the responsibilities of evaluators who use other qualitative methods, except that the first step in a case study is to circumscribe what is the case.

Data Collection

The choice of the case is critical and must be based on carefully considered criteria for what makes the case either uniquely typical or extraordinarily different. However, when the case study method is used for program process monitoring, then the health program is the case. For some effect evaluations, evaluators may select a few individual program participants to be the cases the in order to refine the effect theory based on their experiences and processes of change. For example, Lochman, Boxmeyer, Powell, Wojnaroski, and Yaros (2007) chose one participant in a program for children with disruptive behavior. With the child as the case, they interviewed the parents, teachers, classmates, and the child over a period of several months. In this way, they were able to assess both the program implementation and the program effect on the child. The issue of what constitutes a case becomes more complex in evaluations where multiple institutions or organizations are providing the intervention. This multiplicity of actors necessitates that the evaluator consider whether each organization is a case or whether the organization is the context for the program, thereby making each set of program staff and recipients be the case.

A key feature of the case study methodology is the use of multiple sources of data. Typically data collected as part of a case study include both primary data—generally collected via interviews, observations of behavior, and surveys—and secondary data. Secondary data collection might include review of agency or program documents, review of existing data collected for other evaluation or program monitoring purposes, and review of program-related materials, such as promotional materials, policies, and procedures. Case study then involves considering all these data to arrive at some answers to the evaluation question. The amount of data collected may prove overwhelming to evaluators, resulting in "analysis paralysis" or delays in arriving at sound conclusions.

Examples of case studies used in program planning and evaluation can easily be found. From published reports, the value of such studies becomes evident. Goodman, Steckler, and Alciati (1997) used case study methodology to conduct a process evaluation of state agency programs that implemented the Data-Based Intervention Research program. This program was designed to build the state agency's capacity to translate research regarding cancer prevention into practice. These authors' decision to consider the four state programs as one case reveals the complexity of defining and selecting a case. Their report about capacity building around implementation of cancer prevention and control programs also reinforces the idea that program planning and evaluation occurs at the infrastructure level of the public health pyramid.

In a slightly different vein, Goodson, Gottlieb, and Smith (1999) reported using case study methodology to study the implementation of the Put Prevention into Practice (PPIP) program. They interviewed all staff at the nine clinical sites where PPIP was implemented. Using structured interviews and open-ended questions with staff, they were able to identify site-specific problems with implementation of the program. Again, their report serves as an example of how the case study is ideal for process-monitoring evaluations and subsequent program planning, particularly at the infrastructure level.

Innovative Methods

New qualitative methods and approaches continue to be developed. The qualitative methods reviewed in this chapter have included the major types, which form a broad base for development of other methods. The three additional qualitative methods introduced in this section are examples of the evolution of qualitative methods and their applicability to program planning and evaluation.

Photovoice
Photovoice is a relatively new approach to data collection that involves the use of photography by the participants and analysis of those photographs to understand the phenomena and lives of the participants who took the photographs. The photovoice methodology involves not only taking the photographs as the data collection phase, but then interpretation of those

photographs through dialogue or discussions. The ease in using cameras, especially disposable cameras, makes photovoice an attractive alternative to qualitative methods that rely heavily on language. For this reason, it has been used with individuals with intellectual disabilities (Jurkowski, Rivera, & Hammel, 2008). The interactive, interpretive aspect of photovoice also makes it appealing for use with community groups. In an interesting community health assessment application, Downey, Ireson, and Scutchfield (2008) found that photovoice facilitated community members in identifying solutions and specific action steps for addressing the local health issues.

Narrative Designs

A qualitative approach that is used rarely in health program planning and evaluation entails the use of narrative methods. Narrative methods use text as the data. The text can come from personal sources, such as diaries, and from public or agency sources, such as existing agency records, memos, reports, videos, newspapers, and other print media. Narrative designs focus on the linguistics of the texts and often follow a more straightforward content analysis approach (Krippendorf, 1980).

Narrative designs can be helpful during the community assessment phase for understanding how a community presents itself through the local media and other writings. For process monitoring, such designs can be very helpful in tracking program drift as reflected in writings about the program or program procedures. Narrative analyses might also be useful for identifying outcomes of policy changes, but more recently have been used to understand interpersonal power relationships (e.g., Schow, 2006; Shaw & Greenhalgh, 2008).

The obvious limitation of a narrative design is the inherently limited nature of text sources and the lack of an opportunity to clarify meanings or intent. On the positive side, narrative designs can be less expensive, particularly if the texts are publicly and readily available. In addition, stories, as narrative texts, are easy to obtain during interviews.

Multiple Methods and Triangulation

Each data collection technique has limitations. To compensate for some limitations, it may be helpful to use more than one data collection method. The notion of multiple methods encompasses using a mix of qualitative and quantitative methods, using a mix of quantitative methods, or using a mix of qualitative methods. For example, O'Driscoll, Shave, and Cushion (2007) used individual case studies, participant observation, and in-depth individual interviews to assess the effectiveness of a cardiac rehabilitation program. Their inclusion of both patient program participants and program staff in the evaluation allowed the evaluators to draw a set of integrated conclusions about the implementation of the program.

Use of multiple methods can sometimes yield quite different results, as happened in the study carried out by Quinn, Detman, and Bell-Ellison (2008). They used quantitative survey and qualitative interviews to understand barriers to use of prenatal care. The findings from the two methods were quite different. According to the survey, transportation and child care were the major barriers, whereas embarrassment and other emotional reasons were the major barriers identified in the interviews. Differences in findings from qualitative and quantitative data collection have been found even in the reporting of deaths (Huy, Johansson, & Long, 2007).

In some instances, multiple methods are used for triangulation. The term *triangulation* generically refers to the use of more than one method for the purpose of confirming, disconfirming, or modifying information gained through one of the methods. In some way, perspectives can be reconciled via this approach (Thurmond, 2001), but debates continue on how best to achieve rigorous triangulation (Lambert & Loiselle, 2008). Triangulation has been used to better understand program implementation. An example of triangulation used for program planning is the needs assessment that was conducted for a program in Chicago (Levy et al., 2004). These researchers used focus groups, key informant interviews, observational data, and quantitative data from the BRFSS to arrive at a set of concerns regarding diabetes and cardiovascular disease in a Latino and African American community. The authors demonstrated areas of overlap and disagreement in the data, which contributed to better understanding of both the communities and the optimal programmatic interventions.

The major challenge to using multiple methods is the analysis and synthesis of the data. Although it may seem more straightforward to analyze the data from each source independently, ultimately those findings need to be synthesized and reconciled with the findings based on the data collected with the other methods. In addition, it is important that each data collection method be done as rigorously as possible. Cost and time factors are additional considerations in choosing to use multiple methods. Given these substantial challenges, the multiple methods approach is more likely to be used in evaluation research, or on a very small scale.

SCIENTIFIC RIGOR

Just as with quantitative methods, scientific rigor is important with qualitative methods. The terminology used to describe aspects of rigor is different; nonetheless, the underlying concepts are comparable. The following four elements of scientific rigor in qualitative methods (Lincoln & Guba, 1985) need to be present for the data to be considered of high quality.

Credibility is roughly equivalent to internal validity; it refers to whether one can have confidence in the truth of the findings. Credibility is established through several activities. First, evaluators must invest sufficient time in the process so that the findings can be triangulated. Second, evaluators may use outsiders—that is, individuals other than those who provided or analyzed the data—to gain insights into the meaning and interpretation of the data. This practice is sometimes referred to as peer debriefing. Third, evaluators should refine working hypotheses that are generated during data analysis with negative cases. This activity requires seeking out data that would be evidence that the working hypothesis is not always accurate. With qualitative data, working hypotheses are more like hunches that may be influenced by the researcher's bias. Therefore, in qualitative analysis, efforts are made to both confirm and disconfirm the working hypothesis. The act of seeking disconfirming data ensures that the researcher's biases are minimized in the results. A fourth activity that enhances credibility is to check findings against raw data, by re-reviewing the raw data in light of the findings. Finally, credibility is increased when those who provided the data are asked to review the findings and provide feedback about the accuracy of the interpretations.

Transferability (also known as applicability) is similar to external validity in that the findings ought to have applicability to other contexts and respondents. The main technique to increase transferability is to provide thick (detailed, comprehensive) descriptions in reports so that others can independently assess the possibility of transferability of the findings to other groups. This stands in contrast to the quantitative technique, which focuses on sample selection as a means of increasing generalizability of findings.

Dependability is roughly equivalent to reliability. The notion is that other researchers and evaluators ought to be able to arrive at the same results if they repeat the study or analyze the same set of data. Ensuring dependability is done primarily by leaving a paper trail of steps in the analysis so that others can see that the findings are supported by the data. Another major aspect of dependability is the use of reliability statistics to demonstrate that, given the same set of data, two researchers would arrive at the same coding of the data. The two most widely used reliability statistics in qualitative research are the percent agreement and the kappa statistic; both are determined after the codes for the data have been finalized, including having definitions. Percent agreement is the simple percentage of a given data set that two researchers independently code into the same pre-established categories. The numerator is the number of data units that are similarly coded, and the denominator is the total number of data units to be coded. While this percentage is simple to calculate, it does not take into account the possibility that both researchers might have assigned a "wrong" code to the same data. To compensate for this shortcoming, the kappa statistic can be used (Cohen, 1960). The kappa statistic is based on the ratio of observed (actual) codes used to the expected codes to be used for a given set of data, for any two independently coding researchers.

Confirmability, sometimes referred to as objectivity, connotes that the findings are truly from the respondents, rather than reflecting the researcher's perceptions or biases. As with dependability, the main technique to assure confirmability is to leave an audit trail that others can follow to arrive at the same findings. A variety of techniques to document the researcher's impressions, biases, and interpretations are also available, such as making theoretical memos or taking field notes. Use of such techniques adds to the confirmability of the findings by providing greater assurance that the researcher has taken steps to be self-aware of factors that might have influenced the interpretation of the data, and subsequently the results.

SAMPLING FOR QUALITATIVE METHODS

Qualitative approaches to sampling are guided by a different set of driving forces. The first consideration is the design. Table 15.4 summarizes the general considerations for selecting a sample for each of the qualitative methods. The second consideration is the specific sampling strategy to be used. The purpose of any qualitative design is to understand a phenomenon, so the sample is purposefully selected in reference to that phenomenon. In program planning and evaluation, the phenomenon in the community assessment or planning phases would be a characteristic of the target population that is the focus of the qualitative assessment, whereas in the evaluation phase the phenomenon would be the health outcome of participants or the implementation of the intervention by the program staff.

The need to have a purposive sample means that there is no attempt to make the sample representative of the target population. Thus random selection of a sample is not relevant. Power analyses are also not appropriate because there is no attempt to quantify an effect size or find statistical significance. However, Morse (1994) provides some guidelines in terms of numbers. She suggests at least six participants are needed when trying to understand the experience of individuals, and 30 to 50 interviews are necessary for qualitative studies that focus on culture (ethnographies) and generation of a theory about a health problem (grounded theory studies).

Several different types of purposeful samples are used in qualitative research (Table 15.5). In addition to those that are specific to qualitative research, the sampling strategies for accessing hard-to-reach populations

Table 15.4   Sampling Considerations for Each of the Qualitative Methods Discussed

Method	Sampling Considerations
Case study	Choice of case based on being either "usual" or "unusual," maximum number of cases feasible to conduct
Observations	Ability to sample behaviors or events without altering their quality, need to obtain saturation of categories
Individual in-depth interviews	Need to obtain category saturation, choice of individuals based on theoretical sampling
Focus groups	Representativeness of participants within and across the groups, maximum size of each focus group, minimum number of focus groups needed to capture diversity of views
Survey with open-ended questions	Linked to sampling strategy for the survey, likelihood of write-in responses
Narrative designs	Quantity and quality of existing documents available for review, access to existing documents

(described in Chapter 13) would be appropriate. The qualitative sampling strategies are built around having either homogeneity or heterogeneity of participants. Homogeneity of participants is preferred if the phenomenon is not well understood and is being described for the first time or in-depth for a specific aggregate. To have homogeneity of the sample, either individuals are selected based on a set of inclusion/exclusion criteria or they are considered to be typical. Heterogeneity of a qualitative sample provides a range and points of possible contrast. The latter approach is helpful if the intent of the study is to expand the applicability of the findings.

Heterogeneity of a qualitative sample is achieved through selecting individuals purposively based on their deviation from the norm or purposively so as to maximize variation. If it is unclear what might be "normal" or "deviant," then randomly selecting individuals is an acceptable sampling strategy. The purpose of selecting a sample to have heterogeneity is to uncover as many as possible different responses and perspectives, which then become categories

Table 15.5   Summary of Types of Sampling Strategies Used with Qualitative Designs

Sampling Strategy	Type of Cases Used	Use
Convenience	Participants or cases that are accessible and willing	Saves time and recruitment money
Critical cases	Exemplar participants or cases, cases important in some unique way	Permits generalization to similar individuals or cases
Deviant cases	Highly unusual participants or cases	Reveals the factors associated with unique and extreme conditions and may lead to a new theory or parameters
Maximum variation	Participants or cases with differing experiences	Fosters category saturation with most possible categories
Random purposeful	Participants or cases randomly selected from a large sampling pool	Adds credibility to the sample and thus some indication of generalizability
Typical cases	Usual or normal participants or cases	Leads to a broadly applicable theory or categories but does not address the full breadth of the program effects
Theory based	Participants or cases with the theoretical construct	Elaborates or refines the theory

of information found in the data. Additional individuals are added until no new information is being gained from their participation, a strategy called sampling for *category saturation*. At some point, adding more data from additional individuals will not provide more or new information. This point, referred to as saturation, can be desirable as evidence of having sufficient data to minimize the possibility of missing any key concepts. Sampling for category saturation requires some degree of flexibility in the number of participants, whether cases or individuals, in the evaluation study. Category saturation can be achieved sooner or later than expected, allowing a sooner-than-expected

conclusion to enrollment or necessitating the recruitment of additional participants, respectively.

Recall that the effect theory is a theory about how that the intervention
changes the causal theory. If the qualitative design is being used either to
refine the causal theory of the factors that lead to the health problem or to
assess the intervention theory, then a theoretical sample might be chosen. A
theoretical sample is one that is purposefully chosen to complete or refine a
theory. Theoretical sampling, which comes from the grounded theory tradition
(Charmaz, 2000), entails sampling for ideas and constructs so that theories can
be further developed and refined. To accomplish this, individuals are selected
based on whether they are anticipated to be reflective of or divergent from the
theory. A theoretical sample would, for example, be useful with participants in
a pilot program because those participants ought to have experienced the
same theoretical effect from the intervention. Like sampling for category saturation, theoretical sampling requires flexibility in determining when enough
data have been collected. Key difficulties in implementing a theoretical sample
include knowing who might fit the theory and determining when the theory is
no longer likely to change with the inclusion of additional participants in the
qualitative study.

ANALYSIS OF QUALITATIVE DATA

Numerous texts provide detailed instructions on analyzing various types of
qualitative data, such as the classics by Miles and Huberman (1994), Krippendorf
(1980), Weber (1990), and Lincoln and Guba (1985). These and other texts ought
to be consulted for detailed instructions on the process of analyzing qualitative
data so that scientific rigor is maintained. Remember that program planners and
evaluators, whether engaged in qualitative or quantitative data collection, need
to make every reasonable effort to achieve scientific rigor as a basis from which
claims can be more solidly and confidently made. This section offers a brief
summary of the steps involved in the immersion into the data and surfacing from
the depths of analysis that occurs when working with qualitative data.

A note of caution is warranted. While the steps in this procedure are presented in a sequential order here, most of the steps occur iteratively in real-
world qualitative data analysis. It's a bit like taking two giant steps forward and
then needing to take three baby steps backward before stepping forward again.
This is a normal and expected part of the process of qualitative data analysis.

Overview of Analytic Process

Before analysis can begin, the data need to be transformed into a format
amenable to manipulation and analysis. This effort may involve transcribing

audiotaped interviews or entering text, audio, or visual data into qualitative analysis software. Once the data are reliably and accurately transformed, then analysis can begin.

The first step is to decide what are codable units of data, and then identify those units within the data. Codable units from in-depth interviews can consist of words, phrases, or paragraphs, whereas codable units from observation may be facial movements or interactions. In contrast to quantitative data in which the numerical response to a single question or a lab value are obvious units of data, what constitutes a unit of data is not always so obvious in qualitative data. There is a constant struggle to identify the units of data so that they can be categorized based on their properties. The unit of analysis will vary by method, question being asked, and the underlying perspective from which the question is being asked. Also, the codable unit of analysis can evolve as the analysis proceeds, becoming either larger or smaller in terms of amount or complexity.

The next step is to understand the meaning of what was said, observed, or read. Certain terminology is unique to qualitative methods and its data analysis. Manifest versus implied meanings are critical in qualitative data. *Manifest meanings* are the obvious, unambiguous meanings, whereas *implied meanings* are the unspoken innuendos, metaphors, and references that color the meaning and interpretation. Data analysis relies on making this distinction and being faithful to the decision to code the data based on manifest or implied meanings.

Based on the meanings, a discovery process begins in which groups of data with similar meanings begin to form categories. This process is rather idiosyncratic, with each researcher having a preferred style. Some begin with broad, overarching categories and gradually generate more specific subcategories. Others prefer to begin with many discrete categories; then, based on grouping similar categories, they evolve toward broader, overarching categories. Either approach is fine, as both result in a nested set of categories, not unlike an outline of nested ideas that contains broad topics followed by corresponding, more specific subheadings. The process of generating categories is one of constantly comparing the data to be coded with the data that have already been categorized. Constant comparison is a trademark of qualitative data analysis. The process results in the feeling of being immersed in data, lost among the trees in the forest. As the categories evolve, a paper trail is generated that is necessary to have dependability.

At the point at which sufficient data have been analyzed for categories to develop, the categories are named. This step is likely to occur along with the sorting of data into groups or categories. A category is a classification of concepts in the data. As more data are reviewed for their meanings and grouped accordingly, the properties and dimensions of the categories begin to surface. A dimension implies that the quality of the data exists along a continuum, whereas a property is a discrete attribute or characteristic. As more data are added to the categories, new data are constantly compared with data already in the category and adjustments are made. Table 15.6 shows an example of interview text, the coded units, and the categories to which those data units have been assigned.

When the categories are reasonably well established, definitions of the categories are developed. Based on the properties and dimensions, definitions help establish criteria for whether data belong to that category and are used as the guide for whether new data will be added to that category or a different category. Definitions are considered good if they enable the categories to meet two standard criteria for category development: mutually exclusive and exhaustive. *Mutually exclusive* category definitions allow for data to be in one and only one category; there is no other choice for which category best reflects the data. *Exhaustive category* definitions prohibit the use of "other" as a category; all data have a place, a category in which they belong. Using the concepts of mutually exclusive and exhaustive categories is very helpful as a gauge of definition clarity and for deciding whether more data need to be collected. If considerable amounts of data cannot be categorized, then either the categories need to be changed (broadened or narrowed) or more data need to be collected so that the category properties, characteristics, and dimensions can be more fully understood.

Depending on the qualitative method and perspective taken, a step sometimes taken at this point is to present the findings to the participants in the study. The study participants are offered the opportunity to confirm the results and discuss alternative interpretations of the data. This step adds to the confirmability of the final results.

Typically in the final step in qualitative analysis, researchers generate explanations or working theories based on the data. In terms of program planning and evaluation, this may involve revisiting the process theory or the effect theory or any element of those theories. For example, findings from a qualitative evaluation may cause researchers to revise their view of the key contributing or determinant factors of the health problem or to rethink their perception of which intervention is more effective. In addition, a separate model of the health problem might be developed based on the findings. Ultimately, the results need to be considered in reference to the purpose of the study and the questions that were asked at the outset.

Software

Several software programs are commercially available for use in managing qualitative data and facilitating analysis of such data. The programs commonly used in qualitative research are NUD*IST, Ethnograph, and ATLAS-ti, although

Table 15.6 Example of Interview Text with Final Coding

Interview Text	Final Coding
Interviewer: Okay. Thinking specifically about how case management may have affected you or made a difference to you, how do you think case management has affected your health or your pregnancy or the baby's health? How has it made a difference? **Respondent: It really didn't make me no difference.**	**Outcome code: case management made no difference to me**
Interviewer: You couldn't identify any ways that it made a difference? **Respondent:** No.	
Interviewer: How has case management affected your thoughts or feelings about yourself? **Respondent:** I have had *when I was pregnant. I was depressed and everything,* and <u>talking to my case manager</u> **made me feel better about myself.**	**Risk code:** *expressed psychosocial state, depression* **Intervention code:** <u>talking and listening</u> **Outcome code: increased self-care attributed to case manager involvement**
Interviewer: How did that happen? How did she make you feel better about yourself? **Respondent:** She just told me that don't think about nothing else and let it upset you and just think about what you got inside of you because *I was under a lot of stress* and <u>she said that if I be stressed out too much I could harm the baby.</u> **So, I thought about that, and that was serious. If my pregnancy hadn't been stressed out and depressed like that.**	**Risk code:** *expressed psychosocial state, stress* **Intervention code:** <u>gave information</u> **Outcome code: patient demonstrates a change in knowledge**

several other programs are available. Articles have been written comparing their capabilities (Barry, 1998; Lewis, 1998) and the "Internet Resources" section at the end of this chapter gives links to the websites for these programs. These programs have features that facilitate diagramming relationships among categories, counting units of analysis per category, and coding within coded text. The functions of software for qualitative data analysis include searching for text, text base management in terms of linking text to information about that text, coding and retrieving, support theory building by allowing for higher-order coding, and building networks of concepts in graphic representations.

Software programs can greatly facilitate managing the potentially overwhelming amounts of data. Nevertheless, the conceptual work remains for the evaluator to do. Interpretation of meanings so that codes are applied to appropriate codable units, and ongoing development and refinement of categories, domains, and properties are some of the tasks that cannot be done by the computer software. Also, these programs, like any software program, require training prior to their use.

Issues to Consider

Given the traditional and normal reliance on numbers, one issue when reporting qualitative findings is whether to report numbers—in other words, "to count or not to count." When themes and codes are developed, there is an inclination to count the number of occurrences, or generate percentages related to the codes. However, if data are presented as counts and percentages, these statistics must be interpreted very cautiously; only one or two vocal individuals with many comments could easily change the count or skew the percentages.

The challenge in reporting numbers from qualitative data is determining what is an appropriate denominator. The denominator may consist of either the number of all coded comments or the number of individuals from whom data were collected. Equally important is what is an appropriate numerator: It could be the number of participants who mentioned a category or the number of times a category is mentioned throughout the study. These choices greatly influence how the findings are portrayed and interpreted.

Qualitative methods are notorious for being messy, confusing, and repetitive. While many of these qualities can be minimized using available software for qualitative data management, the nature of the data requires iterative category development. This can prove challenging because the quantities of data are often overwhelming and the various stakeholders and evaluation participants might potentially provide conflicting interpretations of the data. The evaluator, program planner, and relevant stakeholders need to be committed to obtaining and using the qualitative data. Otherwise, the delays and frustrations will overcome the ultimate value of the data, and the data will be set aside to collect dust.

Then there is the cost. When budgeting for collection and analysis of qualitative data, numerous elements must be included as possible expenses. There is travel time and mileage to and from the sites where the data are collected. Interviews that are recorded need to be transcribed and typed verbatim. This activity is roughly equivalent to data entry from a close-ended survey. However, every hour of interview generates approximately three hours of transcription. If independent coders are used to establish reliability of coding data, they may need to be paid for their time and efforts.

A major issue for conducting any qualitative research is the need to have highly trained data collectors and analyzers. Training encompasses not only how to achieve consistent, reliable, and unbiased collection of data, but also how to acknowledge personal preferences and interpretations that may influence the analysis of the data. Training for data collection is important for in-depth interviewing to minimize the interviewer's use of nonverbal or verbal cues that might lead the interviewee to respond in the way he or she thinks the interviewer wants. Humans are very good at reading other humans, and subtle facial movements and body language can alter the response of an interviewee. Training for data analysis is more complicated and is best accomplished by using a team approach. Team members can challenge one another, seek clarification on interpretations of data, and provide checks and balances during the data analysis process.

PRESENTATION OF FINDINGS

As with findings based on quantitative data, the findings based on qualitative data need to be communicated to the relevant stakeholders and presented in a manner that both conveys the scientific soundness of the findings and is understandable. One aspect of conveying the scientific soundness of the findings is to include descriptions of the context in which the data were collected so as to show transferability of the results. Tables can be constructed that show the evolution of category development and can help demonstrate dependability and confirmation. Most important is including the words of the study participants alongside the category; this helps show confirmation. Stories, descriptions, explanations, and statements provided in the words of the participants are more powerful than numbers, and they make the numbers "more human." These statements can be quite powerful as tools for marketing the program and for fundraising. The final step of generating explanation may result in diagrams of relationships among categories that provide a visual means of understanding the overall findings. To the extent that the data can be associated with the logic model of the program or the program theory, the findings will be viewed as more immediately relevant.

ACROSS THE PYRAMID

At the direct services level of the public health pyramid, qualitative methods—and particularly interviews—are used to answer questions about individual perspectives, interpretations, perceptions, and meanings. Observational methods can also be readily used for process monitoring evaluations (Table 15.7). Photovoice is well suited for use by individuals for community assessment data collection.

At the enabling services level of the public health pyramid, qualitative methods are likely to focus on questions about individual perceptions and interpretations as well as on more aggregate-wide perceptions. To obtain individual perceptions for either planning or impact evaluations, in-depth interviews would be appropriate. To ascertain the more common perceptions of members of an aggregate, focus groups would be quite useful.

At the population services level, qualitative methods are more likely to be used during the assessment phase of the planning and evaluation cycle. Qualitative methods can provide detailed and specific information on cultural understandings related to health, illness, and prevention. These population-level, or aggregate-wide, cultural findings can then be used to better design population-level services.

At the infrastructure level of the public health pyramid, qualitative methods have been used for a variety of purposes, using a variety of qualitative

---

Table 15.7 Table of Suggested Qualitative Methods by Pyramid Level and Planning Cycle

Services Level	Assessment	Planning	Monitoring	Outcome Evaluation
Direct	Interview, photovoice	Interview	Observation	Interview, observation
Enabling	Focus group, observation	Focus group	Observation	Interview
Population	Focus group	Focus group	Focus group	Focus group
Infrastructure	Case study, narrative	Case study	Case study	Case study, interview, focus groups

methods. Goodman, Steckler, Hoover, and Schwartz (1993) did a multiple case study to identify ways in which the PATCH program (see Chapter 3) needed to be improved, whereas Duncan and colleagues (2008) conducted a case study to evaluate the implementation of a provider service network in Florida. Bloom et al. (2000) used focus groups consisting of state health department personnel to assess the use of the BRFSS. In other words, the focus group data were helpful in understanding issues related to the information resources of the infrastructure. As these examples demonstrate, qualitative methods can be used at all stages of the planning and evaluation cycle when the focus is at the infrastructure level.

DISCUSSION QUESTIONS AND ACTIVITIES

1. Which qualitative method(s) do you believe would be ideally suited to use at each stage of the planning and evaluation cycle? Justify your answer.

2. If you had a very limited budget but were committed to collecting and using some type of qualitative data to get at the perceptions of program participants, what might your best option be? Explain.

3. List the four criteria for assessing the rigor of qualitative studies. Imagine that you are planning to conduct in-depth interviews of program participants to assess program effects. For each criterion, give one example of how you would address that criterion in your plan for the impact evaluation.

4. Discuss under what circumstances you would and would not use numbers in the presentation of results from each of the types of qualitative methods reviewed.

INTERNET RESOURCES

The Qualitative Report

The meta-site found at http://www.nova.edu/ssss/QR/web.html is maintained by Ronald Chenail at Nova Southeastern University. It offers a long list of links and is fun to browse.

Qualitative Evaluation Checklist

Michael Quinn Patton's Qualitative Evaluation Checklist posted at the Western Michigan University Evaluation Center's website (http://www.wmich.edu/evalctr/checklists/qec/index.htm) summarizes the considerations and steps in conducting a qualitative evaluation.

Qualitative Data Analysis Software

Three commercial software packages are available to assist in the data analysis: ATLAS-ti (http://www.atlasti.com/index.shtml), NUD*IST (http://www.qsrinternational.com/), and Ethnograph (http://www.qualisresearch.com/). At each website, the overview of product features gives insights into the possibilities of qualitative analyses. However, if expense is an issue, you could try CDC's AnSWR software system (http://www.cdc.gov/hiv/topics/surveillance/resources/software/answr/index.htm) for coordinating and conducting large-scale, team-based analysis projects that integrate qualitative and quantitative techniques. The American Evaluation Association has compiled a comprehensive list of qualitative software (http://www.eval.org/Resources/QDA.htm), but a serious comparison is available at http://www.lboro.ac.uk/research/mmethods/research/software/caqdas_comparison.html.

REFERENCES

Affonso, D. D., Shibuya, J. Y., & Frueh, B. C. (2007). Talk-story: Perspectives of children, parents, and community leaders on community violence in rural Hawaii. *Public Health Nursing, 24*(5), 400–408.

Bakeman, R., & Gottman, J. M. (1997). *Observing interaction: An introduction to sequential analysis* (2nd ed.). New York: Cambridge University Press.

Barry, C. A. (1998). Choosing qualitative data analysis software: Atlas/ti and NUD*IST compared. *Sociological Research Online, 3*(3). Retrieved May 29, 2008, from http://www.socresonline.org.uk/3/3/4.html

Bloom, Y., Figgs, L. W., Baker, E. A., Dugbatey, K., Stanwyck, C. A., & Brownson, R. C. (2000). Data uses, benefits, and barriers for the behavioral risk factor surveillance system: A qualitative study of users. *Journal of Public Health Management and Practice, 6,* 78–86.

Charmaz, K. (2000). Grounded theory: Objectivist and constructionist methods. In N. K. Denzin & Y. S. Lincoln (Eds.), *Handbook of qualitative research* (2nd ed., pp. 509–536). Thousand Oaks, CA: Sage Publications.

Clapp, J. D., & Early, T. J. (1999). A qualitative exploratory study of substance abuse prevention outcomes in a heterogeneous prevention system. *Journal of Drug Education, 29*(3), 217–233.

Cohen, J. A. (1960). A coefficient of agreement for nominal scales. *Educational Psychology and Measurement, 20*(1), 37–46.

Downey, L. H., Ireson, C. L., & Scutchfield, F. D. (2008). The use of photovoice as a method of facilitating deliberation. *Health Promotion and Practice.* Retrieved June 2, 2008, from http://hpp.sagepub.com/cgi/rapidpdf/1524839907301408v1

Duncan, P. R., Lemak, C. H., Vogel, W. B., Johnson, C. E., Hall, A. G., & Porter, C. K. (2008). Evaluating Florida's Medicaid provider services network demonstration. *Health Services Research, 43*(1 Pt 2), 384–400.

Farley, T. A., Weriwether, R. A., Baker, E. T., Watkins, L. T., Johnson, C. C., & Webber, L. S. (2007). Safe play spaces to promote physical activity in inner-city children: Results from a pilot study of an environmental intervention. *American Journal of Public Health, 97,* 1625–1631.

Goodman, R. M., Steckler, A., & Alciati, M. H. (1997). A process evaluation of the National Cancer Institute's Data-Based Intervention Research program: A study of organizational capacity building. *Health Education Research, 12,* 181–197.

Goodman, R. M., Steckler, A., Hoover, S., & Schwartz, R. (1993). A critique of contemporary community health promotion approaches: Based on a qualitative review of six programs in Maine. *American Journal of Health Promotion, 7*, 208–220.

Goodson, P., Gottlieb, N. H., & Smith, M. N. (1999). Put prevention into practice: Evaluation of program initiation in nine Texas clinical sites. *American Journal of Preventive Medicine, 17*, 73–78.

Huy, T. Q., Johansson, A., & Long, N. H. (2007). Reasons for not reporting deaths: A qualitative study in rural Vietnam. *World Health & Population, 9*(1), 14–23.

Issel, L. M. (2000). Women's perceptions of outcomes from prenatal case management. *Birth, 27*(2), 120–126.

Jurkowski, J. M., Rivera, Y., & Hammel, J. (2008). Health perceptions of Latinos with intellectual disabilities: The results of a qualitative pilot study. *Health Promotion Practice*. Retrieved June 2, 2008, from http://hpp.sagepub.com/cgi/rapidpdf/1524839907309045v1

Kirk, J., & Miller, M. (1986). *Reliability and validity in qualitative research*. Newbury Park, CA: Sage Publications.

Kissman, K. (1999). Respite from stress and other service needs of homeless families. *Community Mental Health Journal, 35*(3), 241–249.

Krippendorf, K. (1980). *Content analysis: An introduction to its methodology*. Beverly Hills, CA: Sage Publications.

Krueger, R. A. (2000). *Focus groups: A practical guide to applied research* (3rd ed.). Thousand Oaks, CA: Sage Publications.

Lambert, S. D., & Loiselle, C. G. (2008). Combining individual interviews and focus groups to enhance data richness. *Journal of Advanced Nursing, 62*(2), 228–237.

Levy, S. R., Anderson, E. E., Issel, L. M., Willis, M. A., Dancy, B. L., Jacobson, K. M. et al. (2004). Using multi-level, multi-source needs assessment data for planning community interventions. *Health Promotion Practice, 5*, 59–68.

Lewis, R. B. (1998). ATLAS/ti and NUD*IST: A comparative review of two leading qualitative data analysis packages. *Cultural Anthropology Methods, 10*(3), 41–47.

Lincoln, Y. S., & Guba, E. G. (1985). *Naturalistic inquiry*. Beverly Hills, CA: Sage Publications.

Lochman, J. E., Boxmeyer, C., Powell, N., Wojnaroski, M., & Yaros, A. (2007). The use of the coping power program to treat a 10-year-old girl with disruptive behaviors. *Journal of Clinical Child and Adolescent Psychology, 36*(4), 677–687.

Miles, M. B., & Huberman, A. M. (1994). *Qualitative data analysis: An expanded sourcebook* (2nd ed.). Thousand Oaks, CA: Sage Publications.

Morgan, D. L. (1998). *The focus group guidebook*. Newbury Park, CA: Sage Publications.

Morse, J. M. (1994). Designing funded qualitative research. In N. K. Denzin & Y. S. Lincoln (Eds.), *Handbook of qualitative research* (pp. 220–235). Thousand Oaks, CA: Sage Publications.

O'Driscoll, J. M., Shave, R., & Cushion, C. J. (2007). A National Health Service hospital's cardiac rehabilitation programme: A qualitative analysis of provision. *Journal of Clinical Nursing, 16*(10), 1908–1918.

Quinn, G. P., Detman, L. A., & Bell-Ellison, B. A. (2008). Missed appointments in perinatal care: Response variations in quantitative versus qualitative instruments. *Journal of Medical Practice Management, 23*(5), 307–313.

Schow, D. (2006). The culture of domestic violence advocacy: Values of equality/behaviors of control. *Women & Health, 43*, 49–68.

Shaw, S. E., & Greenhalgh, T. (2008). Best research—For what? Best health—For whom? A critical exploration of primary care research using discourse analysis. *Social Science & Medicine, 66,* 2506–2519.

Stake, R. E. (1995). *The art of case study research.* Thousand Oaks, CA: Sage Publications.

Stake, R. E. (2000). Case studies. In N. K. Denzin & Y. S. Lincoln (Eds.), *Handbook of qualitative research* (2nd ed., pp. 435–454). Thousand Oaks, CA: Sage Publications.

Stewart, D. W., Shamdasani, P. N., & Rook, D. W. (2007). *Focus groups: Theory and practice.* (2nd ed.). Newbury Park, CA: Sage Publications.

Strauss, A., & Corbin, J. (1998). *Basics of qualitative methods: Techniques and procedures for developing grounded theory* (2nd ed.). Thousand Oaks, CA: Sage.

Thurmond, V. A. (2001). The point of triangulation. *Journal of Nursing Scholarship, 33,* 253–258.

Veney, J., & Kaluzny, A. (1998). *Evaluation and decision making for health services.* Chicago: Health Administration Press.

Weber, R. (1990). *Basic content analysis* (2nd ed.). Newbury Park, CA: Sage Publications.

Yin, R. K. (2004). *Case study research: Design and methods* (3rd ed.). Thousand Oaks, CA: Sage Publications.

CHAPTER 16

Economic Analyses: The Basics

Cost of a program will always be an issue during planning and implementation, and it might be an issue for evaluation. Therefore, program planners, managers, and evaluators ought to have a basic understanding of the types of program analyses that focus on costs and the relationship of cost to an outcome or impact. The names applied to different types of analyses are not always consistent, although *economic evaluation* seems to be used as an encompassing term for the various types of analyses presented in this chapter. The choice of which type of economic analysis to conduct is based on three criteria: whether two programs that address the same health problem are being compared, whether only costs are being considered, and whether costs and outcomes of dissimilar health programs are being compared. Economic analyses can become very complex, requiring a high degree of knowledge about fiscal and economic methods. These additional knowledge requirements make it a distinct form of program evaluation.

This chapter describes the main types of program economic evaluations so that health program planners can formulate a cost evaluation question in a manner that will lead to the optimal analysis for the situation. Program managers and others who conduct basic program evaluations need to be familiar with the different types of economic evaluations so they can make informed choices. Equally important is being able to understand economic evaluations, especially if a published analysis is being used for making decisions about future programs. This ability makes one a savvy consumer of published health program economic evaluations.

BASIC STEPS INVOLVED IN CONDUCTING ECONOMIC EVALUATIONS

As with any study and analysis, a prescribed set of steps can be used to guide the economic evaluation (Gold, Seigel, Russell, & Weinsten, 1996). The following steps are generic but provide the basis for developing and conducting an economic analysis. The initial steps are similar to the steps involved in any research study and program evaluation, but they diverge when attention to costs and effects is required. Concepts commonly used in economic evaluations are explained as they become relevant in the process.

Define the Problem

The first step is to define the problem. Defining the problem involves being explicit about the purpose of the economic evaluation, as the purpose determines which type of economic evaluation should be done. This is similar to defining the evaluation question or research study question. As will be explained later in this chapter, each type of economic evaluation answers a different set of questions. The target population and the health problem addressed by the program need to be clearly specified. Another familiar aspect of defining the problem is delineating limitations that affect the resources available for the economic evaluation. For example, the experience and expertise available to conduct the cost evaluation may require that a less complex economic evaluation be conducted.

Stipulate Comparison Parameters

Stipulating the comparison parameters means choosing the variables on which the programs or interventions will be compared. This step does not apply to cost descriptions and simple cost analyses but is critical if two or more programs or interventions are being compared. If two programs are not being compared, it is important to explicitly state that the economic evaluation question does not involve comparison and justify the need for conducting a cost description or a cost analysis. If two programs are being compared, it is imperative to clearly identify and justify both of the two programs or interventions being compared and on which dependent variables they are being compared. For comparisons, the two interventions must be fully detailed so that their differences are understood. It is also very helpful to state the goals and objectives of each program being compared. Comparisons can be made between new or innovative programs as well as between a new intervention and the usual standard care or a do-nothing option.

In choosing the interventions to be compared, one must be willing to accept that the innovation or new program may not be more cost-effective than routine care. For example, Hendriks et al. (2008) compared a new multidisciplinary fall-prevention program with the usual care for the elderly. As part of their investigation, these authors randomized patients to the two groups. They found that the new program was not cost-effective when compared with usual care. Such a finding could be disheartening to the evaluator as well as to those who provided the new program. Yet, the findings are important in making future program and health policy decisions.

Develop Decision Rules

As with any evaluation or study, an economic evaluation makes assumptions about the health problem, about the interventions, and about the methods used. If those assumptions are stated explicitly, their potential consequences can then be anticipated and corrections made. The decision rules essentially address the measurement of the variables, the time frame, and the program sample.

One set of decision rules is definitions of key parameters of the economic evaluation. For example, when comparing programs with varying degrees of intensity (e.g., a single, weak intervention versus multiple, intensive interventions) and duration (e.g., annual versus monthly), Torrance, Siegel, and Luce (1996) recommended using in the analysis all intervention levels that are realistically feasible. This is one type of decision rule that needs to be explicit. Another set of decision rules involves the time frame over which the costs and the effects/benefits/utility will be measured. The breadth of program costs to be included also ought to be a decision rule, based in part on the accounting perspective chosen. Lastly, a set of decision rules should focus on the age groups to be included in the analysis. The characteristics of program participants ought to be a point of discussion and decision, particularly if the program effects may vary based on those characteristics in ways that can affect the economic analysis.

A different set of decision rules must focus on interpreting the results of the economic evaluation. Health economists often apply the rule of thumb that $50,000 is the upper limit or maximum that society is willing to pay for one unit of health benefit. While the source and appropriateness of this number have spurred debate, it does provide a reference point for interpreting whether the cost for a unit of benefit or utility is "worth it." In this scenario, the $24,859 for one quality-adjusted life-year that resulted from bilateral cochlear implants (Bichey & Miyamoto, 2008) would be deemed "worth it." For health program planners and evaluators in the process of conducting an economic evaluation for the purpose of future program plans, it would be important to set a priori the upper limit that would be tolerated as a cost for the gains.

Two key variables in an economic evaluation are the costs and the effects. For program decisions using data from economic evaluations, the minimum acceptable amount of effect from the interventions needs to be chosen. Similarly, the program budget limit needs to be set. These two criteria create a matrix (Yates, 1999) for deciding whether a program falls into an ideal cost-effective range, less-than-ideal category, or worst-case scenario range (Figure 16.1). Establishing these cut-offs for budget and effect before conducting the economic evaluation may not be easy, but the process does foster debate, critical thinking, and stakeholder engagement.

Choose an Accounting Perspective

An *accounting perspective* is the theoretical point of view taken, which then guides the decisions as to what factors will be included as costs and as outcomes (Table 16.1). The main accounting perspectives are those of the program participants, the program, the payers, and society. The choice of perspectives is not insignificant. Isaacman and colleagues (2008) found that the cost per life-year gained from pneumococcal vaccination differed by roughly 128,000 euros depending on whether the societal or payer perspective was used. Thus, the key perspectives are reviewed here.

Figure 16.1 Matrix of the Relationship of Program Costs and Intervention Effectiveness

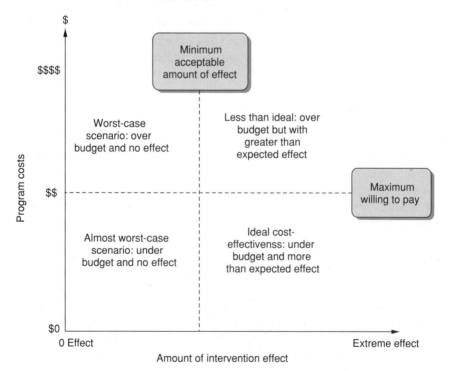

Table 16.1 Accounting Perspectives with Examples of Corresponding Costs and Benefits

Accounting Perspective	Costs	Benefits and Outcomes
Participants	Medical costs, treatment and medication costs, costs of participation	Program-specific impacts, secondary effects on family, quality of life related
Program	Program costs, opportunity costs	Visibility and goodwill (marketing value), increased program or agency funding
Payers	Program costs, loss of revenues, increase in expenditures	Increased revenues or decreased expenditures
Society	Lost taxes, disability support, criminal justice related, etc.	Gain in taxes, reductions in public services (police, fire), reductions in costs to family members related to health problem (lost wages, lost taxes, out of pocket), reductions in costs to support family due to health problem

The simplest accounting perspective is that of the program. From this perspective, only the actual costs of the program and revenues generated are considered. While this perspective is important, it is neither comprehensive nor sufficient. Another perspective is that of the individual participants regarding the costs of and gains from the program's interventions. Costs included from this accounting perspective include out-of-pocket costs and opportunity costs of program participation.

Opportunity costs refer to purchases that cannot be made because of having spent the money on something else. In terms of participants, because they are paying, in some form, for being in the program, they no longer have that money to spend on something else. For example, if someone participates in a diabetes prevention program, then he or she no longer has those hours or that bus fare to go and do something else. In other words, the person does not have the opportunity to spend the money that is going toward program participation. Opportunity costs become critical in decision making, particularly if resources are scarce or severely limited. For example, if a mother takes her child for immunizations, the cost of getting to the clinic and the co-payment may cost her the opportunity (the money) to purchase new clothes for that child. Fiedler and associates (2000), in a cost study of a nutrition fortification program, found that the opportunity costs of volunteers amounted to 41% of personnel costs and 30% of total program costs. The inclusion of opportunity costs in the analysis can alter the final results. Costs, from the point of view of program participants, would include losses or gains in work productivity, the family burden related to the health problem or program, out-of-pocket expenses related to participation, and so forth. For example, to attend an immunization program, a mother's out-of-pocket expenses could include transportation costs, babysitting costs, and the cost of baby Tylenol, as well as losing half a day of work. These findings reinforce the importance of including opportunity costs in the economic evaluation, including the opportunity costs incurred by any volunteers used in the health program.

Another accounting perspective is that of payers or program sponsors. Economic evaluations from this perspective are concerned with direct program expenditures and costs and benefits only of immediate relevance to the payer. Payers may also be concerned with revenues generated or lost due to the program's intervention effects. Most studies of Medicaid or Medicare programs, such as those delivering prescription drug benefits (Roy & Madhaven, 2008), adopt the payer perspective. For large population studies, claims data may be the only cost data available, but they inherently represent the amount paid by an insurer, not the full costs to provide the service. Most providers would argue that Medicaid or Medicare claims data grossly underestimate the actual costs of providing the service. Whether the claims data used to monetize program costs come from federal sources or private insurers, the claims payments represent only the amount that the insurer is willing to pay relative to the charge for the service, not the actual cost of providing the program.

The third key perspective that can be used to determine costs and benefits is that of populations and society. Although this accounting perspective can be complex, it provides a more comprehensive economic evaluation of a program's interventions. From the societal perspective, factors that should be part of economic evaluations include taxes, costs of morbidity, opportunity costs, and, importantly, externalities (explained later in this chapter). The choice to use a societal perspective reflects whether the health problem is viewed as societal problem. This may explain why Doran (2008), in a review of articles on treating opiate dependence, found that most studies used a societal perspective and consistently found positive economic returns on treating opiate dependence.

Each accounting perspective has its advantages and disadvantages, as well as being more appropriate for some economic evaluations than for others. For example, a simple cost description would not include the societal perspective, but a cost–benefit analysis would be deficient if a societal perspective was not taken. For some economic evaluations, it may be appropriate to combine accounting perspectives, within reasonable limits. To avoid a systematic bias in underinclusion or overinclusion of program costs, refer to the service utilization and program theory as guides to what ought to be included as program costs.

Monetize and Compute Program Costs

The majority of costs are related to the program implementation and include the resources utilized by the program and by participants. Detailed program expenditures are used as the basis for computing the indirect and direct costs associated with providing the program, as discussed in Chapter 8. The process theory continues to be a guide for identifying which program costs to include in the economic evaluation (Figure 16.2). Depending on the type of economic evaluation, costs associated with variables in the effect theory—specifically antecedent, causal, moderating, and mediating factors—as well as costs associated with outcomes and impacts, may be included (Figure 16.3).

This step involves attaching a dollar value to those variables. This process is likely to feel odd or uncomfortable, but it must be done if the economic evaluation is to accurately and fully capture the costs and benefits in monetary terms. Costs or expenses to participants are included in the economic analysis and tend to have a known dollar value. Knowable costs for program participants would include new or special equipment (e.g., handrails or cooking utensils), educational materials (e.g., books or magazine subscriptions), transportation, or child care while attending the program. Other costs and expenses may not be easy to monetize. For example, participation in a substance abuse program may cost the participant older friendships based on substance use activities.

Adjust for Time

Time is a factor that affects costs, just as it can affect program outcomes and impacts. Therefore, it is necessary to decide upon a time period during which program outcomes and impacts will be considered, as well as for projecting program expenses and costs. In addition, time changes the value of money and the value of health benefits. Economists have developed procedures for taking time into account. All of these procedures attempt to convert a monetary value either in the past or the future into a current monetary value. The procedures most commonly used in economic analyses of health programs are discounting, adjusting for inflation, and depreciation.

Figure 16.2 Relevance of Process Theory to Economic Evaluations

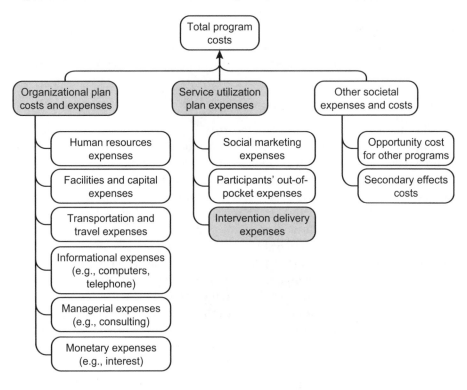

Figure 16.3 Use of Causal Theory to Identify Potential Costs and Benefits Associated with the Health Problem

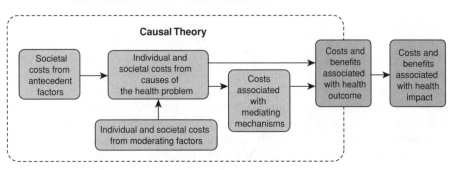

Discounting is the process of converting future health benefits and future dollars to the present value. It involves decreasing the current value by a rate, usually between 1% and 3%, on an annual basis. In a sense, discounting is the reverse of interest. Through this approach, expenses and health benefits that might be expected in 2 or 20 years are all valued on a par with one another. This facilitates interpretation of the values and makes it simpler to see the costs so that decision makers can make choices based on data that are, so to speak, standardized.

Two adjustments for time are typically applied only to expenses or costs: inflation and depreciation. The more familiar of these adjustments is probably inflation. *Inflation* is the rate at which current dollars have a lower value in the future, such that a set number of additional dollars will be needed in the future to have the same value as now. Inflation is applied to program expenses. Adjustment for inflation is readily noted when reports state the year for dollar amounts, such as "$500 (in 1998 dollars)." *Depreciation* is the decreasing value of capital equipment into the future, just as your car or computer becomes worth less the longer you own it.

Each of these adjustments uses a rate. The rate chosen can be an estimated rate, the rate used by the organization providing the program, or the federally established rate. The analyst decides which rate to use in the analysis, which hints at the potential subjectivity of economic analyses of health programs. Despite this area of discretion, each of these adjustments for time follows a standardized procedure and involves the application of standardized economic formulas. Most textbooks on economic analyses provide these formulas. Nonetheless, decisions about the rate selected and the items to which the rates are applied require both theoretical and practical knowledge of the program, its costs, and its potential effects.

Identify and Measure Program Effects

Economic evaluations either use existing data already collected as part of the outcome evaluation or must collect effects data. If effects data are not available, then an outcome evaluation must be conducted, drawing from the effect theory to identify and justify which effects to measure and which measurement tools to use to do so. Program interventions with psychological effects can be used as units for effects. For example, Mandelblatt and others (2008) used units of distress as measured on a standardized scale when comparing the effect of three types of interventions. Although they were able to identify which intervention had the highest and lowest costs per unit of distress decrease, these authors point out that it may be difficult to interpret, given that no standards exist for trials with psychosocial outcomes.

Not all program effects are part of the program theory. Secondary effects, whether anticipated or not, may occur, and the effects can spill over to individuals not participating in the program; these are called *externalities*. An externality becomes a social cost or benefit that resulted from providing the program. Externalities may be indirect or even unanticipated consequences of the program, whether beneficial or harmful. Including them can be important in comprehensive economic analyses that attempt to monetize a broad range of program-related effects, such as from the societal perspective. Externalities are identified by conducting a "thought experiment" in which one imagines possible programmatic effects on the target audience as a whole, irrespective of participation. Identifying externalities is important because they then become effects (if beneficial) or costs (if harmful or in some way costly).

For example, Isaacman and colleagues (2008) conducted a literature review of cost-effectiveness studies of a vaccine against pneumococcal infection. They found that the cost per life-year gained differed for studies that included the indirect effect of herd immunity, an externality. In Layetteville, an economic evaluation of the adolescent violence prevention program using a societal perspective might project the additional births from adolescents not killed due to gunshot wounds and the costs or savings accrued from a different pattern of ambulance use. These effects are examples of possible externalities from the program. Including externalities provides a more comprehensive and thus more accurate economic analysis.

Monetize the Effects

There are many ways to assign dollar values to intangible health program outcomes and impacts, and evaluators planning an economic analysis must decide which of the various methods of monetizing program effects to use. Table 16.2 lists the possible approaches. The choice ultimately depends on the information available and is influenced by the overall accounting perspective of the economic analysis and the level and type of expertise of those doing the economic evaluation. That a variety of methods can potentially be used for monetizing outcomes highlights the potential difficulties in conducting economic evaluations of health programs. One of many possible complications in monetizing outcomes is that not all impacts or benefits are equally important, yet the process of monetizing the impacts and benefits treats them as equal in terms of dollars.

Conduct an Analysis

This step essentially involves doing the math. It is possible to perform the calculations for the more simple economic analyses using readily available

Table 16.2   Approaches to Monetizing Outcomes and Impacts

Approach	Method
Market value (of state of health or ongoing medical treatment for illnesses)	Obtain price for treatments, wages
Client willingness to pay	Observe choices that are made by program participants or members of the target audience
Policy maker's view of the value	Ask policy maker to estimate the dollar value of the impact
Practitioner's view of the value	Ask health professionals to estimate the dollar value of the impact

software, such as Excel. This requires that the spreadsheet must be set up in a manner that includes all key parameters of the economic analysis. More sophisticated economic analyses may require special statistical software.

Conduct a Sensitivity Analysis

A *sensitivity analysis* is the systematic alteration of any parameter of the economic analysis for the purpose of determining the point at which the conclusions would become substantively different (Drummond, Sculpher, Torrance, O'Brien, & Stoddart, 2005). A sensitivity analysis is done as a final step because all of the variables that are to be monetized will have been identified and monetized earlier, as part of the primary analysis. The purpose of conducting a sensitivity analysis is twofold: (1) to identify the parameter that is most influential in altering the conclusion, and (2) to establish the range wherein changes in the costs related to either the program or the outcomes have minimal effect. In conducting any economic evaluation, uncertainties tend to arise regarding factors such as the mortality and morbidity prevented, or regarding the actual costs. Sensitivity analysis helps deal with these uncertainties by allowing the evaluator to examine "what if" scenarios, thereby gaining additional information for decision making. Because it varies and tests the values of key parameters, a sensitivity analysis helps to identify dependence upon assumptions. As a consequence, it provides additional information for determining a break point around which can be important for decision making.

Conducting a sensitivity analysis requires deliberately varying one or more key parameters, one at a time, along a range of values. The economic analysis is then repeated using the new range of values for the key parameter. In a cost-effectiveness study of pneumococcal vaccination of infants and children, Lieu and associates (2000) conducted a sensitivity analysis in which they varied the following parameters used in their economic evaluation: the incidence rate of pneumococcal infection, the rate of serious subsequent infection, the rate of a secondary infection (otitis media), the vaccine efficacy, the cost of vaccine administration, the cost of clinic visits and hospitalizations, the discount rate, the rate at which infants and children were covered by the vaccination, and the cost of medical care and work loss of the parents due to children's adverse reactions to the immunization. By varying each of these key parameters, the authors were able to identify which variable was most critical in altering the results. They found that using assumptions that favored the efficacy and coverage rates altered the "bottom line" recommendation, compared to unfavorable assumptions. Their findings highlight the critical importance of conducting a sensitivity analysis.

Disseminate the Findings

Findings of the economic evaluation need to be distributed to relevant program stakeholders and to policy makers, just as findings from the process and effect evaluations were disseminated. The method of dissemination ought to be suited to the level of rigor used to conduct the economic analysis. In some cases, dissemination can occur through academic venues, such as professional journals, especially if the findings are new or provocative. The assumption is that dissemination, particularly to the stakeholders and decision makers, leads to programmatic decisions based on the findings. Unfortunately, there seems to be consensus that economic evaluations are not used widely in health policy decisions. Prosser, Koplan, Neumann, and Weinstein (2000) have suggested that a lack of understanding about economic evaluations may be one barrier to the use of the findings. Thus, to have a programmatic effect, the dissemination of the findings ought to be accompanied by some education of the decision maker.

TYPES OF COST ANALYSES

Several different types of analyses related to program costs are possible. *Costs* is a generic term used to encompass monetary and intangible expenses related to the program. The determination of what is included as expenses is part of the cost side of the economic analysis and is discussed later in this chapter as part of how to conduct an economic analysis. Types of economic analyses can be classified along two dimensions (Drummond et al., 2005). One dimension is whether one or more programs are under consideration, and the other is whether costs only or costs and effects are included in the analysis (Table 16.3). Classifying economic analyses of programs along these two dimensions helps to discern the types and the subsequent requirements for conducting each type of analysis.

Three types of economic analyses involve comparing one or more programs and a measure of effect, whether outcome or impact. The types of economic analyses described are not mutually exclusive. Program planners and managers and key stakeholders need to be aware of how these economic analyses are done. This knowledge will enable them not only to critique these studies, but also to actively participate in the conceptualization and execution of the more complex economic analyses. Basic information specific to cost-effectiveness analysis (CEA), cost–benefit analysis (CBA), and cost–utility analysis (CUA) is given in following sections (Table 16.4). Shaw (1995) aptly pointed out that outcomes are considered beneficial if they are favorable to the program recipients, but are labeled as costs if they are unfavorable. This perspective applies across all types of cost analyses. This discussion is intended to provide sufficient information about these economic evaluations to allow a program evaluator or program manager to be a savvy consumer of economic evaluations and an informed team member in more sophisticated efforts to conduct an economic analysis of the program.

Table 16.3 Types of Cost Analyses

	One Program	**Two or More Programs**
Costs Only	Cost description Cost analysis Cost minimization	Cost comparison
Costs and Effects	Cost analysis	Cost-effectiveness Cost–benefit Cost–utility

Table 16.4   Summary of Cost-Effectiveness Analysis, Cost–Benefit Analysis, and Cost–Utility Analysis

Type of Analysis	Basic Formula per Program	Outcomes, Impacts, Benefits	Costs, Expenses
Cost-effectiveness analysis (CEA)	$CEA = \dfrac{\text{total cost \$}}{\text{health effect unit}}$	Program direct health impacts	Program direct + indirect costs
Cost–benefit analysis (CBA)	Net benefit = total benefit \$ − total cost \$	Dollar values of program direct impacts + indirect program outcomes + long-term societal consequences, willingness to pay, life expectancy	Program direct and indirect costs + medical costs + non-medical costs + opportunity costs + other societal costs
Cost–utility analysis (CUA)	$CUA = \dfrac{\text{total cost \$}}{\text{utility units}}$	Preferences for health state	Program costs + medical costs + nonmedical costs

Cost Description, Cost Analysis, and Cost Minimization

When only one program is considered and effects are not included, the type of analysis is termed a *cost description*. Cost description is the simplest form of economic analysis in that it is a straightforward presentation of expenses related to the delivery of the health program. Most program managers routinely prepare cost descriptions, particularly for any annual reports that require an accounting of expenses by category or line item. A cost description is best thought of as part of process monitoring, particularly with regard to accountability and the budget aspect of the organizational plan. However, more sophisticated cost analyses might focus on a specific stage in the life cycle of a program, such as the start-up stage. Tangka and others (2008) did just that by estimating the costs associated with starting a colorectal cancer program.

When the cost description includes a breakdown of total expenses by an analytic factor, such as time periods, staff activities, or funding source, it becomes a *cost analysis*. A cost analysis is also useful as a process monitoring tool. It essentially analyzes costs by other elements of either the organizational plan or the service utilization plan. In this way the findings of a cost analysis begin to provide information about the efficiency of a program, using, for example, dollars spent per program participant. These findings can be compared to published reports, benchmarks, or the original program plan to interpret the extent to which the program is more or less efficient than similar programs. Cost analyses can also focus on the costs or savings that result from the health program. For example, Lairson and associates (2008) compared the following costs for participants in a diabetes management program and nonparticipants: costs of office visits, hospital inpatient care, and outpatient care. They reported a significant difference in the outpatient costs but essentially no difference in health outcome measures. Given these findings, it would not have been productive or useful to conduct a cost-effectiveness evaluation.

Cost minimization is an analysis to determine the best ways to provide the program at the lowest cost. This type of analysis ought to be a part of the basic budgeting process, because it allows program managers to select the lowest reasonable expense for a category or to comparison shop for expenses such as supplies and capital equipment.

Program Applications

Published cost descriptions and cost analyses can be used during the planning stage to estimate program expenses for different intervention options. Clearly, cost descriptions and cost analyses are important for process monitoring and for understanding the basic cost parameters of a program. The basic information generated through these analytical approaches is easy for program staff and stakeholders to understand, so it facilitates decision making about the program's future.

Cost Comparison

Cost comparison compares the costs of two or more programs without looking at outcomes or impacts. These comparisons may focus on the costs per participant for the programs being considered or the revenues generated by various programs. Cost comparisons might be done by a single agency with multiple health programs as the basis for deciding which program to continue. For example, Jerrell and Hu (1996) reported on a comprehensive analysis of costs associated with clients in three types of mental health and substance abuse prevention programs administered by one agency: a 12-step program, a behavioral skills program, and case management.

Cost-Effectiveness Analysis

Cost-effectiveness analysis (CEA) always compares the costs of two programs against one type of impact that is measured the same way in both programs. Using this approach, the programs are then compared on the basis of cost per unit of outcome. A cost-effectiveness analysis, as described here, answers the question of whether program A or program B has more effect for the dollars expended. Another way of stating this point is to ask "which treatment or intervention is the best for the money" or to ask, "which program costs less per unit of effect."

A CEA focuses on the cost related to a single, common effect that may differ in magnitude between the alternative programs. It is used to rank alternatives based on their resultant cost-effectiveness ratio (CER). Sometimes the term "cost-effectiveness analysis" is used as a generic category that encompasses CEA, CBA, and CUA. For the sake of clarity, CEA, in this book, refers only to the specific type of economic analysis in which two programs are compared on the basis of one impact indicator.

Costs include all direct expenses and, to the extent possible, indirect expenses related to the delivery of the program or intervention (Table 16.4). Costs may include start-up costs for a new program. The inclusion of indirect program costs, as well as in-kind resources, can alter the results of the CEA. Other costs that are typically part of a CEA are medical costs related to the health problem being prevented by the intervention or program, including both hospitalization costs if the health problem is not prevented and outpatient visits. If the societal accounting perspective is taken, then along with program and medical costs, nonmedical costs such as opportunity and secondary costs will be included. The sum of all these costs is estimated.

On the effectiveness side of the equation, effects of the program are measured in natural or physical units that are common to both programs. Because the effects are common to both programs, they are also quite specific to the health problem being addressed. For example, if two diabetes education programs are being compared with regard to their effects on diabetes prevention and management, the outcomes common to both programs are likely to be blood glucose levels and a score on diabetes knowledge. For the most part, CEA uses outcome measures that are directly and immediately linked to the programmatic intervention. The effect theory and process theories can be very helpful in identifying and justifying which outcomes ought to be monetized in the CEA, specifically the variables included in the intervention and action hypotheses.

The basic formula to be estimated for each program being compared is as follows (Newbold, 1995):

$$\text{Cost-Effectiveness Ratio (CER)} = \frac{\text{(total cost of program A)} - \text{(total cost of program B)}}{\text{(effects of program A)} - \text{(effects of program B)}}$$

The results of this CEA calculation lead to a statement regarding the cost per unit of effect for each program. The CER is the incremental price to get one unit of effect compared to the alternative. A program with a low CER is considered a "good buy."

The formula just given is the basic formula for the CER. However, specific evaluations may derive more realistic applications of the formula. Cost-effectiveness studies need not be limited to existing programs; instead, they can be employed to assess the value or merit of initiating screening tests. The study by Randolph and Washington (1990) is one such example. These researchers used costs associated with screening and treatment and the cure rates to assess the merit of screening adolescent males for *Chlamydia*. A later study by Blake, Quinn, and Gaydos (2008) compared four *Chlamydia* screening strategies used with men and women for cost and effectiveness in preventing pelvic inflammatory disease. These two examples highlight that, as screening methods or interventions improve or change, subsequent CEAs may be needed so as to provide more up-to-date information to program planners.

A possible variation to the CEA is an analysis that focuses on the program-specific outcomes. Sevick and colleagues (2000), for example, conducted a CEA of two exercise interventions for adults. They calculated the cost for each increment of improvement in a set of outcome measures and indicators, such as amount of weight loss, number of additional flights of stairs walked, and blood pressure. The approach is based on another modification of the CEA formula:

$$\frac{\text{Incremental improvement}}{\text{in cost effectiveness}} = \frac{\text{program cost per participant}}{\text{amount of change in a specific outcome indicator}}$$

Program Applications

During the program planning phase, a review of cost-effectiveness reports could help program planners decide which interventions to implement. After the program has been implemented, program personnel can perform a CEA, with some help from a program evaluator. The key would be to have two interventions to compare, such as program versus no program, or old program versus new program. The comparison of outcomes and effects could also be between program participants and nonparticipants. Such comparisons would be appropriate if the program is mature, there is good accounting for the program costs, and outcome data can be collected from the two groups. Alternatively, the comparisons can be among two or more interventions for the same health problem. For example, French and associates (2008) compared four interventions for adolescent substance use disorders. Through a CEA, they were able to conclude that the least costly intervention was also the most effective, but that conclusion varied by length of time post-intervention.

The basic idea underlying the CEA may also be modified to fit the program interventions and expected outcomes. Windsor and colleagues (1990), for example, demonstrated this possibility in an evaluation of a health education program to improve medication adherence. They measured the effect of the program with a reliable and valid scale of adherence. They then used the following simple formula to determine the cost-effectiveness of the intervention: (cost of the intervention) ÷ (percentage improvement on the adherence scale). Although their "cost of the intervention" variable did not include indirect costs, their results were easy to interpret and provided clear evidence in favor of the health education intervention.

Table 16.5 shows the usefulness of conducting an incremental improvement cost analysis. The three hypothetical programs in the table vary in terms of the program cost per participant and the degree to which the three outcome indicators are changed by participation in the program. The cost per outcome objective varies, suggesting that the choice of outcome to be costed and considered is crucial in selecting the "best" health program.

To make choices among intervention options, it is important to balance the amount of effects achieved by the interventions being compared with the costs of the interventions. This yields a matrix (Table 16.6) showing which intervention to choose. If both interventions A and B have the same degree of effect and cost the same, then either intervention is a reasonable choice. But if either the cost or the effectiveness is greater or less for one of the interventions, then one intervention becomes a better choice over the other. The matrix in Table 16.6 shows only two interventions, but the same logic applies if more than two interventions are compared in the CEA.

Cost–Benefit Analysis

Like a CEA, a *cost–benefit analysis* (CBA) compares two programs. In this type of analysis, however, the programs need not address the same health problem. The program effects are compared based on larger societal benefits in addition to the outcomes and impacts of the program. The two dissimilar programs are compared on the basis of cost per dollar value of benefits achieved. Often the program under consideration is compared to a do-nothing option. The intent of a CBA is to determine which of two different programs will have the greater social benefit, given their separate costs. This type of analysis answers questions regarding whether the benefits gained are worthwhile to society, given the costs.

Table 16.5 Example of Simple and Incremental Cost Effectiveness of Three Hypothetical General Health Improvement Programs

	Program A (Usual Care)	Program B (New Program)	Program C (Modified New)
Total program costs	$400	$1000	$700
Number participants per program	100	100	100
Total program cost per participant	**$4**	**$10**	**$7**
Total amount of overall improvement	5%	25%	20%
Overall cost-effectiveness	$800	$400	$350
Overall cost-effectiveness per participant = (cost per participant) ± (amount of improvement)	$80	$40	$35
Incremental Cost-Effectiveness Analyses			
Amount of improvement in outcome objective 1 (increase in perceived health status score)	2 units	5 units	10 units
Cost per unit of higher perceived health status	$2.00	$2.00	$0.70
Amount of improvement in outcome objective 2 (additional minutes of exercise)	3 minutes	20 minutes	15 minutes
Cost per additional minute of exercise	$1.33	$0.50	$0.47
Amount of improvement in outcome objective 3 (diastolic blood pressure decrease)	2 mm Hg	4 mm Hg	4 mm Hg
Cost per mm Hg decrease in blood pressure	$2.00	$2.50	$1.75

Table 16.6   Matrix Showing Ideal Choice Between Programs A and B, Based on
Cost and Effect

Costs: Program A Costs . . .	Effect: Program A Does . . .		
	More than B (A > B)	Same as B (A = B)	Less than B (A < B)
More than B (A > B)	Undecided	Choose B	Choose B
Same as B (A = B)	Choose A	Either	Choose B
Less than B (A < B)	Choose A	Choose A	Undecided

CBA is used to assess the inherent worth of a program, and because of its societal focus, the findings of a CBA are used for policy decision making (Szucs, 2000). This analysis is useful when comparing programs at different levels of the public health pyramid because it can be used to compare dissimilar programs. For example, a CBA could compare the adult immunization program (population level) in Bowe County with prenatal screening for congenital anomalies done by providers in Layetteville (direct services level). In addition, because a CBA compares programs in dollars, programs from different sectors of society can be compared, such as a health program and a military program.

A CBA results in a ratio, expressed in dollars. Outcomes included in a CBA are the benefits (effects) as measured in market value, willingness to pay, or life expectancy. A key feature of a prototypical CBA is that it takes into account all outcomes, thereby considering the broadest possible social consequences of the program. Therefore, all outcomes and benefits must be monetized, including intangibles and benefits of the program. This approach allows for a direct comparison of two dissimilar programs, using dollars as the basis of comparison. Tangible benefits are directly observable and measurable, whereas intangible benefits are indirect, less measurable, and more likely to be secondary benefits. The costs associated with the programs include both the direct programmatic costs and the indirect costs in terms of the program and society. Opportunity costs also can be included in a CBA.

As with the CEA, the program effect theory, and particularly the intervention model, becomes critical as the conceptual and theoretical basis for identifying the direct and tangible program benefits through the CBA. Because the CBA encompasses distal and societal effects of the program, the effect theory becomes a starting point for conceptualizing additional programmatic impacts. The effect theory provides a basis for assigning an outcome as a benefit or as a cost.

The results of a CBA are expressed as a ratio of benefit dollars to cost dollars. The value of this ratio ranges from a negative value to zero or a positive value. If the ratio has a positive value, then the program will provide or is providing a net benefit to society; if the ratio has a negative value, the program will be more costly than the benefits it delivers to society. In short, a program with the higher positive ratio is preferred because it has the greater societal benefit. The formula for the ratio can be expressed as follows:

Cost–benefit ratio =

$$\frac{(\text{dollar value of tangible benefits}) + (\text{dollar value of intangible benefits})}{\text{total costs associated with program}}$$

Some outcomes, such as averted illness, can be valued as either benefits or costs, depending on one's perspective. Averted illness can be a benefit in terms of wages earned, but can be a cost in terms of lost revenue for a clinic. An alternative to calculating the cost–benefit ratio is to use the net benefit. The net benefit calculation avoids the difficulties of determining which costs belong in the numerator and which belong in the denominator of the cost–benefit ratio. The net benefit is calculated as follows:

Net benefit =

(dollar value of tangible benefits + dollar value of intangible benefits) −

(direct costs + indirect costs)

The values of the net benefit of the programs are then compared to determine which program has a greater societal benefit given its costs.

Whether the cost–benefit ratio or net benefit is calculated, ultimately the decision makers are comparing dissimilar programs that have been analyzed on an equal basis. This approach enables decision makers to make difficult choices regarding allocation of resources for one program over another.

Program Applications

Reviews of cost–benefit reports could be helpful during the prioritization phase, as such investigations provide information on which health problem will have larger or smaller costs associated with it if addressed. It is unlikely that program personnel and most program evaluators will perform a CBA, as these analyses are more likely to be done by researchers. Nonetheless, for some health issues, because CBAs are used to establish health policy, it may be important for program staff and evaluators to collaborate with researchers in an effort to influence policies relevant to the health problem.

Cost–Utility Analysis

A *cost–utility analysis* (CUA) measures the outcome of health programs in terms of the potential participants' preference for the health outcome. This makes it the most complex and theoretical economic analysis. Programs are compared on the basis of their cost per unit of preference, called utility. For all practical purposes, such calculations are performed only by researchers. Thus CUAs are less common than either CEAs or CBAs. A CUA is used to answer the question "how much it is worth in dollars to have a particular state of health." Like the CBA, the CUA compares programs with different outcomes.

The outcome considered in a CUA is *utility*—specifically, a preference for a state of health, which is achieved as an outcome from the program. *Preference* or *utility assessment* provides a way to integrate the preferences or values attributed to the worth of life at a given point in time with the quality of life spent in various health states (Patrick & Erickson, 1993). Utility values are obtained through judgment, from the literature, and from program participants. The methods used to ascertain the utility include standardized scales to measure quality of life and preferences, as well as special techniques of standard gamble, time trade-off, and paired comparisons. Paired comparisons used to determine a health state preference might be: Would you rather have severe, chronic hypertension or type 2 diabetes? Would you rather lose your right leg or your left hand? Would you rather lose your left hand or have type 2 diabetes? In addition to preferences, QALYs, DALYs, lives saved, and disability days averted can be used in a CUA. However, the multidimensionality of quality of life and the relative importance of those dimensions of quality of life (Bowling, 1995) add considerable complexity to conducting a CUA.

Conducting a CUA is not appropriate if intermediate program outcomes are of interest or if health utility or quality of life is not measurable. The preferences for health states tend to be related to specific illnesses and, therefore, can be idiosyncratic. Nevertheless, a CUA is a good choice when quality of life is an important programmatic outcome, as would be the case with a program for patients with diabetes or arthritis or for infants admitted to a neonatal intensive care unit. Cost–utility studies are more commonly done as a means of comparing medical treatments for different illnesses, because of the nature of preferences. It is important to recognize that methodological debates about CUA continue as well as concerns about how to make CUA and the use of QALYs more health policy friendly (Ubel et al., 2000).

Nonetheless, the results of CUAs reflect the relative importance of the health program outcome.

As with CEAs and CBAs, CUA findings are expressed as a ratio of the program costs to the level of preference for the health state offered by the program. The formula is as follows:

$$\text{Cost–utility ratio} = \frac{\text{total costs associated with the program}}{\text{utility units}}$$

The results of the analysis, in the form of the ratio, show how much each unit of additional health value costs when the specific program is implemented. As with the economic analyses of programs, the ratio allows decision makers to compare programs on the basis of dollars.

Program Applications

CUAs are difficult to use for planning or policy-making purposes because of the nature of preferences that serve as the basis of CUAs. Gaski and Frick (2008) found that the utilities (i.e., preferences for health states) do not vary by race or ethnicity, except with regard to pain and discomfort. Their study results imply that CUA studies that include a sample from only one racial group are likely to apply to other racial groups as well. In contrast, Gabriel et al. (1999) found that the preference for a health state varied based on the health experiences of those being surveyed. This variation had an effect on the estimated cost–utility value of interventions to prevent osteoporosis in women. Such findings hint at the relative and sensitive nature of preferences and the subsequent difficulty in arriving at one definitive cost–utility ratio.

ASSESSING ECONOMIC EVALUATIONS

Not all publications and reports of program economic evaluations are what they seem or do what their titles say they do. Given this uncertainty, it is important for program planners to become savvy consumers of economic evaluations. This section describes widely accepted criteria for assessing published economic evaluations (Carande-Kulis et al., 2000; Drummond et al., 2005; Gold et al., 1996), which are also used to evaluate economic evaluations (Doran, 2008; Ruger & Emmons, 2008).

The first factor to consider is the framework for the study, with regard to whether the economic question is well defined. A study that is not founded on either economic theory or program theory is likely to contain scientific flaws, especially with regard to monetizing effects and externalities.

Descriptions of alternative programs that are being compared must also be included. These descriptions ought to address the extent to which the effectiveness of the interventions has been established. Preferably, strongly recommended or recommended interventions, practices, or programs are being evaluated. Sometimes, however, a study focuses on a new or alternative intervention that is not yet recommended or strongly recommended as practice. In such a study, the efficacy of the new intervention, practice, or program must then be well established.

The data and methods used in the economic analysis ought to be critiqued. Both the costs and consequences, or programmatic effects, need to be identified for the programs under scrutiny. In addition, the appropriateness of units of measure ought to be critiqued, particularly in terms of the type of economic analysis being done. The dollar values need to be credible for both the program costs and the program benefits, outcomes, and peripheral effects. A carefully done economic analysis will take into account adjustments for time—specifically, discounting, inflation, and depreciation. Moreover, a thorough report will state the base year and type of currency used in the analysis. The type of software used to conduct the analysis should be identified as well.

The results section must be carefully reviewed. In particular, a sensitivity analysis ought to be conducted and the results of that separate analysis included in the report. A well-done report will include a graphical presentation of the results. If any secondary analyses were conducted, the report should describe how they were done and what the findings were.

Finally, program planners should scrutinize the discussion section of the study. This section should acknowledge and explain the limitations of the study. Policy implications of the findings need to be made explicit, and programmatic intervention implications should be addressed. Overall, the discussion section ought not to include new results, but rather provide new insights based on the findings.

ACROSS THE PYRAMID

At the direct services level of the public health pyramid, a CEA is more likely to be used to choose between two comparable programs or treatments for the same health condition. Most medical economic evaluations focus on interventions intended to be delivered at this level.

At the enabling services level, economic evaluations are more likely to be of a CBA or CUA nature, reflecting the intangible aspect of many enabling services. Economic evaluations of enabling services programs are probably the most challenging for several reasons. First, the enabling service is likely to entail considerable intangible benefits, many of which may be difficult to quantify and to monetize. Second, enabling services programs have considerable indirect costs that may not be obvious until the program is carefully reviewed. For example, volunteer time may be a key indirect cost of a less visible component of a larger program. Third, the economic evaluation likely will have considerable and varied family benefits and costs to take into account. This translates into needing to address more secondary costs and benefits, as well as more externalities and opportunity costs for program participants. Fourth, enabling services are often "hidden" within programs, making it difficult to conduct the economic evaluation. For example, providing a referral for high school completion classes can be part of the Special Supplemental Nutrition Program for Women, Infants, and Children (WIC), yet the education referral and attendance may never be measured in the WIC program.

At the population-based level of the public health pyramid, all types of economic evaluations can be used to evaluate programs. A CEA would be appropriate for comparing two screening programs that will be used with a population, such as mammogram versus breast self-examination, vaccine A versus vaccine B for a given infectious disease, or nutritional supplements in flour versus nutritional supplements in bread. A CBA would be appropriate for comparing two dissimilar full-coverage programs. For example, WIC might be compared with a bicycle helmet law, newborn hearing screening might be compared with a new workplace safety regulation, or Medicare might be compared with universal health insurance. A CUA would be appropriate if the overall health of a community is of concern, because this type of analysis takes into consideration general preferences and because the preferences are usually measured in terms that are used to describe the quality of life and the overall health of a community. Examples would be comparing a motorcycle helmet law to no law or comparing a proposed workplace safety regulation to no new regulation.

At the infrastructure level of the public health pyramid, all economic evaluations can help guide health services or health policy decisions. As such, they are most aptly thought of as applying primarily at the infrastructure level. Economic evaluations of the infrastructure level might focus on programs to strengthen the workforce, in which case a simple cost analysis of health personnel would be appropriate, such as the cost of using nurse practitioners or lay case managers to provide a service. Cost analyses indicate how to make the program more efficient as well as how to make the public health sector more efficient.

DISCUSSION QUESTIONS AND ACTIVITIES

1. Compare and contrast CEA, CBA, and CUA with regard to the costs that are included in the analysis. What effects would an underestimation of costs have? What effects would an overestimation of costs have?

2. Conduct a brief literature search for cost analyses or economic evaluations related to diabetes prevention, adult immunizations, violence prevention, child abuse prevention, or congenital anomalies prevention. Which types of economic evaluations tend to be used for each type of program? At what level of the public health pyramid do these economic evaluations tend to occur?

3. Select one of the articles you found in your search of the literature for Question 2. Read the article and critique the report using the criteria provided. What is your overall assessment of the report?

4. Discuss possible methodological, ethical, or moral issues involved in monetizing outcomes.

INTERNET RESOURCES

National Institute on Drug Abuse

The National Institute on Drug Abuse published an online textbook about conducting cost analyses applicable beyond substance abuse treatment programs. Find it at http://www.nida .nih.gov/IMPCOST/IMPCOSTIndex.html.

The Merck Manual for Healthcare Professionals

Because cost analyses are typically done when the intervention or treatment is expensive, pharmaceutical companies often do cost analyses. Merck provides an example (http://www .merck.com/mmpe/sec22/ch328/ch328i.html#CIHEGJHG) in which Table 4 is particularly helpful in sorting out which intervention to choose.

Health Decision Strategies

Free software downloads are available at this website as well as readily available templates and forms that will actually do calculations and graphs related to cost-effectiveness analyses: http://www.healthstrategy.com/.

REFERENCES

Bichey, B. G., & Miyamoto, R. T. (2008). Outcomes in bilateral cochlear implantation. *Otolaryngology, 138*(5), 655–661.

Blake, D. R., Quinn, T. C., & Gaydos, C. A. (2008). Should asymptomatic men be included in *Chlamydia* screening programs? Cost-effectiveness of *Chlamydia* screening among male and female entrants to a national job training program. *Sexually Transmitted Diseases, 35*(1), 91–101.

Bowling, A. (1995). What things are important in people's lives? A survey of the public's judgments to inform scales of health related quality of life. *Social Science & Medicine, 41*(10), 1447–1462.

Carande-Kulis, V. G., Maciosek, M. V., Briss, P. A., Teutsch, S. M., Zaza, S., Truman, B. I., et al. (2000). Methods for systematic reviews of economic evaluations for the Guide to Community Preventive Services. *American Journal of Preventive Medicine, 18*(1 suppl), 75–91.

Doran, C. M. (2008). Economic evaluation of interventions to treat opiate dependence: A review of the evidence. *PharmacoEconomics, 26*(5), 371–393.

Drummond, M. F., Sculpher, M. J., Torrance, G. W., O'Brien, B. J., & Stoddart, G. L. (2005). *Methods for the economic evaluation of health care programmes* (3rd ed.). Oxford, UK: Oxford University Press.

Fiedler, J. L., Dado, D. R., Maglalang, H., Juban, N., Capistrano, M., & Magpantay, M. V. (2000). Cost analysis as a vitamin A program design and evaluation tool: A case study of the Philippines. *Social Science & Medicine, 51*(2), 223–242.

French, M. T., Zavala, S. K., McCollister, K. E., Waldron, H. B., Turner, C. W., & Ozechowski, T. J. (2008). Cost-effectiveness analysis of four interventions for adolescents with a substance use disorder. *Journal of Substance Abuse Treatment, 34*(3), 272–281.

Gabriel, S. E., Kneeland, T. S., Melton, L. J., Moncur, M. M., Ettinger, B., & Tosteson, A. N. (1999). Health-related quality of life in economic evaluations for osteoporosis: Whose values should we use? *Medical Decision Making, 19*(2), 141–148.

Gaski, D. J., & Frick, K. D. (2008). Race and ethnicity disparities in valuing health. *Medical Decision Making, 28*(1), 12–20.

Gold, M. R., Seigel, J. E., Russell, L. B., & Weinstein, M. C. (Eds.). (1996). *Cost-effectiveness in health and medicine*. Oxford, UK: Oxford University Press.

Hendriks, M. R., Evers, S. M., Bleijlevens, M. H., van Haastregt, J. C., Crebolder, H. F., & van Eijk, J. T. (2008). Cost effectiveness of a multidisciplinary fall prevention program in community-dwelling elderly people: A randomized controlled trial. *International Journal of Technology Assessment in Health Care, 24*(2), 193–202.

Isaacman, D. J., Strutton, D. R., Kalpas, E. A., Horowicz-Mehler, N., Stem, L. S., Casciano, R., et al. (2008). The impact of indirect (herd) protection on the cost-effectiveness of pneumococcal conjugate vaccine. *Clinical Therapeutics, 30*(2), 341–357.

Jerrell, J. M., & Hu, T. W. (1996). Estimating the cost impact of three dual diagnosis treatment programs. *Evaluation Review, 20*(2), 160–180.

Lairson, D. R., Yoon, S., Carter, P. M., Greisinger, A. J., Talluri, K. C., Aggarwal, M., et al. (2008). Economic evaluation of an intensified disease management system for patients with type 2 diabetes. *Disease Management, 11*(2), 79–94.

Lieu, T. A., Ray, G. T., Black, S. B., Butler, J. C., Klein, J. O, Brieman, R. F., et al. (2000). Projected cost-effectiveness of pneumococcal conjugate vaccination of healthy infants and young children. *Journal of the American Medical Association, 283*(11), 1460–1468.

Mandelblatt, J. S., Cullen, J., Lawrence, W. F., Stanton, A. L., Yi, B., Kwan, L., et al. (2008). Economic evaluation alongside a clinical trial of psycho-educational interventions to improve adjustment to survivorship among patients with breast cancer. *Journal of Clinical Oncology, 26*(10), 1684–1690.

Newbold, D. (1995). A brief description of the methods of economic appraisal and the valuation of health states. *Journal of Advanced Nursing, 21*(2), 325–333.

Patrick, D. L., & Erickson, P. (1993). *Health status and health policy: Allocating resources to health care.* New York: Oxford University Press.

Prosser, L. A., Koplan, J. P., Neumann, P. J., & Weinstein, M. C. (2000). Barriers to using cost-effectiveness analysis in managed care decision making. *American Journal of Managed Care, 6*(2), 173–187.

Randolph, A. G., & Washington, E. (1990). Screening for *Chlamydia trachomatis* in adolescent males: A cost-based decision analysis. *American Journal of Public Health, 80*(5), 545–550.

Roy, S., & Madhaven, S. S. (2008). Making a case for employing a societal perspective in the evaluation of Medicaid prescription drug interventions. *PharmacoEconomics, 26*(4), 281–296.

Ruger, J. P., & Emmons, K. M. (2008). Economic evaluations of smoking cessation and relapse prevention programs for pregnant women: A systematic review. *Value in Health, 11*(2), 180–190.

Sevick, M., Dunn, A., Morrow, M., Marcus, B., Chen, G. J., & Blair, S. (2000). Cost-effectiveness of lifestyle and structured exercise interventions in sedentary adults: Results of Project ACTIVE. *American Journal of Preventive Medicine, 19*(1), 1–8.

Shaw, J. (1995). Cost benefit analysis in the human services. *Australian Psychologist, 30*(2), 144–148.

Szucs, T. (2000). Cost–benefits of vaccination programmes. *Vaccine, 18*(suppl 1), S49–S51.

Tangka, F. K., Subramanian, S., Bapat, B., Seeff, L. C., DeGroff, A., Gardner, J., et al. (2008). Cost of starting colorectal cancer screening programs: Results from five federally funded demonstration programs. *Prevention and Chronic Disease, 5*(2), A47.

Torrance, G. W., Siegel, J. E., & Luce, B. R. (1996). Framing and designing the cost-effectiveness analysis. In M. R. Gold, J. E. Seigel, L. B. Russell, & M. C. Weinstein (Eds.), *Cost-effectiveness in health and medicine* (pp. 54–81). Oxford, UK: Oxford University Press.

Ubel, P. A., Nord, E., Gold, M., Menzel, P., Prades, J. L., & Richardson, J. (2000). Improving value measurement in cost-effectiveness analysis. *Medical Care, 38*(9), 892–901.

Windsor, R., Bailey, W., Richards, J., Manzella, B., Soong, S., & Brooks, M. (1990). Evaluation of the efficacy and cost effectiveness of health education methods to increase medication adherence among adults with asthma. *American Journal of Public Health, 80*(12), 1519–1521.

Yates, B. T. (1999). *Measuring and improving cost, cost-effectiveness, and cost benefit for substance abuse treatment programs: A manual.* Washington, DC: U.S. Department of Health and Human Services, National Institutes of Health, National Institute for Drug Abuse, Division of Clinical and Services Research.

Section 6

Additional Considerations for Evaluators

CHAPTER 17

Program Evaluators' Responsibilities

A premise throughout this book is that the program planning and evaluation process is a cycle with feedback loops throughout, from assessment and planning through outcome evaluation. Data and information generated by an evaluation do not automatically become a feedback loop; rather, intention and effort are needed to create and maintain the connection between evaluation findings and subsequent planning. Influencing the strength of the feedback loops is a set of evaluator responsibilities—namely, ethical responsibilities, responsibly presenting the data, reporting responsibly, maintaining responsible contacts, being responsible for the evaluation quality, and responsibility for staying current in evaluation practice. These responsibilities of the evaluator, if fulfilled, help ensure that the planning and evaluation cycle continues in a timely and productive manner.

ETHICAL RESPONSIBILITIES

Ethics remains a foremost concern in health care. *Ethics* is the discipline or study of rights, morals, and principles that guide human behavior. Issues become ethical when basic human rights are involved or when dilemmas arise as to what might be the moral and principled course of action. In terms of health program development and program evaluation, the potential for ethical concerns is omnipresent.

Choices regarding who will or will not receive the health program can raise ethical questions. For example, if random assignment is planned, then the ethical question is what to do for those who will not receive the program. Also, the choice of the target population can be subject to ethical questioning. What makes one high-risk or vulnerable group of individuals more or less worthy of receiving a health program can be an ethical issue. It is possible that conflicts regarding the development of a health program are implicitly conflicts of ethical perspectives. The following discussion focuses on the ethics and corresponding legal considerations that are directly related to program evaluation and delivery.

Institutional Review Board Approval and Informed Consent

Ethical issues are most likely to surface with regard to the need to have participants in the evaluation provide informed consent. *Informed consent* is the agreement to voluntarily and willingly participate in a study based on a full disclosure of what constitutes participation in the study and what are the risks and benefits involved in participating. Whether informed consent is used in the evaluation is based on a set of factors: the requirements of the funding agency, the requirements of the agency providing the program, and the intent of the evaluation. If the evaluation will be used only for internal managerial purposes and not to generate knowledge, then the evaluation is not research and informed consent is not required.

In contrast, if the evaluation is done with the intent of generating generalizable knowledge, then the evaluation is considered research. For example, if the findings of the evaluation are to be shared beyond the program agency, as in an academic journal, the evaluation qualifies as research. In that case, evaluators, as researchers, are obligated to comply with federal regulations regarding obtaining informed consent. Universities and healthcare organizations that receive federal research grants have *institutional review boards* (IRBs)—that is, groups that review the proposed research for compliance with the federal regulations governing research involving human subjects. IRBs are composed of researchers, nonresearchers, and representatives from the community at large.

The process of gaining IRB approval for conducting an evaluation is not a trivial issue, but rather warrants serious attention. Even students who are conducting evaluation research need to obtain IRB approval of their research. Three levels of IRB review are distinguished (Table 17.1), with full review being the most comprehensive and involving all members of the IRB. Research may either qualify for expedited review by two members of the IRB or be exempt from IRB review but still required to be registered as human subjects research. Although the exact procedures and forms will vary slightly among IRBs, the responsibilities and reviews are essentially the same because all IRBs follow the same federal regulations—specifically, 45 CFR (Code of Federal Regulations) 46. According to these regulations, informed consent has eight elements (Table 17.2), each of which must be addressed in the consent form. Ideally, the consent form will be written at an eighth-grade reading level. The eight elements can be addressed in brief letters for anonymous surveys or may entail extensive, multiple-page details for studies with risky procedures.

Table 17.1 Comparison of Types of IRB Reviews

Type of Review	Definition Criteria	Process
Full (review by all IRB members)	Involves more than minimal risk, involves knowing the identity of the participants and whether data are sensitive or may put the participant at risk	Requires completing a full IRB application; research must provide copies of all materials (i.e., surveys, consents, recruitment flyers, data abstraction forms, interview questions) that will be used in the research
Expedited (review by two IRB members)	Involves no more than minimal risk and may involve knowing the identity of participants	Requires completing a full IRB application; researcher must provide copies of all materials (i.e., surveys, consents, recruitment flyers, data abstraction forms, interview questions) that will be used in the research
Exempt (from IRB review)	Involves no more than minimal risk, the identity of participants is not known or knowable, routine educational research, food-tasting research	A brief form is completed that describes the research is completed and submitted; usually reviewed by at least one member of the IRB

The highly formalized and bureaucratic procedures involved in obtaining IRB approval often cloud the underlying need to ensure that researchers and evaluators act ethically and that all persons involved in evaluation research be protected from needless harm. Nonetheless, if the evaluation is expected to generate knowledge, the evaluator is obligated to gain IRB approval. IRB approval must be obtained before the evaluation begins, which can be a major issue in the time line of conducting a program evaluation.

Ethics and Evaluation

Marvin (1985) stressed that evaluators have a responsibility to program participants and to evaluation participants to explain how the evaluation has the potential to harm them and future program participants. One point he made is particularly relevant to IRBs and consent forms: If the evaluation has

Table 17.2   Eight Elements of Informed Consent, as Required in 45 CFR 46

1. Statement that makes it clear that the participant is being asked to volunteer to be in a research study (and can withdraw if he or she chooses)

2. Explanation of the purpose of the research

3. Description of the research procedures that details what is expected of the participant (e.g., tasks, length of participation in the intervention and the research, type of data to be collected)

4. Specification of the risks or discomforts that are possible or likely from being in the study

5. Explanation of the direct benefits to the participant, if any are possible or likely, from being in the study

6. Statement of confidentiality and information on how it will be maintained

7. Description of any compensation or payment for being in the study

8. Phone numbers where the participant can get more information about the research, information about his or her right as a research participant, and assistance if there is an injury or other problem resulting from being in the research

potential implications for future programs and their availability, participants have the right to be aware of this fact.

Many health programs are designed for and delivered to children. In such circumstances, the evaluation may need to include collecting data from children. This practice can pose special ethical and IRB problems. Children who are old enough to understand that they are being asked to participate in a study must provide assent to be in the study; this would include their participation in evaluation research. The refusal of either the child or the parent to be part of the evaluation study must be honored. Matters become more complicated when the child becomes older and is increasingly capable of making decisions independently of his or her parents. For example, adolescents in safe-sex education programs may be willing to participate in an evaluation study but may not want their parents to know they are in the program. In this situation, the evaluator must carefully consider the consequences and creatively develop means of including children without denying parental or child rights.

One major consequence of including children in evaluation research is that participation rates may decline when parental consent is required for participation either in the program or in the evaluation. Esbensen and associates (1996) studied the effect of requiring parental consent on participation in an evaluation of a gang prevention program. They achieved a participation rate of 65%, which varied by program site. The researchers were unable to determine the reason that parents failed to provide consent for their children. Johnson and associates (1999) similarly were able to achieve 70% written parental consent but in only 7 of 10 schools involved in a health promotion program. They found that to get parental consent for children to participate in a school program evaluation, a school-based strategy was most cost-effective in reaching the goal of 80% written parental consent. Dynarski (1997) identifies further complications by reminding researchers that consent is needed in experimental evaluations, as occurs when schools are randomized to experimental and control conditions.

Just as children are considered a special vulnerable population, so are many other vulnerable groups for whom health programs are designed and offered. The special circumstances of these groups need to be considered with regard to obtaining consents. For example, Gondolf (2000) found that in evaluating domestic violence programs focused on the batterers, several issues needed to be addressed: maintaining the safety of the victim, tracking in longitudinal studies, and obtaining consent from both the present and past batterers and their corresponding victims. Taking precautions to address these issues resulted in a low refusal rate and few safety problems for participants. Evaluators can use the results of this and similar studies to better estimate the highest possible participation rates and to identify ethical techniques for increasing the participation of children and other highly vulnerable groups in health program evaluations.

Another vulnerable population comprises those in need of emergency care. In anticipation of needing consent for the evaluation of an emergency treatment called PolyHeme, Longfield and colleagues (2008) took the unusual step of assessing the preferences of community members. They found that, despite knowing about the potential benefits of the treatment, 30% would choose not to participate in its evaluation. In population-based programs, the issue of obtaining consent will present challenges that will require creativity and sensitivity to overcome.

Evaluators and program managers also may need to deal with ethical issues related to program staff. Such ethical issues emerge when the health program involves community outreach and the safety of program staff is a major concern. Also, if program staff are participants in the program evaluation, as is likely to occur in process-monitoring evaluations, their rights as study participants need to be taken into account. These rights include confidentiality with regard to the information they provide. Program personnel may themselves face ethical issues with regard to legally mandated reporting of occurrences, such as child abuse and specific infectious diseases (e.g., syphilis, tuberculosis) that must be balanced against their safety or the safety of others involved.

Other factors contributing to ethical issues are financial arrangements, conflicts of interest, level of competence, and deadlines. Each of these factors has the potential to create an ethical dilemma. Another consideration is highlighted by the findings of one study in which evaluators who were employed in private or consulting businesses had different views of what constituted unethical behavior compared to evaluators who were employed in academic settings (Morris & Jacobs, 2000). These results serve as a stark reminder that ethics is both contextual and highly individualized. While principles may be agreed upon, their application may not. Evaluators working closely with stakeholders are likely to encounter a wide range of opinions about ethical behavior. As always, open dialogue and discussion of the ethical issues inherent in the health program or evaluation are the optimal approach to reaching either consensus on actions or comfortable disagreements.

HIPAA and Evaluations

In 2003, the Health Insurance Portability and Accountability Act (HIPAA) went into effect (Center for Medicaid and Medicare Services, 2005; Department of Health and Human Services, 2008). The purpose of HIPAA is to protect personal information related to having received health care. Personal information includes the individual's birth date, any element of an address, dates on which services were received, and diagnoses. Health providers must take specified steps to protect personal identifier information, including having secure fax lines and getting written permission to share personal information with others, whether insurance companies or consulting providers.

The effects of HIPAA on the evaluation of health programs depend on whether the evaluator is an employee of the organization and the evaluation is part of routine care or whether the evaluator is an outsider and the findings of the evaluation will be made public in any way. In the first situation, the evaluation is likely to be small scale and involve an existing program being conducted by program staff. Because personal information about clients or patients is not being shared, evaluators need not take any additional steps with regard to the HIPAA regulations. This situation is similar to the one in which an informed consent would not be needed because the evaluation is not research. However, if client data will be provided to an external evaluator or if the evaluation is federally funded (National Institutes of Health, 2003), then the HIPAA regulations require that each client be informed that his or her information is being provided to others and give a signed authorization for that information release. As implementation of the HIPAA regulations becomes part of the routine functioning of healthcare organizations, evaluators will likely find invaluable those key individuals who can provide guidance on how to meet the regulations.

HIPAA regulations apply only to a specific group of healthcare organizations, typically hospitals, clinics, and physician offices. They do not apply to organizations that do not provide medical care. Thus health programs provided by the latter organizations do not fall under the scope of the regulations, and evaluations of programs in exempt organizations do not require steps beyond the basic ethical considerations discussed earlier.

RESPONSIBLE SPIN OF DATA AND INFORMATION

It is incumbent upon the evaluator to disseminate information about the evaluation to complete the feedback cycle. Several considerations influence the dissemination of program evaluation findings. The first concern focuses on making a persuasive argument based on the data. Once a set of persuasive statements about the program is developed, the next consideration is the logistics of the report format. Finally, evaluators must consider the possibility that the evaluation results will be misused. Each of these considerations is discussed in this section.

Persuasion and Information

A major factor determining the effectiveness of feedback loops is the persuasiveness of the data and the resulting information. Although the word "persuasion" has negative connotations, the reality is that for change to occur and for decisions to be based on evaluation findings, individuals with decision-making authority need to be persuaded by the "facts." Unless the statements made based on the process evaluation and outcome evaluation data are persuasive, no feedback loops will be possible; rather, the program will produce only discrete, disconnected, and unused information.

When using statistical results, Abelson (1995) suggests that five properties of statements govern the degree to which those statements are persuasive: effect magnitude, articulateness, generalizability, interest level, and credibility. *Magnitude* of the intervention effect is the amount of change attributable to the program. The amount of change that can be attributed to the program influences the extent to which the statistical data are perceived as persuasive. One way to think about this issue is to note that people are more inclined to believe good news and, therefore, larger intervention effects increase the persuasiveness of evaluation findings. A corollary of this idea is that people are less likely to persuaded by small program effects, regardless of the potential clinical significance of a small effect. While it would be unethical to conduct an outcome evaluation that is highly biased in favor of the program, the design and methods need to be such that the largest effect theorized can be identified.

Another property of a statement is the degree to which it is *articulate* in explaining the findings. Articulate statements have both clarity and detail. This speaks directly to the quality of the written or verbal report, sometimes referred to as style. Being articulate may require not using statistical terminology in reports intended for stakeholders and policy makers. Recipients of the findings must perceive that the report is clear, regardless of whether the producer of the report feels it is clear. Clarity can be achieved through style, language, use of graphs, and careful delineation of ideas and issues. Similarly, consumers of the evaluation report may have a different need for details compared to the producers of the evaluation report. One strategy for arriving at the optimal level of detail needed to be persuasive is to have someone not involved in the evaluation review the report and make suggestions about what needs to be included. In other words, evaluators should involve a few stakeholders in the development of any written reports that will be disseminated to their peers.

The third property of a statement that contributes to its persuasiveness is the *generalizability* of the conclusions. The wider the applicability of the findings, the more likely those findings are to be persuasive. The notion that having highly generalizable findings makes the findings more persuasive runs counter to a more popular line of reasoning in the health field—namely, that results must be tailored to the unique characteristics of the program participants, especially race, ethnicity, sexual orientation, and such. While it is imperative to consider the effect of the unique needs and perspectives of the program recipients to have an effective program, when it comes to influencing decisions, policy makers want information that will make the decision widely applicable. As a consequence, they often seek results that are generic, rather than specific. In addition, there is an intuitive sense that if something applies to many, it must reflect some underlying truth. Whether this line of reasoning is accurate is less important than acknowledging that as human beings we may instinctively think this way.

The fourth characteristic of persuasive statements is the degree to which the findings are *interesting* with regard to challenging current beliefs. When the findings are a surprise, more attention is paid to them. Similarly, if the findings make important claims or deal with important behaviors, the statements will receive more attention and be more persuasive. Another way of thinking about this characteristic is that if the evaluation does not answer the "So what?" question or merely confirms the obvious, the findings will be less persuasive. Findings that are surprising, unexpected, or not immediately explainable and those that are important become sound bites that are used to get attention and influence perceptions.

Lastly, if the findings have *credibility* in terms of being based on rigorous and sound methods and a coherent theory, the findings will be more persuasive. The bottom line: If the evaluation methods, design, data collection, or analyses are flawed, the findings lose credibility and persuasiveness. Of course, a coherent theory is also needed for the findings to have credibility and persuasiveness. A coherent theory such as a causal theory explains the findings in terms of relationships among the program intervention and outcome and impacts. Such a theory decreases the possibility of claims that findings happen by chance.

Patton (1997) has suggested that both the strength of the evaluation claim, like the first of Abelson's statement properties, and its importance to the decision makers are crucial to the evaluation being of value. If we extend Patton's two dimensions to encompass intervention effect and interest values, the result is a matrix demonstrating that the influence of these characteristics on decision making varies (Table 17.3). Unimportant claims that are not interesting and that reveal a low level of intervention effect based on weak rigor are quickly forgotten. Claims that are important and interesting, are based on good science, and show large program effects are readily used as the basis for decision making. The matrix hints at the challenges that must be overcome to generate claims that will be used in decision making, including subsequent program or evaluation decisions.

Information and Sense Making

Steps taken to turn data into persuasive information are important, but so is the process by which sense is made of information. *Sense making* (Weick,

Table 17.3   Effect of Rigor and Importance of Claims on Decision Making

Strength of Claim	Quality of Claim	
	Major Importance, High Interest	**Minor Importance, Low Interest**
High Rigor and Effect	Ideal for making decisions	Becomes "factoid"
Low Rigor and Effect	Cause for concern, need to study further, tentativeness to decisions	Ignored, forgotten, unspoken

Source: Adapted from Patton, 1997.

1979, 1995) involves attributing meaning to information. Understanding the psychological processes used by individuals to interpret information in order to make decisions is the other side of the persuasion coin. Data become information only when they are given meaning. The process of giving meaning involves various human perceptual and judgment-making processes; these processes, in turn, ultimately influence the decision-making process and, therefore, are important for health program planners and evaluators.

Several well-recognized phenomena are now widely accepted as affecting decision making. These include the unconscious use of a set of heuristics in making judgments (Tversky & Kahneman, 1974) and the use of hindsight bias and consequences to make judgments (Chapman & Elstein, 2000; Fischhoff, 1975), which is also called retrospective sense making (Weick, 1979, 1995) or the one-of-us effect (Hastorf & Cantril, 1954). Each of these cognitive processing phenomena has potential consequences for program planners and evaluators.

For example, Lipshitz, Gilad, and Suleiman (2000) studied the effect of having information about the outcomes on the perception of events. They found that the perception that the subject was "one of us" was dramatically altered depending on whether the subject's success or failure was met with reward or punishment. The findings from their study underscore the importance of the sociocultural context of decision making, especially with regard to situations in which there are clear failures and successes and when both rewards and sanctions are possible. These findings have relevance to the presentation of evaluation information. They suggest that if the evaluator is *not* viewed as "one of us," then failures of either the program or the evaluation are more likely to be met with sanctions. In other words, evaluators who become aligned with the stakeholders are less likely to experience repercussions. This same psychological phenomenon applies to program staff: If the policy and organizational decision makers view program staff as "one of us," then the program staff are less likely to experience sanctions if the program is not successful.

Culture is another factor that can affect interpretation of data. Culturally based values, ways of thinking, and experiences influence the meaning attributed to results. One key area in which this factor may become evident is in discussions about which program changes need to occur. Just as there is a need for cultural competence in the design of the health program, so there is a need for cultural competence in terms of organizational competence to make or guide the implementation of program changes based on data about the program theory or the effect theory.

A recognition of the cognitive elements in interpreting data, whether related to decision making or culture, highlights the intricate nature of facts and interpretations. It is easy to believe that having factual data will always result in a detached, logically derived decision. In reality, evidence from decision science and psychology (not to mention one's own experience) does not fully support this proposition. Evaluators and program planners need not only to attend to the science of their work, but also to apply the science of decision making and attribution.

REPORTING RESPONSIBLY

Report Writing

Evaluators are required to generate written reports and perhaps to make oral presentations of the findings. The notions of persuasiveness and the malleable nature of interpretations are part of the context for these reports. Typically, the format of a report is tailored to the evaluation and overall situation. In some instances, however, the format is very specific and the evaluator has minimal flexibility in the report format, as is the case with state or federal grants. Typically, reports related to federal programs are submitted over the Internet, using predetermined forms that place strict limits on the number of words or characters. If the evaluator is not the one submitting the forms, it will be critical to work with program personnel in advance so that they have the information required for reporting to the funding agency. In addition to the reporting required by the funding agency, the evaluator may be asked to prepare a longer narrative report.

To the extent possible, a report ought to relate findings to the program process and outcome objectives. This linkage might utilize a table format, in which each objective is listed and the corresponding evaluation results are presented. Such a table will provide a visual context in which the audience can clearly see in which areas the program was more and less successful in meeting its objectives.

Evaluation reports generally contain an executive summary, background on the program and evaluation, a description of the program, a description of the evaluation, and a summary and recommendations. The content and style used for writing the report ought to be tailored to its audience. Gabriel (2000) has argued that because of the ever-evolving nature of the evaluations of health programs, evaluation reports and reporting strategies ought to forgo the usual research format that emphasizes data analysis and instead focus on providing evaluation information to the decision makers and program stakeholders as expediently and accurately as possible.

An *executive summary* is a one- or two-page synopsis of the program, its evaluation, and the recommendations. This portion of the report is most likely to be copied and distributed and, therefore, is likely to be the most widely read part. It ought to contain enough information to convince any reader that the program and evaluation designs were appropriate. The length of the executive summary depends on its anticipated use and reporting requirements.

As mentioned earlier, evaluators often will be asked or required to give an oral presentation of the evaluation plan or results. The first consideration when preparing such a presentation is the audience: Will it be staff, program participants, policy makers, or other researchers? The answer to this question will influence the content to be covered as well as the choice of which details will be of greatest interest to the audience. Use of software such as Microsoft PowerPoint can greatly facilitate generating an outline of the presentation and can simplify making appropriately designed slides. The material on each slide should be displayed in large print, with no more than one idea per slide and no more than seven or eight lines of text. Audiences have also become accustomed to receiving handouts of the presentation, but carefully consider what is on the handout and whether it is wise and timely to make that information widely available. If the evaluation has been done in a manner that has involved the stakeholders throughout the process, there should not be any surprises, and release of the information will not be an issue. In less ideal situations, caution may be in order.

The use of charts and graphics is important when writing reports. The old adage that a picture is worth a thousand words is true: Exhibits are more likely to be remembered than text. While not every number needs to be graphed, having no graphic representations makes reports dense, potentially boring, and less persuasive. All exhibits—whether graphs, charts, figures, or tables— ought to contribute to the ease of understanding and remembering critical points, rather than only being fancy additions that demonstrate the author's skill with a software program. The rationale for including the exhibit needs to be made explicit. The choice of what is presented graphically is in part a way to influence perceptions, attention, and hence decision making.

A list of suggestions for creating good graphics, drawing upon the recommendations given by Good and Hardin (2006), appears in Table 17.4. Findings that are surprising, confirming, alarming, or interesting are appropriate choices for being illustrated with exhibits. Readily available software makes generating exhibits and integrating them into written reports quite easy. Exhibits should follow convention regarding which variable is on which axis. For example, time is best plotted on the horizontal axis (x-axis). It is essential that some explanatory text accompany all exhibits, as not all readers will be able to interpret graphic presentations. For some reports, it may be necessary to be creative in the presentation of findings. For example, Dyer, Goodwin, Pickens-Pace, Burnet, and Kelly (2007) used a Venn diagram to convey the

Table 17.4   List of Ways to Make Graphs More Interpretable

- Only display graphs for ideas that are more easily explained with visual aids. Limit graphs to those that show key variables and crucial ideas.

- Use only as many dimensions in the graph as there are dimension in the data. For this reason, do not use three-dimensional bar graphs.

- Place the labels where they do not interfere with seeing the data. For example, keep all axis labels and tick marks on the outermost sides.

- Carefully select the range of the axis values to be realistic and reasonable. Choose a range of values closest to those in the data.

- Use numerical labels only if the data are numerical. For categorical or nominal data, give the category title.

- Create line graphs only if the data points reflect a trend.

- Give your graphic a full title that explains the contents of the graphic. Titles need not always be short.

- Careful choice of variables and scale is much more important than choice of color scheme. Spend most of your time choosing and adjusting the numeric information.

proportion of individuals with abnormal assessment scale scores and to illustrate how proportions of individuals with overlapping (concurrent) abnormal scores were distributed. Their use of multiple overlapping circles was needed to show that of the 22% of individuals with depression, 8% also had inadequate activities of daily living and impaired cognitive functions.

Making Recommendations

Making recommendations, whether in a report or verbally, can tax the interpersonal and political skills of an evaluator. Recommendations can focus on the positive aspects that were identified through the evaluation as well as on areas needing change or improvement. They must be based on, and be a direct and clear outgrowth of, the evaluation data. Recommendations ought to be linked to the program theory and should address the organizational and service utilization plan (Figure 17.1), identifying specific elements in need of improvement. Likewise, the recommendations can address elements of the program theory (Figure 17.1) by specifying which of the hypotheses seem not to be supported by the evaluation data and indicating alternative hypotheses

Figure 17.1   Making Recommendations Related to the Organizational and Services Utilization Plans

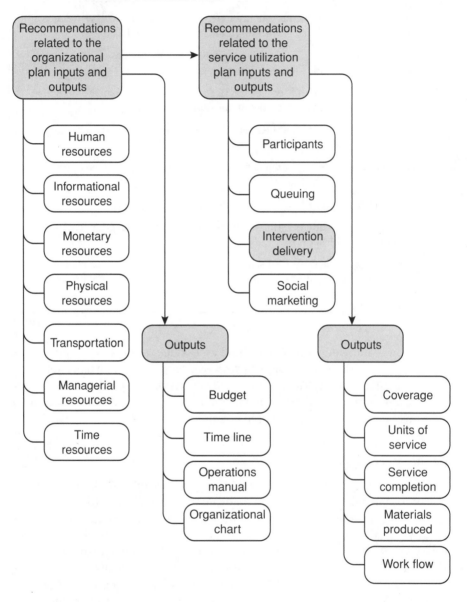

that could be used to explain the findings. Framing the recommendations in accordance with the way the program was conceptualized will help program managers and other stakeholders make decisions regarding what needs to be or can be done and in what order of priority (Figure 17.2). Also, recommendations that are linked to elements of the program theory are more likely to be readily understood and hold higher credibility. The following information regarding recommendations frames the "dos and don'ts" suggested by Hendricks and Papagiannis (1990) within the context of program theory.

Throughout the development and evaluation of the health program, recommendations can be collected so that good ideas and insights are not lost or forgotten. Also, a wide variety of resources can be the basis of making recommendations, including existing scientific literature, program staff, and program stakeholders. Drawing on such sources for explanation or justification

Figure 17.2   Making Recommendations Related to the Program Theory

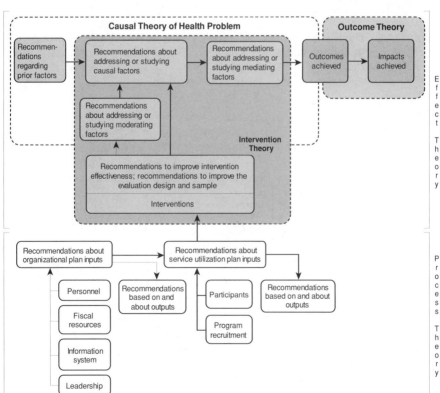

of the recommendations adds to their credibility. Obviously, it is important to work closely with the program decision makers, including during the process of developing the recommendations. This approach will minimize the possibility of surprises being included in the report, thereby decreasing the risk of being perceived as undermining the program. Working with the decision makers also begins to build support for the recommendations.

Recommendations ought to make sense in the larger context in which the program and the evaluation occurred, including in the social, political, and organizational contexts; in the context of the technical knowledge available when the program was conceived; and throughout the planning and evaluation cycle (Figure 17.3). Recommendations that show knowledge of the contextual influences can more easily be accepted as applicable and may lead to changes in various elements of the program theory. Recommendations that are realistic in the view of the stakeholders are more likely to be accepted and implemented. Of course, this does not negate the need to make appropriate recommendations that may take time to implement or that could be implemented

Figure 17.3   The Planning and Evaluation Cycle with Potential Points for Recommendations

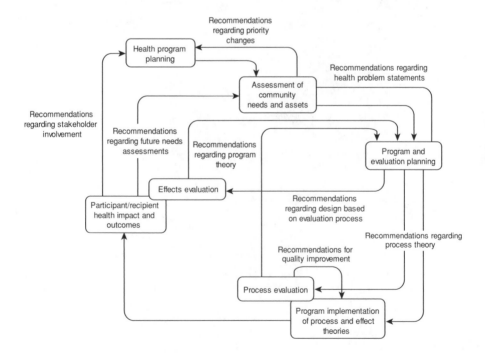

under different circumstances. Not all recommendations need to be equal in terms of the effort required to implement them, or in terms of specificity and generality. Decision makers generally prefer choosing from a set of recommendations, so that they maintain their positions as decision makers.

Recommendations that require a fundamental change, such as to the program theory, are less likely to be accepted or implemented than recommendations that call for less extensive change. The former recommendations are best made in an incremental format so that they are simplified and, hence, more acceptable and useful to the decision makers. It also helps to provide some accompanying statements or insights into future implications of the recommendations, such as potential benefits or implementation strategies. Again, this type of information facilitates the decision making regarding which recommendations to act upon. Of course, recommendations that are easy to understand will receive more attention and acceptance. Techniques for improving the ease of comprehension include categorizing the recommendations in meaningful ways, drawing a boundary between the findings and the recommendations, placing the recommendations in a meaningful and appropriate position in the report, and presenting the recommendations in ways that the decision makers are accustomed to receiving information.

Misuse of Evaluations

Given the pressures to sustain programs and to meet funding mandates, evaluation results may sometimes be misused. Misuse can occur in many ways, but is generally understood to consist of the manipulation of the evaluation in ways that distort the findings or that compromise the integrity of the evaluation. Misuse can occur at any point during the evaluation process, beginning with an inappropriately chosen design that will bias findings, and extending to interference with data collection and the outright alteration of the evaluation findings (Stevens & Dial, 1994). Evaluators, program management, program staff, stakeholders, and program participants involved in an evaluation can all be susceptible to a variety of pressures that may result in a less than unbiased evaluation. These pressures include biases based on resource constraints and self-interest, as well as external political and funding agency pressures. Pressures can also come from within the organization providing the health program. Such pressures affect not only the evaluation design and execution, but also the manner in which the results are interpreted, used, and disseminated or suppressed.

Patton (1997) has argued that increases in the use of evaluation information are accompanied by increases in the misuse of that information. This relationship is a function of the increased opportunity for the pressures leading to misuse to be present. Program planners and evaluators must recognize that misuse can be either intentional, such as falsifying client satisfaction responses, or unintentional, such as not having enough time to distribute client satisfaction surveys on busy days. Sometimes the pressures for misuse are subtle and responses are almost subconscious; in fact, the intention might even be to help the program. Such complexities add to the difficulty of detecting and avoiding misuse.

One way to minimize the potential for misuse is to involve program stakeholders and educate them about the evaluation and its appropriate use. For example, it may be important not only to publicize favorable findings, but also to acknowledge unfavorable findings and the plans to address those findings. In addition, sharing with the stakeholders and program staff the standards to which evaluators are held by their professional organization may help them realize that the use of evaluation is not just a funding or sustainability issue, but also an ethical issue.

Broader Dissemination

Most recommendations and reports are intended for internal program use and are distributed only to key program stakeholders and staff. In contrast, broader dissemination of lessons learned can be important for the dissemination of the program. For programs that were the subject of evaluation research because they were novel or experimental, the findings from those evaluations ought to be disseminated broadly as a contribution to the science and the literature. Equally important is dissemination of information to ensure program fidelity and to serve as general guidelines for subsequent program development. One question to consider is what influences the dissemination and uptake of program intervention ideas. Brownson and associates (2007), in seeking to answer this question, found a difference between state health department practitioners and local health department staff in terms of implementation of recommended programs. Thus there is no one way to ensure broad dissemination and program uptake.

Broader dissemination includes making the report more widely accessible—for example, at the program website or the website of the evaluator. It also includes publishing the findings in academic and practice journals so that a broader audience can become aware of the effectiveness of the interventions as well as the issues involved in implementing the program. Having the evaluation published in peer-reviewed and practice journals helps ensure that the evaluation findings become part of the evidence to be used in future program development efforts. However, as Gorman and Conde (2007) point out, a conflict of interest may arise when the published program evaluation was conducted by the program developer. Accordingly, the consumer of published evaluation reports ought to be sensitive to this possibility.

Involving and Negotiating with Program Partners

To more broadly disseminate the findings from either the process or effect evaluations may first require some negotiation with program partners. Specifically, in addition to addressing the ethics of obtaining informed consent for participation in the evaluation, evaluators will need to negotiate authorship, publication outlet, and manuscript content before submitting a manuscript for publication. The negotiation on these and similar points will go more smoothly if program partners and stakeholders have been involved throughout the evaluation and report preparation phases. Even so, because egos and reputations may be at stake, additional attention and negotiations may necessary.

Expansions and Replications

Related to dissemination is the diffusion or replication of programs, as well as the sustainability or expansion of existing programs. Fisher et al. (2007), for example, reported that the findings from 14 demonstration projects related to diabetes self-management would be disseminated in hopes of the programs being implemented more broadly across clinical settings. In contrast, the study by Hill, Maucicone, and Hood (2007), which explored adaptations of programs, is a stark reminder that limits on time and resources pose serious threats to the replication of programs in a manner that maintains fidelity to the interventions. As a program moves into a new planning cycle, reassessment of the local capacity to deliver the program may be in order. For example, Alfonso and others (2008) conducted a capacity assessment to determine the sustainability of a physical activity program for children. Through community involvement, they were able to identify strategic activities necessary for program sustainability. Their work reinforces the cyclic nature of program planning.

RESPONSIBLE CONTRACTS

Organization–Evaluator Relationship

The relationship between the evaluator and the organization is one that requires attention, whether the evaluator is an employee or an external consultant. Several factors can influence or shape this relationship. For example, if the evaluator is a third party between the program or organization and the funding agency, third-party dynamics come into play. That is, two parties may form a coalition against the third. The most likely scenario would be for the program manager to align with the funding agency in any dispute with the evaluator. Another factor influencing the evaluator–organization relationship is the different levels of priority given by the evaluator and the organization to the health program and the possible changes in these priorities. Such differences in priorities can lead to different time lines, different expectations, and different levels of commitment in terms of attention and resources. Yet another factor affecting the relationship between the evaluator and the organization is differences in professional and organizational cultures and in the language used to describe the health program and the evaluation. Divergences in any of these areas can become a source of tension and conflict, especially if the divergence is not explicitly acknowledged. This list of possible factors affecting the relationship of the evaluator and the organization of the health program, although certainly not exhaustive, reveals the complexities of the relationship, which deserve attention and merit the development of strategies and dialogues to optimize the relationship.

Another area of possible divergence is the broader purpose of the evaluation. Owen and Lambert (1998) have suggested that evaluation for management is different from evaluation for leadership. They claim that evaluation for management focuses on individual units or programs for the purpose of making ongoing adjustments with an emphasis on performance and accountability; this is essentially a process-monitoring evaluation. In contrast, evaluation for leadership focuses on the whole organization, with a long-term perspective and collection of information across programs.

Owen and Lambert (1998) also note that the roles of evaluator and organizational development consultant become blurred, particularly if the evaluator is asked to provide recommendations. In fact, Patton (1999) has argued that evaluators have numerous opportunities to act as organizational development consultants. He explains that, because programs are embedded in organizational contexts, improving programs may require attention to that organizational context. Patton found, through a case study, that the attainment of project goals is not necessarily related to the extent to which the program contributes to the fulfillment of the organizational mission. In other words, some programs are very good at doing the wrong thing when viewed from the perspective of the organization's business strategy. Being aware of this potential paradox and addressing it is one way in which evaluators contribute to organizational development.

Evaluators may see themselves, or be seen by others, as agents for organizational change. As change agents, evaluators need to be conscious about how change occurs; a prerequisite for change is organizational readiness. The type of organization being changed is a further consideration—namely, whether it is a small, community-based, not-for-profit agency or a large federal bureaucracy. Evaluators can influence organizational decision making by first having affected or changed the perceptions held by those who are decision makers for the program. This can occur through the recommendations made at the end of an evaluation, or through continual rather than sporadic involvement with the program. Education of stakeholders throughout the planning and evaluation cycle, and through personal perseverance with regard to dissemination of information and accessing decision makers, can also contribute to some degree of organizational change. In the end, the evaluator's skills in generating an understanding of what is needed from the organization must be matched to the organizational type, culture, and readiness for change.

An early point of discussion between the planner/evaluator and the hiring organization needs to focus on who owns the data that are gathered and analyzed throughout the planning and evaluation cycle. Generally, planners and evaluators who are hired as consultants have very limited proprietary rights over the data. The contract with the hiring organization will specify who owns the data and what can and cannot be done with it. An external evaluator needs some leeway and latitude so that potentially unfavorable findings can be seen by those who need to know about them. Getting the information to the decision makers is essential if the evaluation—whether a process-monitoring or effect evaluation—is to serve as an effective feedback loop that fosters the development of the health program and the organizational functioning. Evaluators who cannot express concerns to key decision makers will be frustrated and are essentially divested of their proper responsibility. Ownership of data and dissemination of findings can become not only an internal political issue but also an ethical issue in terms of getting the results to decision makers and to making public the research findings, which can influence choices. The underlying issue is that evaluators may have a different perspective and interpretation of the evaluation results than members of the hiring organization; this divergence may lead to conflict and tension.

The organization is also a context for ethical dilemmas. Mathison (1999) has suggested that there are minimal differences in the ethical dilemmas faced by internal and external evaluators. However, the two parties live in different environments, which inevitably influence their actions or responses to ethical situations. Ultimately, evaluators need to be clear on their relationship with the organization and their role vis-à-vis ethical factors.

Health Policy

The interface between program evaluation and health policy can be intricate and complicated. There are two general situations in which health policy becomes the focus of action. One situation arises when an independent program evaluation has been done and the stakeholders are attempting to use the evaluation findings to change health policy. VanLandingham (2006) suggests that two strategies are needed to increase the use of evaluation results for making policy changes. One strategy is to develop communication networks that allow for exchange of information with legislative stakeholders, including to enable their input into the evaluation design and process. The other strategy is to effectively communicate the evaluation results in a manner that is readily understandable and actionable, as was discussed earlier. Actionable evidence is a potential sticking point, as Julnes and Rog (2007) note. Each source of evidence, whether from outcome research, literature synthesis, or practice, has imperfections that make action based on that data less than foolproof. These sorts of flaws create a barrier to using evaluation results for policy making or legislation.

The other situation in which health policy becomes the focus of action arises when the evaluation is done under contract to a governmental agency of a government-sponsored program. In this situation, there can be pressures related not only to the way the evaluation question is framed, but also to the methodology used in the outcome evaluation (Chelimsky, 2007). At the heart of these pressures is the political agenda for finding supportive or disconfirming evidence for the program. The pressures to uphold current policy or to provide actionable findings for making policy change can be most easily seen with population-level programs that are governed by health policy, such as Medicaid and Medicare, SCHIP, WIC, and other federal programs. Given the longevity and popularity of these programs, the pressures might be relatively small when compared to evaluations of discrete, discretionary, and controversial programs, such as the Just Say No program or abstinence-only programs. Program evaluators who are faced with these pressures may need to make both politically and personally uncomfortable decisions about how to proceed.

RESPONSIBLE FOR EVALUATION QUALITY

There are three main approaches to assessing the quality of a program evaluation. One approach is to determine whether the evaluation met the Program Evaluation Standards of the American Evaluation Association (http://www .eval.org). The Joint Commission on Standards for Educational Evaluation has created standards for evaluation practice (see Table 1.2); these standards of utility, feasibility, propriety, and accuracy remain cornerstones for assessing the quality of health program evaluations. To achieve the feasibility standard, the evaluation must be developed and implemented with the same careful planning as was required to develop and implement the health program.

Evaluations must be conducted in ethical and legal ways that are unbiased and sensitive to the vulnerability and rights of all program and evaluation participants, which requires attention to ethical, legal, and moral parameters. Lastly, evaluations must collect appropriate and accurate data that are consistent with the purpose of the evaluation and the health program being evaluated. According to this perspective, the scientific rigor of the evaluation is only one of four criteria by which a health program evaluation can be assessed.

A second approach is to confer with the users of the evaluation for their perspective on its usefulness. Evaluations need to be useful in meeting the needs of the program stakeholders, program audiences, and funding agencies. This requires communication, dialogue, and negotiation. Evaluations must be feasible in terms of cost, political and diplomatic factors, and time lines.

The third approach is to assess the evaluation in terms of its scientific rigor. The elements of a rigorous evaluation were presented throughout this textbook. One element is that the conceptual foundation of the evaluation should be explicitly stated, including the use of biological, social, psychological, or other theories relevant to the program effect theory (Chapter 6) and references made to previous evaluations of the same health problem. Another element is that the evaluation question should be clearly stated and should focus on identifying the effects of the program (Chapter 11). This emphasis on effects and outcomes is consistent with the purpose of meta-evaluations and evidence-based reviews to identify the most effective intervention for the stated health problem. Next, the evaluation design must be valid, credible, and feasible (Chapter 12). In other words, the scientific rigor of the design must be evident in the published findings or the report. A high-quality evaluation of outcomes also includes attention to multiple health domains of the outcome, using existing reliable measures (Chapter 13) and multiple modes of data collection when necessary or scientifically justified (Chapters 13 and 15). The attention to multiple domains stems from the multiple components and multiple facets of health that might be affected by the health program. An optimal design includes random assignment to the program but does not compromise the provision of the health service to those not receiving the program. It also includes careful selection of program sites and careful attention to incentives for participating in the evaluation. Lastly, the data analysis methods must be appropriate for the data collected and the evaluation question (Chapter 14).

Mohan and Sullivan (2006) summarize key characteristics, explicit or implicit across the various standards, that apply to evaluators: maintain independence, report conflicts of interest, maintain confidentiality of information, and keep records of the evaluation process. Of course, each of these elements can be addressed to varying degrees, and rarely will any one evaluation address all elements to perfection. These criteria also provide an outline that evaluators can follow to avoid evaluation failure and that ought to serve as a reminder of the challenges inherent in program evaluation.

The term "meta-evaluation" has been used since at least 1982 (Feather, 1982). One type of meta-evaluation focuses on programs either funded by or provided by a particular agency; such an evaluation seeks to understand the overall effectiveness of programs associated with that agency. Agency-based meta-evaluations are done using existing evaluations conducted by programs related to that agency. Major philanthropic foundations and large public health agencies are the types of agencies likely to engage in this type of meta-evaluation.

RESPONSIBLE FOR CURRENT PRACTICE

RE-AIM and Other Models

The discipline of evaluation continues to evolve, with the constant emergence of new concepts, updates to approaches, and development of new models that synthesize key elements. Throughout this textbook, the intent has been to provide a historical and general overview of program planning and evaluation, without advocating for any particular model. Responsible evaluation practice includes staying current with these developments in the field both to enhance one's own evaluation practice and to be able to respond to questions about the "latest and greatest" models and trends. The value of models of planning and evaluation is that they allow the user to quickly sort ideas, tasks, and considerations into recognizable patterns that can be easily remembered.

One such model is RE-AIM, which stands for Reach, Effectiveness, Adoption, Implementation, and Maintenance. The RE-AIM framework can be used to organize a flowchart of program activities (Farris, Will, Khavjou, & Finkelstein, 2007) or to compare two programs on summary indices (Glasgow, Nelson, Strycker, & King, 2006). The RE-AIM framework is intended for individual behavioral change programs. As such, it is more difficult to apply to programs at the population or infrastructure levels of the public health pyramid.

Meta-analysis

Meta-analysis is the analysis and synthesis of findings from previous studies in an attempt to draw conclusions across a variety of data sets and samples about the strength of relationships among variables or the effectiveness of an intervention. Meta-analysis is very similar to evidence-based approaches to medicine, in which the optimal, most effective intervention is sought based on a synthesis of existing research. In fact, the methods for conducting meta-analyses are similar to those for generating evidence-based practice guidelines.

The steps in a meta-analysis for program development—especially for intervention selection—begin with a comprehensive search for existing evaluations on the health problem or intervention of interest. The advent of electronic databases of published evaluation research makes it easy to search for existing evaluations from which to draw conclusions about effective interventions and programs. Once all relevant research has been located using a variety of techniques (Cooper, 1998), a systematic review of each publication is conducted. From the information abstracted about the studies reviewed, a synthesis is done that results in conclusions based on all relevant research or evaluations. The conclusions drawn from meta-analyses and evidence-based reviews are valuable because the techniques used in such assessments overcome the pitfalls inherent in relying on only one study or evaluation to make decisions. In addition, when meta-analytic statistics are used in conjunction with the review, the meta-evaluation results are adjusted for variations in the sample sizes of the original studies or evaluations.

Meta-analyses certainly have a place in health program planning and evaluation. For example, Boyd and Windsor (1993) did a meta-analysis of prenatal nutrition programs and later of smoking-cessation programs among pregnant women (Windsor, Boyd, & Orleans, 1998). According to Cooper (1998), both of these studies would be considered systematic literature reviews rather than meta-analyses, because they did not present any summative statistics across the evaluations. Nonetheless, the use of meta-evaluation and evidence-based approaches has led to some proactive thinking about health programs. For example, Robinson, Patrick, Eng, and Gustafson (1998) proposed a framework for reporting evaluations of the use of interactive health communications, such as websites. The purpose of their framework is to systematically develop a body of information that can be used to determine the effectiveness of the interactive health communications. Because such coordinated efforts are not likely to be widely adopted, reliance on the diverse evaluation studies is likely to remain the primary source of meta-evaluations and evidence-based reviews.

Whether meta-analyses are conducted using extensive published evaluations or in-house reports, they are a means of synthesizing information across programs, across agencies, or across recipient populations. A major step in conducting meta-analyses and evidence-based reviews is to determine the quality of the evaluation research included in the systematic review. A wide variety of tools and criteria have been developed for use in systematically evaluating the quality of the intervention and evaluation research. West, King, Carey, & Lohr (2002) summarize these tools and the corresponding criteria into 11 items. Because published reports vary in what may be reported as well as in how rigorous the evaluation was, it can be very helpful to have a standardized tool to assess the reports and then summarize the literature.

ACROSS THE PYRAMID

At the direct services level of the public health pyramid, the concern is with how the processes discussed in this chapter ultimately affect the quality, type, and existence of the direct services health program. Most of the processes discussed occur at the infrastructure level but can subsequently affect decisions regarding what is done at this level of the pyramid. Nonetheless, informed consent from program and evaluation participants is most likely to be obtained at this level of the pyramid because health programs at the direct services level involve individuals who are accessible for obtaining consent. Meta-analyses, along with evidence-based reviews, are likely to focus on direct services and programs, as they are widely studied and evaluated.

At the enabling services level, obtaining informed consent for participation in the health program and evaluation may be feasible and, therefore, necessary. The interpretations and sense making of groups is different from that of individuals or of populations. This may be an important consideration in reporting the evaluation findings. Also, aggregates and groups are often the recipients of enabling services and programs, making their participation both feasible and helpful in generating recommendations.

At the population-based level, the issue of informed consent becomes blurred with the implementation of health policy, because consent is almost always implied by the passage of the health policies. Nonetheless, as Davis and Lantos (2000) point out, ethical considerations pervade population-level services. These authors caution that if sanctions are attached to a failure to comply with required services, such as immunization, harm may be done. Unfortunately, the nature of the harm is likely to be overlooked by policy makers when health policy is formulated and evaluated, because policy makers tend to focus on the benefits. Because population-based services are so closely linked to health policy, the processes that occur at the infrastructure level are critical in determining the nature and scope of health programs at this level of the pyramid. However, the growing body of evaluations of population-based health services, often couched as health policy studies, can lead to meta-evaluations and evidence-based practice for population-based services.

At the infrastructure level of the public health pyramid, although sense making occurs within individuals, the collective processes by which organizations and policy makers achieve a shared understanding and interpretation of evaluation findings leads to policy decisions regarding health programs. Policy adoption and program implementation are two possible uses for evaluations

(McClintock & Colosi, 1998). Recommendations are given to the decision makers, and decisions regarding health program implementation are made. At some point in this process, the organizational, contextual issues become evident. This evolution is reflected in the findings from Brownson, Ballew, Dieffenderfer, et al. (2007) that, although state health officials may be aware of effective programs, they may not have authority, budget resources, staffing, or legislative support to implement those programs. Also, approaches to improving organizational processes are essentially infrastructure processes that have consequences for programs at the other levels of the public health pyramid. Decision makers, who are part of the infrastructure, may need to reconcile differences between organizational process improvement and evaluation with regard to perspectives and recommendations. Lastly, procedures for dealing with ethical issues and IRB and HIPAA procedures must emanate from the infrastructure level and be consistently applied throughout the pyramid levels.

DISCUSSION QUESTIONS AND ACTIVITIES

1. At each level of the public health pyramid, identify at least two factors that can affect the acquisition of informed consent from those involved in providing evaluation data about a health program.

2. What might be some effective strategies to prevent the various misuses of evaluations that were described?

3. In what ways might evidence-based practice (of any of the health disciplines) benefit from a meta-evaluation of programs to address a given health problem?

4. Using evaluation findings as part of feedback loops to improve or sustain health programs is predicated on a set of assumptions about humans and decision makers. What might be some of the assumptions that underlie this perspective? What, if anything, can be done to overcome, address, or deal with those assumptions to create more effective feedback loops?

INTERNET RESOURCES

Health Insurance Portability and Accountability Act

There are several websites specific to the HIPAA regulations, such as federal websites (http://www.hhs.gov/ocr/hipaa/ and http://www.hipaadvisory.com/REGS/HIPAAprimer.htm) and, perhaps not surprisingly, a Wikipedia entry (http://en.wikipedia.org/wiki/HIPAA).

Human Studies

A number of websites focus on the protection of human subjects, including those operated by the Department of Health and Human Services (http://www.hhs.gov/ohrp/) and various universities, such as the website operated by the University of Minnesota (http://www.research.umn.edu/irb/_.

RE-AIM Model

The official website for RE-AIM is found at http://www.re-aim.org/; it has many useful resources.

Research Quality

Various resources exist to help check on overall quality. For example, this paper by West and colleagues deals with assessing the quality of research: http://www.ncbi.nlm.nih.gov/books/bv.fcgi?rid=hstat1.chapter.70996. The Key Evaluation Checklist by a renowned evaluation center is also helpful throughout the research process: http://www.wmich.edu/evalctr/checklists/kec_april05.pdf.

REFERENCES

Abelson, R. P. (1995). *Statistics as principled argument*. Hillsdale, NJ: Lawrence Erlbaum Associates.

Alfonso, M. L., Nickelson, J., Hogeboom, D. L., French, J., Bryant, C. A., McDermott, R. J., et al. (2008). Assessing local capacity for health intervention. *Evaluation and Program Planning*, *31*(2), 145–159.

Boyd, N. R., & Windsor, R. A. (1993). A meta-evaluation of nutrition education intervention research among pregnant women. *Health Education Quarterly*, *20*(3), 327–345.

Brownson, R. C., Ballew, P., Brown, K. L., Elliott, M. B., Haire-Joshu, D., Health, G. W., et al. (2007). The effect of disseminating evidence-based interventions that promote physical activity to health departments. *American Journal of Public Health*, *97*, 1900–1907.

Brownson, R. C., Ballew, P., Dieffenderfer, B., Haire-Johu, D., Health, G. W., Kreuter, M. W., et al. (2007). Evidence-based interventions to promote physical activity: What contributes to dissemination by state health departments. *American Journal of Preventive Medicine*, *33*(1 suppl), S66–S78.

Center for Medicaid and Medicare Services. (2005). The Health Insurance Portability and Accountability Act of 1996 (HIPAA). Retrieved May 29, 2008, from http://www.cms.hhs.gov/HIPAAGenInfo/Downloads/HIPAALaw.pdf

Chapman, G. B., & Elstein, A. S. (2000). Cognitive processes and biases in medical decision making. In G. B. Chapman & F. A. Sonnenberg (Eds.), *Decision making in health care: Theory, psychology, and applications* (pp. 183–210). Cambridge, UK: Cambridge University Press.

Chelimsky, E. (2007). Factors influencing the choice of methods in federal evaluation practice. *New Directions for Evaluation, 113*, 13–33.

Cooper, H. (1998). *Synthesizing research* (3rd ed.). Thousand Oaks, CA: Sage Publications.

Davis, M. M., & Lantos, J. D. (2000). Ethical considerations in the public policy laboratory. *Journal of the American Medical Association*, *284*(1), 85–87.

Department of Health and Human Services. (2008). Office for Civil Rights—HIPAA. Retrieved May 29, 2008, from http://www.hhs.gov/ocr/hipaa

Dyer, C. B., Goodwin, J. S., Pickens-Pace, S., Burnet, J., & Kelly, P. A. (2007). Self-neglect among the elderly: A model based on more than 500 patients seen by a geriatric medicine team. *American Journal of Public Health, 97*(9), 1671–1676.

Dynarski, M. (1997). Trade-offs in designing a social program experiment. *Children and Youth Services Review, 19*(7), 525–540.

Esbensen, F.-A., Deschenes, E. P., Vogel, D. E., West, J., Arboit, K., & Harris, L. (1996). Active parental consent in school-based research: An examination of ethical and methodological issues. *Evaluation Review, 20*(6), 737–753.

Farris, R. P., Will, J. C., Khavjou, O., & Finkelstein, E. A., (2007). Beyond effectiveness: Evaluating the public health impact of the WISEWOMAN program. *American Journal of Public Health, 97*(4), 641–647.

Feather, J. (1982). Using macro variables in program evaluation. *Evaluation and Program Planning, 5*(3), 209–215.

Fischhoff, B. (1975). Hindsight ≠ foresight: The effect of outcome knowledge on judgments under certainty. *Journal of Experimental Psychology: Human Perception and Performance, 1*, 288–299.

Fisher, E. B., Brownson, C. A., O'Toole, M. L., Shetty, G., Anwuri, W., Fazzone, P., et al. (2007). The Robert Wood Johnson Foundation Diabetes Initiative: Demonstration projects emphasizing self-management. *Diabetes Educator, 33*(1), 83–84, 86–88.

Gabriel, R. M. (2000). Methodological challenges in evaluating community partnerships and coalitions: Still crazy after all these years. *Journal of Community Psychology, 28*(3), 339–352.

Glasgow, R. E., Nelson, C. G., Strycker, L. A., & King, D. K. (2006). Using RE-AIM metrics to evaluate diabetes self-management support interventions. *American Journal of Preventive Medicine, 30*(1), 67–73.

Gondolf, E. W. (2000). Human subject issues in batterer program evaluation. *Journal of Aggression, Maltreatment and Trauma, 4*, 273–297.

Good, P. I., & Hardin, J. W. (2006). *Common errors in statistics (and how to avoid them)* (2nd ed.). New York: John Wiley & Sons.

Gorman, D. M., & Conde, E. (2007). Conflict of interest in the evaluation and dissemination of "model" school-based drug and violence prevention programs. *Evaluation and Program Planning, 30*(4), 422–429.

Hastorf, A., & Cantril, H. (1954). They saw a game: A case study. *Journal of Abnormal Psychology, 49*(1), 129–134.

Hendricks, M., & Papagiannis, M. (1990). Do's and don'ts for offering effective recommendations. *Evaluation Practice, 11*(2), 121–125.

Hill, L. G., Maucicone, K., & Hood, B. K. (2007). A focused approach to assessing program fidelity. *Prevention Science, 8*(1), 25–34.

Johnson, K., Bryant, D., Rockwell, E., Moore, M., Straub, B. W., & Cummings, P. (1999). Obtaining active parental consent for evaluation research: A case study. *American Journal of Evaluation, 20*(2), 239–250.

Julnes, G., & Rog, D. J. (2007). Current federal policies and controversies over methodology in evaluation. *New Directions for Evaluation, 113*, 1–12.

Lipshitz, R., Gilad, Z., & Suleiman, R. (2000). The one-of-us effect in decision evaluation. *Acta Psychologica, 108*(1), 53–71.

Longfield, J. N., Morris, M. J., Moran, K. A., Kragh, J. F., Wolf, R. & Baskin, T. W. (2008). Community meetings for emergency research community consultation. *Critical Care Medicine, 36*(3), 731–736.

Marvin, G. (1985). Evaluation research: Why a formal ethics review is needed. *Journal of Applied Social Sciences, 9*, 119–135.

Mathison, S. (1999). Rights, responsibilities, and duties: A comparison of ethics for internal and external evaluators. *New Directions for Evaluation, 82*, 25–34.

McClintock, C., & Colosi, L. A. (1998). Evaluation of welfare reform: A framework for addressing the urgent and the important. *Evaluation Review, 22*(5), 668–694.

Mohan, R., & Sullivan, K. (2006). Managing the politics of evaluation to achieve impact. *New Directions for Evaluation, 112*, 7–23.

Morris, M., & Jacobs, L. R. (2000). You got a problem with that? Exploring evaluators' disagreements about ethics. *Evaluation Review, 24*(4), 384–406.

National Institutes of Health. (2003). Impact of the HIPAA privacy rule on NIH processes involving the review, funding, and progress monitoring of grants, cooperative agreements and research contracts. Notice NOT-OD-03-025. Retrieved May 28, 2008, from http://grants2.nih.gov/grants/guide/notice-files/NOT-OD-03-025.html

Owen, J. M., & Lambert, F. C. (1998). Evaluation and the information needs of organizational leaders. *American Journal of Evaluation, 19*(3), 355–365.

Patton, M. Q. (1997). *Utilization focused evaluation* (3rd ed.). Thousand Oaks, CA: Sage Publications.

Patton, M. Q. (1999). Organizational development and evaluation. *Canadian Journal of Program Evaluation* (Special Issue), 93–113.

Robinson, T., Patrick, K., Eng, T. R., & Gustafson, D. (1998). An evidence-based approach to interactive health communication: A challenge to medicine in the information age. *Journal of the American Medical Association, 280*(14), 1264–1269.

Stevens, C. J., & Dial, M. (1994, Winter). What constitutes misuse? *New Directions for Program Evaluation, 64*, 3–14.

Tversky, A., & Kahneman, D. (1974). Judgment under uncertainty: Heuristics and biases. *Science, 185*(4157), 1124–1131.

VanLandingham, G. R. (2006). A voice crying in the wilderness: Legislative oversight agencies' efforts to achieve utilization. *New Directions for Evaluation, 112*, 25–39.

Weick, K. E. (1979). *The social psychology of organizing.* Reading, MA: Addison-Wesley.

Weick, K. E. (1995). *Sensemaking in organizations.* Thousand Oaks, CA: Sage Publications.

West, S. L., King, V., Carey, T. S., & Lohr, K. (2002). *Systems to rate the strength of scientific evidence.* Rockville, MD: Agency for Healthcare Research and Quality. AHRQ Publication 02-E016. Retrieved May 2, 2008, from http://www.ncbi.nlm.nih.gov/books/bv.fcgi?rid=hstat1.chapter.70996

Windsor, R. A., Boyd, N. R., & Orleans, C. T. (1998). A meta-evaluation of smoking cessation intervention research among pregnant women: Improving the science and art. *Health Education Research, 13*(3), 419–438.

Index